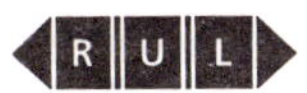

Foreign Body Prevention, Detection and Control

Practical Approaches to Food Control and Food Quality Series

Series Editor: Keith G. Anderson

Also available

1 **HACCP**
A practical approach
S. Mortimore and C. Wallace

2 **Crisis Management in the Food and Drinks Industry**
A practical approach
C. Doeg

3 **Food and Drink Laboratory Accreditation**
A practical approach
S. Wilson and G. Weir

Companion volume

Quality Management Systems for the Food Industry
A guide to ISO 9001/2
A. Bolton

Foreign Body Prevention, Detection and Control

A practical approach

P. Wallin
Technical Manager
Spillers Pet Foods
New Malden, UK

and

P. Haycock
Former Director
Goring Kerr plc
Windsor, UK

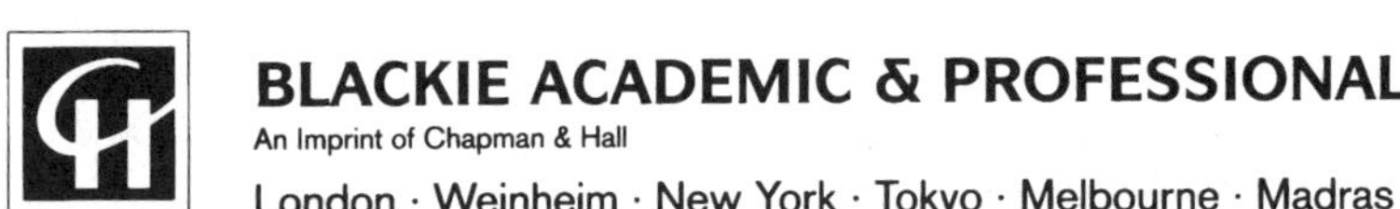
BLACKIE ACADEMIC & PROFESSIONAL
An Imprint of Chapman & Hall
London · Weinheim · New York · Tokyo · Melbourne · Madras

Published by Blackie Academic & Professional, an imprint of Thomson Science, 2–6 Boundary Row, London SE1 8HN, UK

Thomson Science, 2–6 Boundary Row, London SE1 8HN, UK

Thomson Science, 115 Fifth Avenue, New York, NY 10003, USA

Thomson Science, Suite 750, 400 Market Street, Philadelphia, PA 19106, USA

Thomson Science, Pappelallee 3, 69469 Weinheim, Germany

First edition 1998

Thomson Science is a division of International Thomson Publishing 

Typeset in 10/12pt Palatino by Saxon Graphics Ltd
Printed in Great Britain by TJ International Ltd, Padstow, Cornwall

ISBN 0 7514 0416 0

A catalogue record for this book is available from the British Library
Library of Congress Catalog Card number: (to follow)

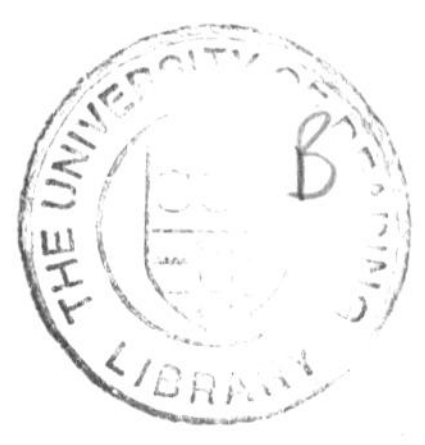

Printed on acid-free text paper, manufactured in accordance with ANSI/NISO Z39.48-1992 (Permanence of Paper)

Contents

Biographical notes

Peter J. Wallin
Dr Peter Wallin is Technical Manager for Spillers Petfoods. He studied Chemical Engineering, is a Chartered Engineer and a Royal Academy of Engineering Visiting Professor in Engineering Design at Brunel University. Previously he worked as a controls and process engineer for two major food equipment companies and was head of the engineering and manufacture department at Leatherhead Food Research Association until 1996.

Peter Haycock MIFST
Peter Haycock was first introduced to what is known as HACCP 30 years ago when he joined a subsidiary of an American company producing components for the aerospace industry. Part of his responsibilities as technical manager for the subsidiary included the overall management and development of the quality control department.

This was followed by 17 years' experience in the metal detector, X-ray and vision industry as a main board director of Goring Kerr PLC, a leading supplier of detection equipment to the food and other industries. His responsibilities included application advice and user training throughout the world. He was a member of the group which produced the Campden & Chorleywood Food Research Association Technical Bulletin No 88 on the 'Identification and control of foreign bodies' and 'Guideline for the prevention and control of foreign bodies in food'. He is a member of the Council of the Institute of Food Science and Technology.

Series Editor's foreword

Since I was first involved in a foreign body prosecution nearly 40 years ago, providing defence material for the manufacturer concerned from the Leatherhead Food Research Association, I have had a keen interest in the prevention and detection of foreign matter in food. The magistrates in that case, I am certain, made the wrong decision then because they did not understand the technical evidence and I am sure that some magistrates still make similar wrong decisions today. It can be difficult for a food business to appeal with internal pressures to avoid the attendant publicity and the 'no smoke without fire' perceived by many customers. The statistics of incidences of foreign matter are difficult for the non-technical person to follow, as are the cost–benefit consequences of prevention. An authoritative book on the prevention and detection of foreign bodies can surely only be of assistance to all concerned, especially with the development of the 'due diligence' defence in the United Kingdom.

Having worked with both Campden & Chorleywood and Leatherhead Research Associations in these areas over many years, I was delighted to secure the services of two authors to write this book who I believed would be able to put a proper context around such difficulties. I was also very pleased to have Tony Heaney, who was chairman of a Campden Working Party on the topic and an old Unilever colleague, write a foreword.

There is plenty of uncollated material on various aspects of foreign body prevention and detection neither available to the world at large, nor readily accessed by a literature search. In this book Peter Haycock and Peter Wallin have shared with us a great deal of experience and collective wisdom, not to mention singular skills of their own. These attributes, together with their keenness and good humour, made it a pleasure to work with them and between us (about 98% them and 2% me) I really believe that we have produced an excellent book which may stand as a textbook for students, a handbook for food engineers and technologists, a reference book for prosecution or defence in litigation, but above all provide the only comprehensive generally available source of information on its subject.

This book makes an invaluable addition to our *Practical Approaches* series and for example should be of assistance in carrying out hazard analyses and setting up prevention and control systems. It is also rather a good read for anyone interested in the subject. My own son, who is a mechanical engineer with Rolls Royce Associates and has nothing to do with food control matters, picked up the proof one evening when visiting and sat down and read through about half of it.

Of particular interest are the observations on future developments and the capabilities of equipment to go far beyond the basic function of foreign matter prevention and detection. Already, the thinking business is recognising the need to take these malfunctional factors into account when making decisions about future investment. What value a machine that can see and video record foreign matter against real time (due diligence?) and can also tell you counts and monitor dimensional tolerances compared with the straight-through ferrous metal detector from the past? We hope that the Appendices will prove valuable, dealing as they do with providers of inspection and sorting systems, sources of specialist assistance and summarising available methods of prevention and control. I really, really commend this book.

Should any readers have suggestions for future books in the series we shall be pleased to hear from them. Also if there are any revisions or needs for inclusion or expansion that occur to readers, we shall be pleased to hear of them

Professor Keith Anderson
Epsom Downs
March 1998

Foreword

Today consumers have very high expectations of the quality of the food they purchase, unaware that most primary food materials have to be cleaned and prepared to make them suitable and safe for consumption. This may simply involve washing or more complex processes such as filleting or heat treatment. The industry invests extensively in machinery, processes and controls to ensure that the products offered to the consumer are free from foreign body contamination. Unfortunately, in spite of the technology and procedures, incidences of contamination can occur but at a very low frequency.

Foreign body contamination in particular is an emotive subject and is often misinterpreted by the consumer as an indication of carelessness by the food processing industry. Reports regularly appear in the UK national press of prosecutions for foreign body contamination in food and very occasional product recall notices only confirm existing prejudices.

I welcome this book. It is the first time a textbook has been written which deals with all the detection and separation techniques available and the control systems and investigation procedures to support them. Technical articles on metal detectors and occasionally on other relevant technologies have been published from time to time. Except for the Campden & Chorleywood Research Association's Guidelines document No 5, *Guidelines for the Prevention and Control of Foreign Bodies in Food,* there has not been an authoritative consolidated source of information on all the available technologies. This book attempts to fill that gap.

The authors are acknowledged experts in the field and use their vast experience of the subject to highlight the benefits and limitations of the equipment and technology currently available. The misconceptions of what can and cannot be practically achieved are discussed. The text covers the potential sources of contamination and the preventative measures applicable to minimize it by the use of Good Manufacturing Practices and quality management systems.

The contents of this book form a sound basis for the training of personnel involved in the food industry both in manufacturing and enforcement. It also provides an excellent overview of the subject for those with an interest in food safety from the consumer's point of view.

Dr Tony Heaney
Company Regulatory Affairs manager
Birds Eye Wall's Ltd

March 1998

About this book

This book is aimed at a wide spectrum of readers who are involved in food and drinks manufacturing and associated businesses. It is especially intended for those involved in the industry and is a very practical book which should be useful to all those responsible for functions such as:

- Production
- Quality assurance
- Engineering
- Maintenance
- Auditors and inspectors
- Those in research and development
- Equipment suppliers to the food industry
- The food student

The book provides essential information relevant to a line operator but detailed enough to assist the company director or those in higher education. It includes an introduction to foreign body prevention and detection, including background information on definitions of key terms, legal requirements, risk assessment and 'Good Manufacturing Practices'. If the reader is employed in the food industry it is considered essential that he/she grasps an understanding of the basics of inspection and of how inspection systems function including their limitations.

The book reviews and educates the reader on all the currently used technologies; the scientific background to the technology by which the systems operate is explained in easy to understand layman's terms. In order to appreciate the technology the reader is informed of the working principles, historic problems, how and where systems should be installed, and the safety, maintenance and management aspects associated with such systems. The major technologies covered in detail include metal detection, physical separation, magnets, vision systems and X-ray machines.

New and emerging technologies are reviewed to give the reader an appreciation of what the future could hold. The technologies are examined so as to expose any present limitations on their potential use, and where and how the technologies could be best applied. Illustrations are given to aid the reader.

The book also includes other related important aspects of inspection, such as central reporting and information technology (including the use of ISO 9000), and external influences, such as tampering and crisis management, thus giving the reader a full and rounded appreciation of the subject.

The reader will be sufficiently informed so as to be educated in foreign body inspection, and to acquire sufficient knowledge on the subject be able to manage, specify and procure a system. There are design issues that are covered which will be of assistance to those designing as well as specifying machines.

The appendices are a useful source of information including contact details regarding companies selling inspection systems and organizations offering contamination identificaiton services. References aid the reader to appreciate the subject allowing one to gain access to key documents.

Acknowledgements

Dr Ian Wells (Boxmag Rapid)
Chris Caine (Loma Ltd)
Peter Binns (Heuft UK)
David Harverson (Pulse Technology Ltd)
Ben Stanborough (Sortex Ltd)
Steve Hemming (Sortex Ltd)
Mark Auty (Leatherhead Food Research Association)

1

Introduction

1.1 General

The objective of this book is to discuss the major sources of foreign body contamination in food and the preventative measures applicable to minimize the risk of foreign body contamination reaching the consumer. The capabilities and limitations of the machines used to remove foreign body contamination are dealt with in sufficient detail for them to be understood by technologists and scientists from disciplines other than engineering. The use and application of quality control systems, in particular Hazard Analysis and Critical Control Point (HACCP), are discussed in principle. HACCP and its application to the food industry is the subject of a companion volume: *HACCP: A Practical Approach* by S. E. Mortimore and C. Wallace.

A subsequent objective of the book is to discuss the establishment of control procedures for foreign body contamination detection machines based on performance as opposed to some common practices that have been adopted based on older less reliable equipment.

Finally, the impact of digital technology and the automatic provision of performance records and its impact on quality systems is discussed.

1.2 Complaints and the market size

The importance and emphasis placed on the prevention of foreign bodies in food by the manufacturer and the consumer is confirmed by the frequency of articles on the subject in the food trade press and the unfortunate frequency of reports in the national and local press of manufacturers being pursued through the courts when a member of the public has found a perceived foreign body in a food product.

Examples of the types of complaints are the following reports picked at random from recent press reports:

- Peanuts recalled for metal contamination resulting from engineering work
- Hypodermic needles in cold meat, reported as arising from pigs eating needles dropped by farmers after treating the animals
- Glass in crisps resulting from a machine failure during manufacture
- Doughnut containing a spring

The public, of the UK at least, finds foreign body contamination in food products and complains about it. How many complaints are satisfactorily dealt with by manufacturers is unknown, what is known are the reports which get through to the enforcement authorities which are summarized in Table 1.1 of extraneous matter in foods made as food complaints under the 1990 Food Safety Act in the UK.

The tables given in Appendix IV show the results of prosecutions over a 3 year period in the UK. From these it can be seen that prosecutions for metal contamination is the most common, while bakery products are the most frequent type of food subject to complaints. Over the period the recorded fines have totalled £176 130 the highest being £40 000, the lowest £350 and an average of £3830.

Table 1.1 Food complaints – extraneous matter

	1992	1993	1994
Fresh and frozen foods			
Eggs	26	21	34
Fish	284	284	321
Fruit and vegetables	741	622	757
Meat and poultry	712	661	677
Milk (liquid)	979	915	770
Manufactured food			
Bread and confectionery	1503	1430	1465
Cereals, bread, flour and flour products	2870	2790	2366
Cocoa and cocoa preparations	239	195	159
Fruit and vegetables (canned and processed)	1678	1710	1596
Ice cream and desserts	295	310	336
Processed meat and fish and products	2450	2382	2563
Milk products and cheese	738	631	680
Oils and cooking fats	48	67	37
Preserves, jam and marmalade	393	357	324
Ready prepared foods (including sandwiches)	1406	1499	2051
Soups, broths and sauces	261	245	327
Tea and coffee	93	88	81

Information courtesy of The Chartered Institute of Environmental Health

The figures have to be considered in light of the size of the food industry within the UK, a market of £37 billion, employing nearly 10% of the working population and accounting for nearly 10% of the Gross Domestic Product of the UK. There are of the order of 8000 manufacturing units, three-quarters of whom have sales of less than £1 million.

Until the BSE crisis the meat sector was the largest individual sector measured in monetary terms followed by the bread, biscuit, cake and cereal sector, with the fruit and vegetable sector close behind. In total, these three sectors account for nearly 60% of the market. The fourth largest sector is the dairy industry.

The industry is experiencing a period of rapid change. Table 1.1 shows increases in complaints associated with convenience foods, e.g. sandwiches and ready made soups. Sandwiches were a novelty only a few years ago, while today they are a standard product not only in supermarkets but in garages, newsagents and convenience stores as well as being a significant export item. The sale of ready to eat products, from complete meals to constituents that can be mixed to the consumers choice, e.g. pasta and sauces or prepared salads, is increasing. This reflects the reduction in the time available of the working population to prepare food and changes in eating habits. This increase in the consumption of prepared and part processed food has gone hand in hand with the consumers expectation for everything to be perfect and, in the context of this book, completely free from foreign body contamination, no matter what the source.

The industry manufacturing cleaning and removal equipment to minimize the incidence of complaints, particularly in the handling of ready to eat products, has responded to the changing needs of the user. New technology is being continuously introduced to improve both the level of sensitivity and the types of contaminant that can be removed. Great strides have been made to improve the data recording capabilities of the equipment. The basic principles of all the current technology are discussed in detail together with the changes which are likely to occur in the future.

1.3 Definition of a foreign body

A foreign body is a piece of solid matter present in a (food) product that is undesirable. It may be *intrinsic*, e.g. hair or bone in an animal product, or a stalk or pit in a vegetable product, or an *extrinsic* foreign body, e.g. an insect or piece of metal derived from somewhere in the process from field to finished product.

The size of the contaminant is irrelevant, as long as the consumer can identify it, by definition it is a foreign body. Bearing in mind just how sensitive the mouth is, how easily we feel a hair if it gets into our food or a tiny piece of aluminium foil, the smallest size the consumer can detect is already approaching the point of being invisible to the naked eye. This situation may be aggravated by the classification of mites to being foreign bodies, insects which can only be seen by the aid of microscopes.

1.4 Summary of the methods of foreign body detection and separation

Detection methods available as practical devices include:

- Metal detectors
- X-ray machines
- Optical-based systems

These three methods are the only practical techniques to detect foreign bodies within food products. Magnets while not precisely 'detection' devices have applications within the process akin to detection equipment, unlike sieves, washers and sprayers, settlers and flumes, aspirators, abraders, and grinders which are exclusively separators. Not automatic, but commonly used, although often not properly applied, are human inspectors.

All the detection devices depend on recognizing differences in response to some part of the energy spectrum between a contaminant and the product but there is no system able to detect every contaminant regardless of size and type. The reason may be the reaction to the energy source is the same, e.g. cherry stones have the same response as the flesh of the cherry when examined by X-ray, or stainless steel below a certain size is indistinguishable by a metal detector. It may be the contaminant is too small to generate a detectable response.

Table 1.2 summarizes where the different detection systems will generally be found to work in practice. There will of course be exceptions in specific instances. As can be seen there are a whole series of contaminants that it is very difficult if not impossible to detect using current technology. For these the only solution is the adoption of the best 'Good Manufacturing Practices', a term which in this context includes HAACP and similar systems and approaches, the keeping of records, and a philosophy of continuous monitoring.

A comprehensive summary of applicable separation methods at various stages of the food manufacturing and distribution process is given in Appendix III.

1.5 System utilization

Table 1.3 is based on the statistics available to the author (refer to biographical notes of P. J. Haycock. While the numbers may have a

Table 1.2 Detection methods summarized

Contaminant material	Magnets	Metal detectors	X-ray machines	Optical systems
Iron/steel	*	*	*	
Non-ferrous		*	*	
Metals				
Stainless steels		*	*	
Bone			*	
Glass			*	*
Stone			*	*
High density plastics			*	*
Plastics				*
Insects, dirt, debris, oil, paper, wood.		GMP		

degree of inaccuracy, the comparative size of the estimated annual sales indicates the acceptance and usage of the various technologies. The number of manufacturers of magnets is shown for the UK only as no data has been found for all the world markets.

The cost factor is an important element of what is reasonable as the decision to invest £100 000 will be quite different in an enterprise with sales of £1 million and one with sales of £50 million.

1.6 Legal position

Consumers expect the food they purchase to be free from foreign body contamination as well as meeting their expectations of quality in general, although the way consumers react when they find foreign bodies in food varies from country to country. Consumers in the UK are far more likely to take their complaints to the enforcement authorities than other Europeans, even though within the

Table 1.3 System utilization

	Magnets	Metal detectors	X-ray systems	Optical systems
Cost (£)	< 1500	< 15000	> 30000 < 200000	> 6000 < 250000
Number of manufacturers	4[a]	20	6 (growing)	10
Estimated annual sales (units)	10000	3500	125	400

[a] UK manufacturers only.

European Common market the standards manufacturers have to achieve are the same and based on the same EEC directives. American consumers will use the failure as an opportunity for litigation while in other parts of the world the consumer will not do much more than remove the contamination or complain to the shop.

In the UK food manufacturers have to meet the requirements of the 1990 Food Safety Act. This Act was derived from the EC Directive 89/397/EEC. The UK Food Safety Act is supported by Codes of Practice published by the government. The application of the Act and the Codes of Practice within the UK are controlled by Local Authority Environmental Health Departments whose activities are co-ordinated by a central body (LACOTS) who in turn publish guidelines on the way the law is to be interpreted and applied.

Code of Practice No. 1 states:

> *District Councils should investigate and take legal proceedings in all cases of mould or foreign matter (such as glass or metal shavings) found in food.*

As previously stated, foreign body contamination is treated very seriously in the UK, the papers regularly report cases of contaminants found in food and the records of the Chartered Institute of Environmental Health for 1992 (Table 1.1) show there were approximately 15 000 complaints for extraneous matter reported to the enforcement authorities. How many complaints are dealt with directly by the manufacturers and shops is unknown.

Based on the author's experience, in the rest of the EEC, with the possible exception of Ireland, foreign body complaints rarely if ever reach the courts or the press. In the USA foreign bodies are more likely to give rise to civil claims for damages.

1.7 Sources of contamination

Contamination can arise from a very wide variety of causes. Some are naturally occurring within the product, while others are introduced somewhere in the process of converting an agricultural product to a finished product on a consumer's plate which includes the introduction of contamination once the product is in the hands of the consumer.

This variety of contaminants is almost endless. Just considering metal contamination it is quite easy to identify over 75 types or sources of metal that can get into the product at all or various stages of production.

Table 1.4 demonstrates just how complex the situation is in respect of one contaminant which fortunately has the greatest range of options available for its detection and removal. Other examples of contamination problems which are a common cause of foreign body contamination are stones in vine fruit, shells in edible nuts, bones in chicken and fish, foreign seeds and grains in harvested crops, etc. A further specific area of potential contamination by foreign bodies is in the use of recycled containers.

Similar tables of potential sources for other contaminating material could be produced. Some of these are not detectable, e.g. plastics which appear in so many guises today, showing that the most important factor in the prevention of foreign bodies in food is the adoption of good manufacturing practices in the widest sense as previously defined.

This applies to all establishments regardless of their size. However, the law recognizes that the smaller enterprise cannot economically bring the same weight to bear in this area as a large multinational. It does, however, expect that even the smallest enterprise considers the risks inherent in its process and takes all reasonable precautions to prevent them.

Because metal detectors are so widely used and relied upon by the food industry, and considering metal contamination continues to be a major cause of complaints, the technology is given detailed consideration in Chapter 9. The author's experience (refer to biographical notes) has identified that metal detection is seen as something of a black art, probably because users, particularly those without any prior experience, are surprised and disappointed to learn that a metal detector cannot be guaranteed to detect each and every metallic contaminant. The complex reasons for this are dealt with.

1.8 The importance of records

Hazard and risk analysis form the basis upon which equipment and process controls are specified. The operation and performance of the equipment and process controls has to be monitored, and the results recorded. The results are used for continuous improvement and the records kept for future reference if this becomes necessary.

For the small operation it may be that the information is taken and recorded manually while in the larger organizations there is an increasing use of electronic data capture. The design and implementation of a manual system, while not necessarily simple, is comparatively straightforward as it can be made up of discrete components dealing with individual aspects of the process in isolation from other parts of the process and in many cases without the need for a central combined report.

In the case of larger operations, while each step may be considered individually, the impact of each step in the process will need to

Table 1.4. Some sources of metal contamination

Raw material	Processing	Maintenance	Human	Cleaning
Nails from pallets and boxes	instrument components	conduit and fittings	jewellery, rings, watches, etc.	bristles from wire brushes
Ingested metal from animals	broken mincer blades	electrical wire	dental amalgam	cleaning machine components
Harvesting machinery parts	broken saws	fasteners	pins, needles, safety pins, etc.	clips, staples pins from cleaning materials
Clips from packaging	nuts, bolts, rivets, washers and other fasteners	inspection devices	coins	wire wrapping from cleaning materials
	packing material	plugs, sockets and parts	keys	cleaning material containers and lids
Storage bin components	pneumatic fittings	shards from cleaning and fitting	metal foils	
Staples from packaging	flexible hose connectors	solder	spectacles and component parts	
Can pull rings	conveyor components	swarf from machining	lighters	
Wire strips from can opening	embossing wires from chocolate moulders	tools	pens, pencils and components	
Transport machinery components	light fittings	trunking and fittings	clips from boards	
Veterinary instruments	belt joining clips	welding rod	staples paper clips	
Ear tags from animals	broken knives	welding spelter	drawing pins	
Butchers tools and gloves	rust		'Lucky' pieces	
Wire wrapping	swarf worn from mills		buttons	
Knives and tools	thermocouples		belts and clips	
Containers	wear swarf from screw conveyors		tools	
Caps, lids and closures	wire from woven wire conveyor belt			
Syringe needles from animals	wire heater elements			

be considered in association with the total process and some form of central reporting system implemented.

A great deal of this work can now be carried out automatically with the data being stored and analysed electronically.

The impact of the microprocessor has been so great and the rate of development of both hardware and software so rapid that new developments can be made obsolete almost before they have time to be adopted. As yet there are no industry standard solutions to the question of electronic quality control monitoring and data storage for a complete process. Developments so far are by individual manufacturers who deliver equipment which has the facility to record its status and performance, and to deliver this as an electronic output in real-time or on demand.

There are two basic types of systems available for some of the detection equipment. The simplest being a printer connection, either stand alone or through a network to a central point where the information is printed or stored. The more complex being management information systems capable of collecting data from more than one type of equipment, presenting it in the form of reports in real-time, archiving the data for future use or storing it for further processing using standard software packages. Both of these systems only work with the data from a specific manufacturer's equipment; the only information they will accommodate from other equipment is simple on/off data from sensors.

To implement a completely integrated quality monitoring and reporting system across a production process requires specially written software, including interfaces to convert the different data formats to a standard format.

1.9 Non-food applications

Because of the importance of packaging and packaging materials in the food manufacturing and distribution process, the applications of special purpose detection techniques for these industries has been included. The application of risk assessment and HACCP is of equal importance in this industry.

2

Risk assessment and HACCP

2.1 Introduction

Any food manufacturer or handler has to provide a safe food product ensuring that it is not contaminated with any foreign bodies or objects and that it is safe and fit for human consumption. Within the food chain there are many different points at which food can potentially become contaminated, which makes it an ever increasing challenge. A food company is usually involved in one or more stages of the supply chain, which takes food from the field and provides a finished food product in our shops and ultimately on the table. A typical chain of food handlers and producers may include:

- The farmer
- Primary processor
- Main food processor
- Distributor
- Wholesaler
- Supermarket

In most countries it is the legal responsibility of the person at the end of the chain, supplying the food to the consumer who has to ensure that the food is safe. However, the safety of food has to be protected through the whole chain so as to allow the provision of food safe and fit to eat. There are now moves by many authorities and governments to spread the legal responsibility to all those involved in the supply chain. This includes all those in the chain from the farmer to the consumer. In some countries the chain is short and, therefore, easier to manage than in other countries. Generally, there has been an increase in the length of the supply chain as consumers have opted for ready prepared meals as opposed to purchasing basic produce and preparing the meal in the home.

Complaints are usually addressed directly to the final supplier of the food, in most cases it is the retailer who supplies the consumer. The retailer refers the complaint back to the food producer who will then investigate to find out who in the chain was responsible. If it is a major incident or problem it will normally be referred to the authorities who will carry out an investigation. They will usually hold an inquiry to discover who was responsible and then take whatever legal action is appropriate. They may in the event of a major contamination introduce revised legislation to prevent a re-occurrence of such an incident.

As the food chain has become longer the management of food safety has become more crucial to ensure that food reaches the consumer in a form that is safe to eat. The concerns over the safety of food have also increased as consumers have become more educated – there is also a greater awareness of food-related illnesses and any food contamination issues can be widely publicized by the world's media in a matter of minutes.

In order to ensure safety, controls have to be put in place and methods adopted to reduce or eliminate the possible risks of contamination. Many countries have now adopted either laws, regulations or directives relating to food safety and hygiene. Many of these regulations also encourage or prescribe the use of HACCP.

2.2 Food safety

As mentioned, food safety has to be paramount for any food manufacturer or food handler. Although this book focuses on physical food contamination, the techniques and approaches to overall food safety are highly relevant. The key areas of concern over food safety include:

- Microbiological
- Pesticide residues
- Physical contamination
- Adulteration

There has been considerable concern over food safety in the world and the World Health Organization (WHO) has published material to assist nations to improve their food safety through evaluation programmes. The WHO monitors the cases of food-related illnesses around the world and, in particular, in developing countries. Food-related illnesses still remain a major cause of illness in the developing world.

In the developed world many of the advances in the food industry have been towards the manufactured and consumer convenience foods. These forms or types of foods have brought about their own problems. The kinds of technologies utilized in the production of convenience foods can actually increase the potential risk of food contamination particularly as many foods are minimally processed and only re-heated in the home. The potential for contamination from foreign bodies or objects has also increased due to the:

- Increased number of processing stages
- Machine automation
- Increased handling through the chain
- Packaging

It is, therefore, essential that food manufacturers use rigid evaluation techniques to ensure that any risks are minimized so that the likelihood of contamination is most improbable.

2.3 What is HACCP?

HACCP is an abbreviation for Hazard Analysis and Critical Control Point. It was originally developed for the US manned space missions by NASA where it was a requirement to ensure that their food would remain safe to eat throughout the duration of their missions. The systems were developed in collaboration with Pillsbury who then explored the technique further applying it to commercial food processes. HACCP is now used by most food companies, and is regarded as an effective, rational and systematic approach to the identification and assessment of potential hazards. Initially focused on microbiology the application of the technique has now been broadened to include all types of hazards. The approach allows one to identify the hazards or risks associated with manufacturing, distribution and retailing of food products, and to define an effective and specific method by which to control these risks.

A hazard can be defined as a potential cause of harm, a possible threat to food safety or a danger that might occur such as food spoilage or a cause of illness. Critical Control Points (CCPs), which are distinguishable operations, can be identified where there is a risk and if loss of control occurred there would be a reasonable chance or probability of creating an unacceptable level of risk. The CCP is normally a procedure, process, location, etc., at which a control can be effected to minimize or prevent a hazard occurring. Therefore, HACCP is a preventative method of ensuring safe food production, which is an essential tool to be used by a food producer or food handling company. Although primarily used as a safety tool it can also be utilized in conjunction with good manufacturing practice to ensure a factory operates efficiently producing quality products.

HACCP has been widely adopted by many food companies around the world, and is accepted as a primary approach and method of food safety. It has been endorsed and recommended by all the major authorities. Although in most countries it is not obligatory to utilize a HACCP system, it is usually advised that one should implement a HACCP system. Within the EU the need for this type of approach is embodied in the legislation. The Food Safety Act 1990 in the UK states under Section 21 that:

> *... it shall ... be a defence for the person charged to prove that he took all reasonable precautions and exercised all 'due diligence' to avoid the commission of the offence by himself or by a person under his control.*

Although HACCP in itself does not make the food inherently safe, it does provide a means to self-evaluate and audit the operations carried out, and to identify the CCPs, so they can be monitored. The CCPs should be related to overall food safety and, therefore, cover more than just food contamination. The preventative measures required to ensure food is not contaminated with foreign objects can be carried out using the HACCP process. A foreign body contamination of a food is a potential hazard for which effective controls can be put in place.

The use of HACCP was one that has taken the emphasis away from traditional product and ingredient sampling and laboratory testing to the approach of greater control within manufacturing and the food supply chain.

2.4 Examples of HACCP

In order to develop a complete HACCP programme for a business, an individual factory unit or a production line it is necessary to carry out the following steps of evaluation:

- Describe the product
- Develop an overall table or flow diagram of all the key stages in the process, the raw materials and the equipment used within the process
- Assess each of the production stages to identify potential hazards and list the preventative measures used to control such hazards
- Decide which hazards are critical – develop a 'decision tree' diagram
- Evaluate each individual hazard to decide on the specific control(s) which could be used.
- Implement the monitoring programme for each of the CCPs identified

- Establish record keeping and procedures to ensure CCPs are effectively monitored and there is evidence of effective monitoring

In order to decide if there is a hazard associated with a particular ingredient, process step, item of equipment, etc. one has to go through a decision process as indicated in Figure 2.1.

The WHO produced their own similar chart of a HACCP systems as indicated in Figure 2.2.

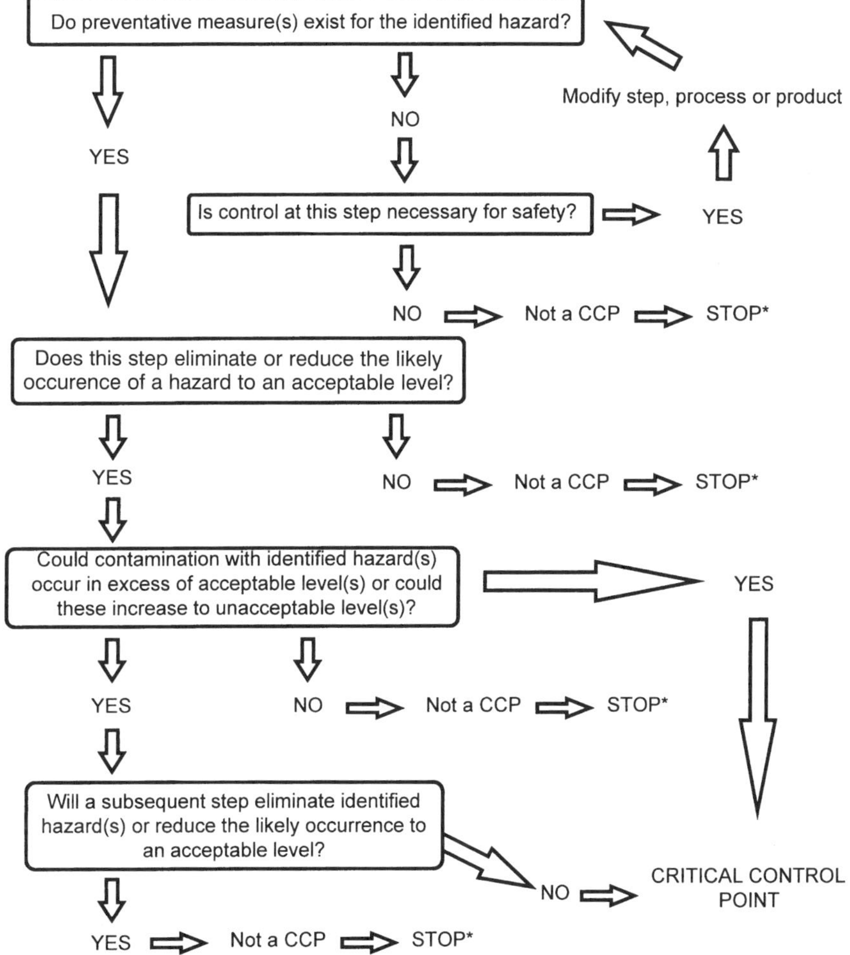

Figure 2.1 Codex Alimentarius Commission (1991). Adapted by Mitchell (1992) – decision process to determine CCPs.

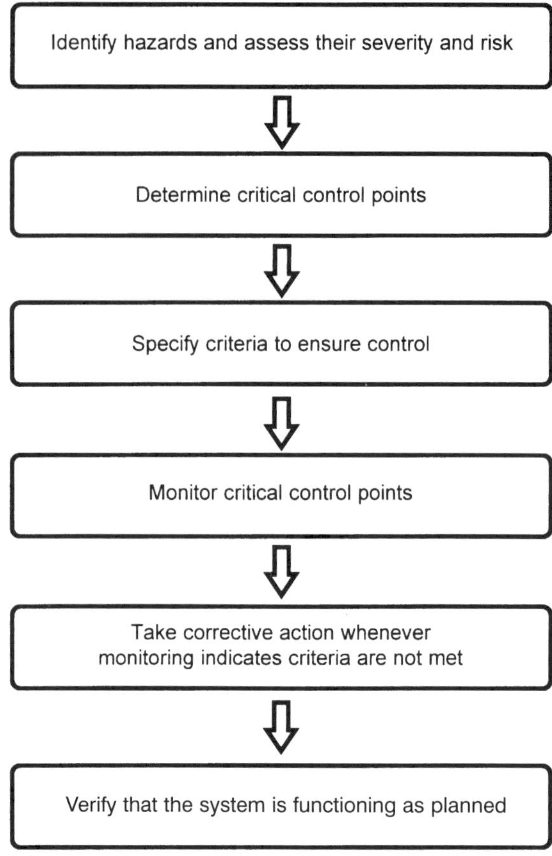

Figure 2.2 WHO model for determination of CCPs.

In order for one to appreciate what a HACCP analysis is and how it can be implemented two examples have been developed below.

2.4.1 *A sauce product*

The first example is that of a sauce product which is heat processed in a glass jar. The sauce is one that will be used as a sauce to cook meat in. The first step is to develop a process flow diagram showing the major steps in the process. This then enables one to identify all the materials that are used in the product including packaging see Figure 2.3.

Within the process fresh vegetables are added to a base sauce mix which contains tomato, water, a thickener and other preservatives, and some flavourings such herbs and spices. All the ingredients are

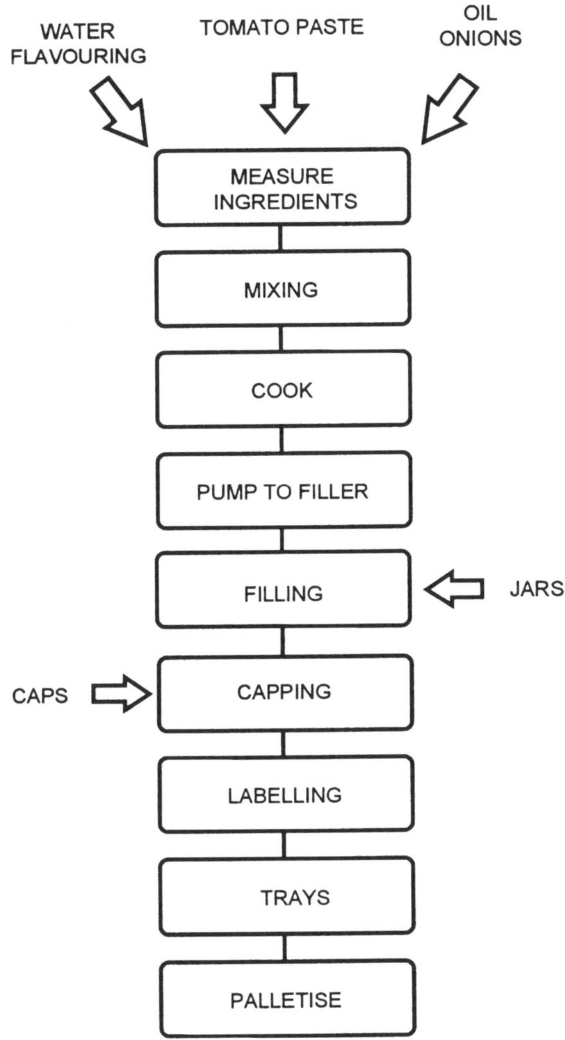

Figure 2.3 Process diagram for a sauce process.

mixed for the appropriate time and then the mix is filled into glass jars. Lids are placed on the jars and the jars are then heated to the required temperature by passing though a hot water spray/pasteurization tunnel for a set time and then cooled down. The jars are then labelled and coded, and placed either on trays which are then wrapped or into cases which are then sealed.

One has to decide which steps within the process prevent the major hazards and how critical these are in ensuring the food is produced safely. For the process described the most critical steps are:

- Inspection of raw materials
- Pasteurizer temperature and f_0 or P value
- Time in the pasteurizer
- Inspection of glass jars
- Inspection of tops

Table 2.1 identifies the critical control point relevant to this particular manufacturing process.

When packaging the product into glass containers there is a high risk that some of the containers may crack or break and, therefore, some means of inspection is vital. It is possible to use automated forms of inspection with glass jars – there are many very sophisticated vision systems that can be used. The systems can be used to inspect the glass jars prior to filling and to look for cracks or flaws in the glass that could fracture on heating.

Although it is not a legal obligation or a requirement of HACCP to utilize the latest inspection technology, it can sometimes be of help in a court case as a means of defence.

2.4.2 *Ready to eat breakfast cereal*

This example is that of a ready to eat breakfast cereal. Once again one needs to develop a process flow diagram as shown in Figure 2.4 to ensure that all the process steps are fully considered.

Raw materials are ground and blended, and water is added to obtain the required moisture level. The cereal mix is then extruded and a coating applied. The coated product is then dried in an oven and cooled. The product is weighed using a multi-head weigher and filled into plastic bags followed by a wrap-around carton. The cartons are placed in cases, palletized and stretch-wrapped. The pallets are transferred to the storage warehouse or sent directly out. The critical hazard points in the process are:

- Contamination of raw materials
- Temperature in the extruder
- Moisture content after the drier
- Quality and control of coatings
- Build up of coating or product debris in machines
- Inspection prior to packaging
- Condition of the filling machine
- Inspection and control of packaging materials – in particular the primary packaging

The reasons for these critical points are highlighted in Table 2.2. One has to be careful not to select too many critical control points otherwise their importance can be disregarded. It is important that a sys-

Table 2.1 Sauce production CCPs

Process staff	Hazard	Preventative measures	CCP	Critical limits	Corrective actions
Raw materials					
Water	foreign boodies	filter to remove contaminants	yes	within specification	
	chemical	sample and analyse			
	microbiological	GMP			
Vegetables	foreign bodies	sieve/screen to remove contaminants	yes	no foreign bodies	re-sort
(onions, tomatoes)	mould	sampling and analysing			
carrots, etc.)	microbilogical	GMP			
	chemical residues	GMP – pesticides, heavy metals, etc.			
Minor ingredients	foreign bodies	sieve/screen to remove contaminants	yes	no foreign bodies	re-sort
(starch, sugar,	mould	GMP – sampling and analysing			
herbs and spices,	microbiological	GMP			
etc.)	chemical residues	GMP – pesticides, heavy metals, etc.			
Process					
Mixer/heating	cross-contamination	cleaning	yes	Temperature ± xx°C	do not fill
	metal/contaminants	GMP		pH ± x	re-process
	microbiological	check product temperature and pH			
Filling	microbiological	GMP – Cleaning	yes	Temperature± xx°C	do not fill
	metal/contamination	metal detector			
Capping	inspection	regular checks	yes		
	steam supply	hygienic design of system			
Cooling	microbiological	product temperature		temperature ± xx°C	test
	cooling contamination	check cooling water		water specification	
Jars	contaminated packaging	chemical analysis	yes	no foreign bodies	do not use
	dirty container	washing of jars			
	broken glass	inspection – visual			
Final product	foreign body contamination	glass	yes	zero	reject product

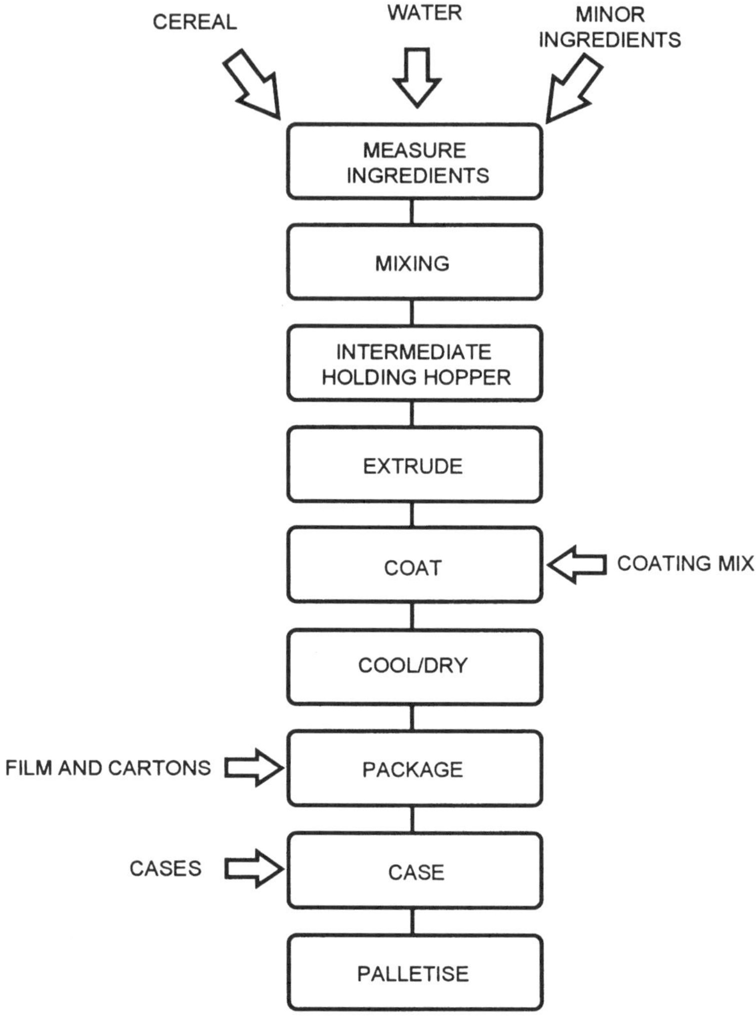

Figure 2.4 Process diagram for a breakfast cereal.

tem is developed to ensure these CCPs are monitored on a continuous basis.

A HACCP analysis is never complete as, on a regular basis, one should always review the HACCP system, as products and processes change, and therefore hazards change. This is particularly significant if coatings or ingredients change. There are also continuous improvements in the methods, instruments or equipment used for control. It maybe new equipment is available that could eliminate

Table 2.2 Cereal production CCPs

Process step	Hazard	Preventative measures	CCP	Critical limits	Corrective actions
Raw materials					
Water	foreign bodies chemical microbiological	filter to remove contaminants sample and analyse GMP	yes	within specification	
Cereals	foreign bodies mould microbiological chemical residues	sieve/screen to remove contaminants optical sorting system sampling and analysing GMP	yes	no foreign bodies	re-sort
Minor ingredients		sieve/screen to remove contaminants GMP	yes		re-sort
Nuts and fruit	foreign bodies mould microbiological chemical residues	sieve/screen to remove contaminants optical sorting system sampling and analysing GMP	yes		re-sort
Sugar		GMP			
Process					
Mixer	cross-contamination (in particular nuts)	cleaning GMP	yes		
Extruder	microbiological	correct residence time temperature moisture	yes		
Coater	build-up of caramelized or congealed solids which could fall into product	regular cleaning hygenic design of system	yes		
Cooler/dryer		final moisture control	yes	less than *xx*%	re-process
Packaging	contaminated packaging	chemical analysis	yes		do not use
Final product	foreign body contamination	metal detection	yes		

certain hazards or new suppliers that have new systems to ensure their materials are not contaminated.

One must ensure that the total process is considered and that no part is left unexamined. The packaging materials can often hold many potential risks and these have to be carefully examined.

2.5 Risk assessment

It is interesting first of all to define what the word risk means. Risk, as defined in the dictionary is – *jeopardy* or *hazard*. It is generally regarded that a risk relates to the chance, likelihood or probability of a particular hazard occurring.

It is planning for the unexpected which is always the most difficult. Some eventualities are easy to predict and past experiences can enable us to have some prior knowledge of the likelihood of an event occurring. However, many events are impossible to predict and combinations of events are almost impossible to foresee. It is sometimes the unexpected that does occur. It is how one is able to minimize risks that is important.

In order to decide what priority to place on certain issues that are involved in the manufacture of food the use of risk assessment techniques and tools can be most useful. Risk assessment allows one to quantify or categorize risks. The main categories of risk are:

- Life threatening
- Danger to consumers
- Company threat
- Affect on product sales or brand share

The usual approach to assessing risk is to use decision tree structures or a series of questions.

2.6 Examples and techniques of how to assess risks

One of the greatest problems faced is how to identify where risks lie and what likelihood they have of occurring. We all know that there are a number of fatal car or aeroplane crashes a year and yet most of us still use these forms of transport because we believe the probability of being involved in such an accident ourselves is remote. There are also ways we can limit that risk – an airline will frequently maintains its planes, use qualified mechanics and approved parts.

One step is to identify the risk areas, the next is to then limit the potential or probability of that risk occurring and the third step is to minimize the effect of a risk should it occur. Some events can be catastrophic and some have long-lasting memories. Some events that aroused much publicity include:

- Flixborough – UK
- Three Mile Island – USA
- Bhopal – India
- Chernobyl – Russia (Ukraine)
- Farley's baby food – UK
- Perrier – France
- Kings Cross Fire – UK
- *Herald of Free Enterprise* – English Channel

Often a failure or a series of minor failures can lead to a major disaster. Although any one individual event might be insignificant, the combination could be deadly. What can we learn from the above tragedies.

- It is not always the obvious which will pose a risk
- One has to have a system to check and identify all potential risks
- The effect of combined risks needs to be considered

Risks are difficult to quantify because there is often no past experience to go by and use to assess statistically the probability of that event occurring or re-occurring. New methods of control will aid in the prevention of risk. As one is able to measure more parameters on-line and continuously monitor equipment within a food factory, one is then able to use this information to detect when anything abnormal is occurring.

2.7 Minimizing risks

In life we know if there are risks. If one flies in an aircraft there is a limited risk of it crashing. If one drives on the road there is a risk of an accident. Obviously what one likes to do is to minimize these risks. With aeroplanes they have an air worthiness certificate and are regularly tested, the maintenance crew will always be routinely checking the aircraft, and there are checks prior to each flight by the flight crew. Whilst flying there are key instruments to monitor the plane and indicate any abnormalities. With a motor car, in most countries, there is an annual road worthiness check and one should also maintain the car regularly – checking brakes, tyres, etc. These checks are carried out to meet certain standards.

In the food industry the same type of approach can be taken. Factories should be well maintained and checks or audits should be made regularly. It is best that audits are carried out by trained and qualified auditors and by a third party. Often in-house auditing leads to complacency. HACCP is a system that is applied by most food companies to specific food processing or handling issues; however, the technique can be taken further into the engineering and maintenance systems that are used to keep the factory operational. Many major food incidents have stemmed from poor maintenance – a filter blocking, insufficient ventilation, poor cleaning or an equipment failure.

2.8 Malicious tampering

There has been a marked increase in the number of reported cases of malicious tampering. This is where a product has been deliberately spiked or contaminated by someone or an organization. In the past this type of event was not such a serious matter as news travelled slowly and often did not reach the national press. Nowadays an event can be publicized world-wide within 24 hours. This has a significant impact on a business and for global companies can have devastating consequences. The reason for such action by an individual or a group could be:

- Extortion
- An employee or group with a grudge against the company
- A prank or practical joker
- A politically minded group

They would hope that the food company or retailer would hand over a sum of money in return for the action to stop. Tampering can take place in many different forms. Some of those reported include:

- Glass in baby foods
- Hypodermic needles in soft drinks
- Needles in fruit
- Chemical contaminants in various products

To have total protection against any threat of tampering would be impossible, particularly where humans are involved. Some companies have seen that people issues need to be taken seriously, and some have even gone to the extent of carefully screening all new employees and even using psychologists to assess their mental position. An even more extreme measure which some companies have had to resort to is the use of methods such as closed circuit television to observe employees. This is often used where pilfering is also suspected. However, once the product has left the confines of the factory there is the distribution chain to contend with and the retailer, and through this chain there could be many more people who could gain access. Therefore, all those handling food in the chain have to be just as vigilant. Some specific actions that could be taken to reduce the risk of malicious tampering include:

- Employee–employer relations
- Employment selection methods and criteria
- Observing any unusual actions or behaviour

It is essential to know where the source of the contamination is likely to have occurred as early as possible. Analysis of the foreign object is advantageous as it can often reveal, and sometimes pin point, the origin of the contaminant. Using the techniques above to be as certain as possible it could not have occurred in the factory allows one to potentially focus the search on a restricted area.

2.9 Crisis management

One of the primary objectives of any company in crisis management is to prevent an incident becoming a crisis. For any problem that occurs one wishes to ensure that it does not become a crisis by dealing with the situation in a controlled and manageable manner. Once a situation is out of control it is very difficult to bring it back under control.

Because many companies now operate globally in the resourcing of their raw materials or in supply of final products, a potential crisis has to be dealt with on a 24 hour basis. An issue could arise anywhere around the world and at any time day or night. To control any crisis on a global basis it is likely that a multi-lingual capability will need to be readily available. It is most important that these skills are the best because any misunderstanding could be potentially extremely costly. Some practical aspects to managing a crisis are:

- Establish a crisis team before one occurs
- Define the roles of the team (who will do what, who will make decisions, level of responsibility, etc.)
- Put into place a crisis plan of action
- Ensure all necessary communications are in place
- Provide back-up plan for potential failures in communication

A crisis management team needs to be one that is trained in handling such potentially damaging events. One has seen that some companies have been lost or destroyed through the poor handling of a major crisis. The team should have the right mix of people to cover all the key elements that could occur in a crisis and they also require the right authority levels to be able to make key decisions happen (including getting the CEO out of bed!). Some of the general requirements include:

- Management skills

- Communication – press and media
- Links with laboratories to carry out quick analyses
- Ability to work under pressure

Staff should have experience in dealing with the media and being able to communicate effectively. The media is always looking for a story and the ability to curtail further media investigations is vital by giving the right answers such that speculation is ended. The need within an organization for a crisis to be reported quickly is one that often eludes a company, but clear reporting and trust in junior staff to inform their senior managers and directors without fear of reprisals is required.

In a crisis decisions need to be taken by the appropriate level of management and, therefore, protecting colleagues by not reporting major problems will lead to untrained or junior staff controlling major issues and possibly acting either against or not in line with company interests.

When a foreign body or foreign bodies are the cause of a crisis, discovering the identity of the contaminant is key (different analytical methods are covered in Chapter 5). Establishing what the object is and where it has come from makes it far easier for the crisis management team to control the situation. Often there is a great deal of damaging speculation.

Although smaller companies often find it more difficult to handle crisis situations because of the lack of resources and trained personnel, they do have an advantage in that there are fewer staff involved in the chain and the best people to deal with the situation can usually be contacted quickly.

In dealing with an event or issue it is important that whoever is dealing with it has all the relevant information available to them as quickly as possible. The use of information technology and being able to communicate with people quickly can be an immense advantage in this situation. It is important that all communication is via secure means and that there is protection against phone tapping or interception of communications, as many people will go to extreme measures to secure exclusive stories for their publications. Arrangements with telephone companies to provide additional telephone lines at short notice is advisable. In case there is such a crisis, mobile communications are also useful to have available.

References and further reading

Abbott, H. (1991) *Managing Product Recall*. Financial Times/Pitman, London.
Abbott, H. (1992) *Product Risk Management*. Financial Times/Pitman, London.

Baird-Parker, A. C. and Mayes, T. (1989) Application of HACCP to assure microbiological safety. *Food Science and Technology*, **3**(1), 23–26.

Bryan, F. L. (1992) *Hazard Analysis Critical Control Point Evaluations – A Guide to Identifying Hazards and Assessing Risks Associated with Food Preparation and Storage*. WHO, Geneva.

CCFRA (1997) *HACCP: A Practical Guide*, 2nd edn. Technical Manual No. 38. Campden and Chorleywood Food and Drink Research Association, Chipping Campden.

Codex Committee on Food Hygiene (1993) *Guidelines for the Application of Hazard Analysis Critical Control Point (HACCP)*. WHO, Geneva, WHO/FNU/FOS/93.3 II.

Dillon, M. and Griffith, C. (1996) *How to HACCP*, 2nd edn. MD Associates, Grimsby.

Doeg, C. (1995) *Crisis Management in the Food and Drinks Industry, A Practical Approach*. Chapman & Hall, London.

HMSO (1991) *Food Safety Act*. HMSO, London.

ICMSF (1988) *Micro-organisms in Foods 4. Application of the Hazard Analysis Critical Control Point (HACCP) System to Ensure Microbiological Safety and Quality*. Blackwell Scientific Publications, Oxford, UK.

Mortimore, S. and Wallace, C. (1994) *HACCP: A Practical Approach*. Chapman & Hall, London.

Pierson, M. D. and Corlett, D. A. (1992) *HACCP Principles and Application*. Van Nostrand Reinhold, New York.

3

Good Manufacturing Practice (GMP)

3.1 Introduction

The concept and approach of GMP has been used by many companies for many years. However, it is still a subject which is talked about often but not always acted on, or if acted on, is only implemented in part. It is the attention to detail which is important. GMPs cover all aspects of the food manufacturing process. The building design is a fundamental aspect.

There is an initial investment that is required to ensure good GMP and some ongoing costs; however, as history continues to show, prevention is better and cheaper than cure. In operating a food factory one has to be aware of the risks and potential risks of contamination. Any techniques or methods of operation that can reduce that risk are essential.

3.2 Pest prevention, control and detection

It is virtually guaranteed that any food factory will face problems from pests, vermin and insects. It is a common problem but it is a subject where there is often misinformation or poor knowledge. One of the reasons for this is the wide variety of animal pests; some common ones are classified in Table 3.1.

Some of the potential pests listed in Table 3.1 are more common than others, and are often very much dependent on the location of the factory and the food products or ingredients being used or produced. These different pests can be quite ingenious, particularly if they know there could be a good supply of food. Many vermin have been known to scale great heights or tunnel to great depths to avoid

Table 3.1 Categories of types of typical pests

Phylum	Class	Species
Chordates	birds	perching (pigeons, sparrows, starlings, etc.), owls, gulls
	mammals	rodents (mice, rats, voles, squirrels), rabbits, bats, carnivores (foxes, dogs, cats, badgers), moles and shrews
Arthropods	Insects	silverfish, flies, crickets, locusts, grasshoppers, earwigs, cockroaches, termites, lice, beetles, weevils, moths, bees, wasps and ants
	spiders	spiders, mites and ticks
	centipedes	approximately 1500 species
	millipedes	approximately 7000 species

preventative measures. They can also become immune to poisons or deterrents.

The prevention of pests and vermin entering the factory is the key solution to the problem. There are a variety of preventative measures which can be taken and these include:

- Filling in of all non-functional openings
- Fitting fully sealing doors, windows and vents
- Protecting air intake points with filters or grills
- Protecting drains and other facility intakes and exits

Even after all these measures pests are very persistent and will still attempt to get into the factory by any opportunistic means. Once in the factory, one requires methods of detecting that any pests are present. There are a range of detection methods which can be used to detect and trap insects and rodents. Baited traps can be used for some, although one has to select baits that are appropriate for the food industry (food safe, toxicity, aromas, etc.). Pheromones are used to trap many insects as they are attracted to these odours, they are then caught by entry into pots or on sticky cards. The pheromones are specially formulated chemicals that give off specific odours that attract insects as they are similar to those used naturally for insects to attract each other.

Ultraviolet (UV) lights can be used to attract a wide variety of flying insects and then an electrocutor or electronic fly killer, a wire grill onto which they land or touch has an electric current flowing through it, used to kill them. These types of system have to be designed properly to ensure they do not cause debris to drop from the collector tray located under. The systems should be placed strategically within the factory so as to eliminate the insects prior to them causing any contamination. One also needs to ensure that the systems are maintained and regularly inspected. Tubes require regular replacement which should be the subject of a written procedure and records kept of the change. Regular inspection of the catch tray contents and the recording of the contents by weight, for example, should be made and recorded as part of the quality control programme.

Insects can reside in stored products – beetles, mites and moths are some of the common insects that often adapt to live off the particular food they reside in. Not only do the insects themselves create a problem but the larval stages they go through can produce additional problems. The typical types of materials that can become infested include cereals, pulses, dried fruits, oil seeds, herbs and spices.

3.2.1 *Birds*

Birds can often be a real pest in and around factories or warehouses but unlike other pests there are certain types species which are protected by law in the majority of countries. Therefore any eradication must comply with the law and any restrictions laid down by local authorities. The more common methods used to encourage birds to leave premises or to eradicate them include:

- Gassing
- Shooting
- Trapping
- Baits – poisoning, sterilizing and narcotics
- Mists
- Surfactant sprays

There are in addition national restrictions to some of the methods listed above as they are not all permissible in many countries. In many cases eradication may be difficult or not possible in which case methods or scaring have to be used such as scarecrows, acoustics or pyrotechnics. Birds nests can also present a problem particularly in warehouses and these have to either be left until the fledglings have flown or be removed with care. Not only are the birds themselves a problem but the droppings are obviously problematic. They can fall in open containers or equipment or even drop onto clean products.

The nests can pose a major problem as they encourage other insects who harbour in the nest. During feeding birds carry insects as feed and these can be dropped in flight. Another problem are feathers which can be lost in flight and can find their way into foodstuffs.

There are a wide range of birds that can cause a nuisance. The more common ones include pigeons, starlings, sparrows, seagulls, owls and house martins. Birds differ from many other pests in that their roosts are sometimes many miles away from where they feed and this makes their eradication or control more difficult. In order to prevent roosting or perching in many cases it is possible to use proofing such as nets. Most birds come for any potential food so the removal of any food sources or adding a repellent to a bird food source can assist. Materials such as plastic compounds can be used to coat ledges – these reduce the grip of a bird and will cause it to feel insecure and find another perch.

3.2.2 *Rodents and other mammals*

Rodents relate to the group of animals that are 'gnawing animals', and they have large projecting front teeth which are used for gnawing food and materials to make their nests from. This group can cause major disruption. They can cause food contamination by droppings, hairs, eating foods, and damaging storage containers and infrastructure. They also can potentially spread a range of diseases. Because they have such strong teeth, rats, in particular, can eat through a range of materials such as cables, wood and plastics.

Most rodents eat all types of foods but will particularly search out cereal products. They rear their offspring in nests. They have litter sizes of about five to 12 and can produce three to seven litters a year. They are usually detected in a factory by their droppings and the damage they cause. It is also possible to identify them from their footprints. They will build their nests in holes in walls, cavities, service ducting, drains, etc. Rats and mice can crawl through small cracks as small as 10 and 6 mm, respectively. They will usually feed at night time and, therefore, are not seen. One of the most common methods of eradication is to set traps which are baited with poison. The rodent will enter the trap, eat the poisoned food and then die in the trap.

Other rodents and mammals that can cause a nuisance include domesticated foxes that look for food in the refuse and waste but at night time can find their way into stores if doors are not secure. Squirrels will also enter into premises, although they are more selective about the types of foods they will eat. Wild or uncontrolled dogs and cats can also present a problem both in terms of contamination and hygiene. Protective measures are usually effective in keeping these larger mammals out of the factory.

3.2.3 Wasps, bees and flies

The problems encountered from wasps bees and flies are usually in the summer or warmest months of the year. The best form of defence is to prevent them entering the premises in the first place. One preventative measure is to use screens on all openings – the screen aperture size should be such as to allow air to pass through but prevent any insects passing through.

Wasps are a major pest to a number of food manufacturers, particularly those such as soft drink, bakeries, preserves and confectionery manufacturers who have large and frequent deliveries of sugar and other sweeteners, and particularly during the summer months when wasps are active. The wasps will swarm around the inlet systems and if there is inadequate defences soon enter into the product or through any openings and into the factory. Wasps can breed very rapidly in the summer months with the queen laying 20 000–30 000 eggs. The eggs only take 14–30 days to develop into adult. During winter months there is not a problem as the workers and males all die off. The wasps live in the nest and, therefore, the best method of dealing with the problem is to locate the nest. If the nest cannot be located then one has to rely on insecticidal bait being taken back to the nest. Traps and insecticutors are useful where there are only a few wasps, but for larger numbers they are less effective.

Bees are not such a common problem. Probably the most likely encounter is when they swarm and decide to find their new habitat inside a warehouse or food factory. In this case the colony will have to be tackled by a trained beekeeper who be able to come and collect the colony and return them to the hive. Often the beekeeper will use smoke to calm the bees, allowing for an easier transfer back to the hive.

Flies are a common source of contamination and, in particular, the spread of germs. Flies are filthy pests which carry and transmit many harmful diseases. However, as flies cannot digest solid food they tend to land on foods and vomit on them so that the active enzymes in their vomit can pre-digest the food prior to consumption. This method of eating sounds repulsive but it is difficult to detect where they have been eating.

For flies, as mentioned previously, the use of UV light traps are popular. They use UV emissions with wavelengths or 250–400 nm, produced from mercury vapour or fluorescent tubes to attract the flying insect. The power rating of the light must be more than 20 W in order to emit sufficient 'black' light. The light source is surrounded by a high voltage, 4500 V, low current, 9 mA, electric grid which when the flying insect makes contact it is electrocuted. Once killed the insect falls into a tray located under the lamp. The design of the system is important because if the dead insects are not caught they could fall onto open processing equipment below. These types of units can only be used where the area is not classed as an explosion proof area due to the sparking from the system.

3.2.4 Cockroaches and mites

Cockroaches can present a serious problem as they can contaminate foods but also are notorious for spreading diseases. They tend to inhabit drains and rubbish. One has to beware of sewage systems because they will use these as a means of entry by emerging through the drainage system. This also has the added problem that they can be heavily contaminated from the sewer. They leave an unwanted smell and taint on foods where they have contaminated it. They are more difficult to detect than other insects because they are nocturnal; however, close inspection at night time will soon reveal their presence. The cockroach breeds through producing nymphs that can reach adulthood in 8–12 weeks. The offspring from one couple can be as many as 10 000. There are different types of cockroach native to the different continents.

In order to treat factories or buildings where there is evidence of cockroaches, one has to find out where they shelter. Generally they are very difficult to find, but one can use substances such as synthetic pyrethrins which can be used to stimulate the cockroaches and encourage them out of hiding, which is usually in cracks, crevices or other suitable hiding places. Once the hiding places are known it is then possible to treat them – this will normally be by applying a synthetic pyrethoid or organophosphorous insecticide.

Mites are very small insects which are normally very difficult to see with the naked eye; however, some can be detected from the 'minty' odour they emit which can taint the infested food. They are members of the arachnid group. There are a wide range of species but the most common species found in foodstuffs are *Glycyphagus*, *Tyrophagus* sp. and *Acarus* sp. Mites tend to live in and on stored commodities foodstuffs such as grains and oilseeds. They can live in certain specific foods. One of the most common is the flour mite, *Acarus siro*. The optimum breeding conditions for the flour mite are 21–27°C and a relative humidity of 80%. Mites can be detected through a number of means, and mite traps can be used to pinpoint the source of infection and the extent of the infestation.

It is very difficult to see them as they are the size of dust particles and they can be spread easily, being conveyed by moderate air flows, walking or being swept by brushing. They prefer a damp environment, so if a store is kept at the correct conditions mites should not infest. The common method of dealing with such an infestation problem is to fumigate with either phosphine gas or methyl bromide. The chemical pirimiphos-methyl can be used, but in most countries is closely regulated as to its area of application, storage containers, etc., along with the residual level in the food material. Other commercial insecticides are Actellic D liquid and Actellic.

Many mites are killed through the processing or handling systems within a mill or processing plant. If the correct sieves or types of screens are used they can remove the mites. The control of temperature and humidity can assist in reducing the mites' chances of survival.

3.2.5 *Ants*

Ants can be a major nuisance and can cause contamination of foods very rapidly due to their acute sense of smell, in particular in detecting their main liking of sweet foods such as honey and jams. Some ants also eat proteins such as cheese, blood and meats. Ants are usually a problem during the warmer months of the year (in colder climates). They can live outside or inside and find a habitat usually under stones, in paving cracks or among plant roots. During their feeding part of the lifecycle they tend to forage for food and this is when there is the highest risk of contamination in the food factory. The ants set up trails and will search out food sources. They are quite adept at climbing pipes and following pipe routes or finding their way through cracks. After the summer the ants swarm, which is when the flying ants are seen. Depending on where the nest is located, this can produce a further risk of contamination. The 'swarming' is part of the lifecycle, and involves both females and males. It usually lasts only for a few days. The two main types of ants that cause a problem are the common black ant and the garden ant. Another species is a tropical ant called Pharaoh's ant. In a colony there is normally one queen and the larvae are cared for until they pupate.

In order to treat a problem of an ant infestation it is best to locate the nest(s) and treat these. The nests can be treated with sprays around the location in case there are other undetected nests. There are also dry formats that can be used to reach less accessible locations. Another method is to use baits which are carried back to the nest. These baits are either protein-based or sugar solutions laced with an appropriate insecticide.

3.2.6 *Beetles*

Beetles belong to a group called dermestidae and present many potential problems. Some species feed only on animal matter, others only on vegetable matter and some on both. Within the cereals and baking industry there are a number of common beetles such as the red flour, biscuit, 'drug-store', spider and saw tooth beetles. The beetles tend not to survive winter conditions unless they are in heated locations. Infestations may be treated by the use of fumigation or suitable insecticides.

3.3 Eradication of pests

For most pests it is difficult to eradicate them completely, but is possible to control them. Infestations of certain vermin have to be eradicated and it is normal to call in the expert to handle this. There are a range of eradication methods for specific types of pests.

Other types of eradication can be more involved and mean sealing up the premises and defumigating. This can cause operational problems as the area will be out of action for several days and the materials also have to be treated. It is important to ensure that the building fabric is suitable for fumigation. In Table 3.2 there are some different forms of insecticide.

The insecticides are usually organophosphorous compounds in nature. With fumigation one has to ensure that the building is suitable. Porous structures or building fabrics such as breeze blocks can often be problematic as the gas can be absorbed into the building materials. It is possible to shield off areas using impermeable membranes such as plastics. If there is any doubt about how to treat an infestation it is advised that your pest control company is asked to deal with the situation.

There are specialist pest control companies that provide services for the eradication of pests. Any reputable pest control company

Table 3.2 Different forms of insecticide

Form of insecticide	Concentration	Application
Dusts	1–1.5%	for inaccessible harbourages or locations beneath or inside building structure or within machinery
Smoke	lidane smoke generators	use on ships for flying insects in empty warehouses
Fogs	oil spray (pyrethum)	this can be used within food premises for immediate impact on flying insects
Sprays (oil based)	0.25–1.0%	used for food residues that are in difficult locations but not to be used on foodstuffs
Powders (wettable)	0.5–1.0%	can be applied to hideaways where food is not present

employs experts who can determine which pests are present and which methods of eradication or control are possible and the most effective. Some companies provide a complete service and will manage all aspects concerned with pest control for a food company.

3.4 Building design

Often the building design is considered unimportant to the food manufacturer. This is not so as it plays a vital role in determining the safety and quality of food produced, and will affect the bottom line of the company. Food is produced in many different types of facilities, but all have to be safe, hygienic and fit for their purpose.

3.4.1 Factory location

The location of the factory can have a significant impact on the integrity of the factory and the potential contamination of food processed or stored at that location. The potential risk from the surrounding environment can be significant. If another manufacturing site, which is located near to a food factory, starts processing dry dusty materials such as rubble compounding, minerals or cement in an open environment, this could have a major impact or risk on the factory. The prevailing wind direction is a very important factor as it could increase the likelihood of airborne dust and contaminants being carried from another site and entering the factory either through the air intake or through other openings. Certain preventative measures can be taken in order to seal, but this is expensive and does not always prevent taints in the form of volatiles entering.

The food company then has to lodge complaints with the local authorities to prevent such a risk occurring. The factory should be sited on land which is not likely to flood and away from any sources of airborne contamination such as chimney stacks or exhaust vents from other factories.

As we know it is impossible to make food premises completely airtight and, therefore, where there is a potential risk from airborne contaminates from the surrounding local environment it has to be taken seriously. There are some means of redress through the local authorities or courts if the contaminants contravene the local or national environmental laws.

Some older factories face different environmental problems as often they may have be sited next to a potential hazard or risk such as a river where there can be many rodents that are keen to use the factory as a source of food supply. Many animals will go to extreme lengths to burrow, swim, jump or climb any preventative measures that are taken to stop them entering.

3.4.2 *Factory layout*

The layout of the factory is important in preventing or deterring the potential contamination of foods. A factory which is cramped and lacking in space has the added risk in that something may fall over or be dislodged and other process equipment in close proximity could become contaminated. This type of cross-contamination incident is all too common in poorly designed factories.

Segregation of working areas is most important to ensure that there is no cross-contamination from one area to another, one product to another and from raw ingredients into the product. Raw, untreated foodstuffs should be kept physically separate from treated clean product. Most factories are designed now such that the higher risk areas are segregated, in particular the area where a treated product is being filled into its primary container or pack and even more so when there is no further processing such as heat treatment. This area as well as providing a high microbiological risk can also present a high general contamination risk as in some processes it is the only time when the food product is exposed to atmosphere. It is, therefore, important in this type of high risk area that the air is treated appropriately and that the people working in this area are well trained and appreciate the potential risks.

Air circulation should be such as to prevent the carry over of airborne contaminants. One method is to ensure areas are categorized and then use a higher air pressure in the highest risk area.

3.4.3 *Interior finishes*

Most factories are not new and some are quite old. Some of the older buildings, particularly those not specifically designed as food premises, can have many potential problems. Older buildings often have internal wall cavities or voids which can present ideal locations for vermin and for dirt and dust to collect. These are best dealt with by either structural changes if suitable, filling or sealing.

The design of the food factory building can have a significant effect on contamination prevention. One of the major causes of contamination that results from building fabrics is the shedding of material, this can come about through various causes such as:

- Flaking paint
- Rusting steelwork
- Build up of deposits of dust and dirt
- Cracks, etc.

The selection of building materials can have a significant impact to overcome some of these common problems. The selection of paints and their application can assist and many of the paint manufacturers have addressed some of the issues relating to flaking paint. Traditionally food factory walls were tiled to a certain height, normally about 1.5–2 m, and then painted above that height. The preferred method by many food producers and handlers now is to clad the walls, and this has shown some marked improvements. The cladding (more commonly known as composite panels) can be bought in various forms and can be supplied as insulated panels. Some of the common types of exterior finish to the panels are glass reinforced fibre, polyvinyl chloride, sheet stainless steel and Plastisol. The insulation material requires careful selection to ensure that it has the correct fire resistant properties, and that it is both safe from a fire and a food safety point of view. There are a variety of core materials and one of the most common ones now is mineral wool because it is non-combustible. However, one needs to ensure the use of non-shedding materials which are well bonded.

Mastics or rubberized sealants are useful to bond and seal the panels. An even better option is the use of welded stainless steel sheets as cladding, thus providing an impregnable layer which can be thoroughly cleaned. For most applications this proves to be an expensive option.

Floors need to be such that they do not crack, as cracks can provide insects with an excellent hiding place. To avoid the risk of cracks one should consider the following:

- The foundation of the floor – is it solid?
- Is floor suitable for point loadings?
- Appropriate sealing of the top surface – tiles, epoxy, etc.
- Designed for cleaning and drainage
- Floor needs to be designed with appropriate falls for drainage
- Damp course needs to be in place

The Food Hygiene Regulations 1995 require that the layout, design, construction and size of food premises should be such as to permit adequate cleaning and/or disinfection. They should be protected against the accumulation of dirt, contact with toxic materials, the shedding of particles into food and the formation of condensation or undesirable mould on surfaces.

The use of glass in the building fabric should be avoided wherever possible, and where used must be such that there is no potential risk of breakage and possible risk of contamination.

3.4.4 *Working environment*

In most factories people are required to operate machines, carry out tasks, etc. The conditions are most important in order for people to work effectively and efficiently in a healthy environment. The major factors that affect performance are temperature, lighting levels and humidity. Research has been carried out to determine how people are affected by these conditions. Table 3.3 shows some recommended lighting levels for different working environments. Illuminance is measured in lux where a lux is equal to 0.093 lumens per square metre. A lumen per square metre being equivalent to 1 foot candle.

In particular, lighting levels are important in the food industry where inspection work is carried out. It is also important that the ratios of illuminance for adjacent areas are not too high where people are transferring from one area to another, so as to minimize eye strain and adjustment time.

Glare can be experienced in a number of different ways. One example is looking directly at bright objects such as light filaments – usually lights have shades fitted to prevent this. A contrast in lighting levels can be a problem which is associated with poor lighting design due to positioning of lamps, shades, etc. Reflected glare when light is reflected off objects, often producing glinting, is a problem in many food factories due to the presence of highly reflective stainless steel surfaces and the presence of water.

As food processing equipment is regularly moved and relocated it is important that lighting levels are regularly reviewed in order to ensure that the optimum conditions abound, particularly where inspection is taking place or in an area of high risk. Lights should be

Table 3.3 Recommended lighting levels for different working environments (Occupational Health and Hygiene, 1995)

General activity	Typical location	Average illuminance (lux)	Minimum illuminance (lux)
Movement of people, machines and vehicles	lorry parks, corridors, circulation routes	20	5
Movement of people, machines and vehicles in hazardous areas; rough work not requiring any perception of detail	construction site clearance, excavation and soil works, docks, loading bays, bottling and canning plants	50	20
Work requiring limited perception of detail	kitchens, factories, assembling of large components, potteries	100	50
Work requiring perception of detail	office, sheet metal worker, bookbinding	200	100
Work requiring fine perception of detail	drawing offices, factories assembling electronic components, textile production	500	200

protected so as to ensure there is no possible contamination of foods if they break. The surround units should be made of plastic and designed so as to prevent any glass falling from them if there is a breakage.

Noise levels are also important as they can produce damage to hearing, but at lower levels can also affect concentration. Governments set specific exposure levels to sound above which ear defenders must be worn.

The air temperature, air flow and wet bulb temperature in the work environment affects people's work and their performance. At sub-zero temperatures there are cold stress tolerance levels. When outdoor clothing is worn, the tolerance times at –12°C is a period of 6 hours whilst at –57°C it reduces to approximately 0.5 hours. The optimum temperature for factory work is 18.3°C for light work and 12.8–15.6°C for heavy work. An acceptable level of relative humidity is best between 30 and 70%. As it is necessary to have a high risk area at a higher air pressure this could create a high air velocity. Velocities above 0.5 m/second cause people to feel a draught and be uncomfortable, and therefore potentially affect their performance.

3.4.5 *Immediate factory surroundings*

The location of a factory is important – many older factories have been sited historically. The location and type of food factory will determine the likely species of vermin and insects that will be attracted. Around the outside of the building it is advantageous to place gravel, normally a depth of several centimetres is sufficient, and a strip width of a few 100s of centimetres. The purpose for this is that many rodents do not like to walk on gravel and hence they will not cross this boundary. However, some animals will go to great extent to try and enter factories, and they will burrow under fences and bite through woodwork. It is important if in a rural area to ensure perimeter fencing is appropriate to keep out unwanted pests.

It is important to keep rubbish, in particular waste food materials, well concealed as these will often attract insects, birds and vermin, as many have very acute odour receptors.

3.4.6 *Entrances and exits*

Doors into and out of production areas should not open directly outside as this can allow airborne contaminants to easily enter each time the door is opened. If there is a two-door entry system, materials or any other items entering the production area can be checked and if necessary transferred to more appropriate containers before utilization in the production area.

Many rodents and insects enter the factory through openings. These may be doors, windows, air bricks, drains, etc. There are many methods of protection. Brushes can be fitted around doors and other openings which prevent insects crawling under or through cracks.

Sealing can be carried out using mastics or other appropriate sealant around drains and openings in walls so as to prevent any entrances for vermin. Care should be taken to ensure that in blocking holes there is adequate ventilation to prevent build-up of carbon monoxide or other gases produced from combustion or reactions.

3.4.7 People

As people are a major potential source of contamination within food factories it is vital that this risk is minimized through general good manufacturing practices which include:

- Personal hygiene – general cleanliness
- Health – no infectious diseases, etc.
- Hair – protection, no hair clips, etc.
- General clothes – appropriate protective clothing or change of clothing
- Footware – change, protective, washing or sterilizing
- Appropriate washing facilities – sterilizing
- Removal of rings, jewellery, etc.
- Clothing designed to be non-shedding – no loose ends, buttons, etc.
- Detectable pens, etc.

Generally the minimum of change for staff entering a food production area should include – hair net to prevent any hair falling into products, a snood for those with beards and a hat. From hair there is the risk from the bacteria *Staphylococci*. It is a major issue with many customers if they find hair in any foodstuffs. A change of footwear into shoes or boots which are easily cleanable is advisable along with the correct cleaning procedures and facilities. It is often appropriate in high-risk factories to have a footwear cleaning systems in operation where boots are automatically cleaned and sterilized prior to entry into the factory. The degree of cleaning or sanitation and changing will depend on the risk. Colour-coded footwear can be used in different areas of the factory to indicate the level of risk and ensure there is no cross-contamination. It may be sufficient to wear overshoes if outside footwear is to be worn in the factory. However, overshoes are not recommended for routine use as they wear very rapidly and once holed are inadequate.

In wet production areas a foot bath should be used on entry. For this to be effective it requires routine checking and cleaning. The foot bath has to be well designed – easy to empty and fill, deep enough, sited in the right place. Trays containing sponges can be useful but in many cases they are not routinely cleaned and, therefore, can add to the spread of contamination, If they become contaminated everyone passing through them will also become contaminated and a rapid spread of contamination will arise.

Protective coats should have pockets on the inside so as to prevent anything falling out of them. Jewellery such as watches, rings, necklaces, hair clips, bands, earrings, etc., should be removed as these can easily fall off or break and end up in the food products being processed or manufactured. Pens, which are often used in a factory, should be metallic such that they can be detected by the metal detectors employed in the factory (they should be tested before being approved for use). Finger nails should be well looked after, clean and manicured. Often nails can be bitten or fall off, therefore short, well manicured nails reduce any risk.

Gloves are often worn where food is to be directly handled. This barrier method is an effective one if managed correctly. Rules have to be set as to when to use gloves, for how long, what products to handle, etc. If used incorrectly they can aid the spread of contamination.

What is vital is that personnel change their clothing when entering the factory and change back whenever they go outside. One of the major sources of contamination is from dirt and dust carried in on workers shoes and clothing. Clothing should be laundered regularly by an approved laundry company.

3.4.8 External building

The external structure and appearance of the building can present some potential problems. Features such as skylights, located in the roof to allow in additional light, can also let in other unwanted creatures and contaminants. Skylights can also leak and if they do any contaminated water drips will possibly land on food products below. Glass windows in the roof are a major potential hazard as they could potentially break and then fall into food products below, they should be avoided or at the minimum replaced with non-breakable plastic.

Pigeons and other birds can be a problem if they find places to roost on the roof on ledges on the building. They have a habit of dropping faeces, feathers and other undesirable matter which can then find its way into the factory. The building should be designed so it does not have suitable ledges, etc., for birds. Protective measures should be taken to stop birds landing if the building does have possible perching locations.

3.5 Machinery and equipment design

The design of machinery and processing equipment systems can present potential food safety risks if not carried out correctly. The major sources of problems tend to be the disintegration of components, conveyor belts, contact parts and leaks, and the use of non-appropriate materials of construction such as brass, copper or glass.

3.5.1 Processing machinery

Equipment design can be a major concern as the machinery parts will normally contact or be in close proximity to the foodstuff being processed, handled or packaged. There has been a considerable amount of work carried out on the hygienic design of food processing equipment.

The European Union funded a project carried out by the European Hygienic Equipment Design Group (EHEDG). This group developed a systematic approach to the evaluation of the cleanability of in-line pieces of equipment. Although it was predominately for equipment which in cleaned-in-place (CIP) it has also issued guidelines for open processing equipment. The guidelines include some specific design issues concerning a range of food processing machine components.

Recently there has been the development of machinery directives. These new European directives cover specific types of machines, and include their design operation and cleaning. There is also now a requirement to use food grade oils and lubricants in machines as the lubricant can sometimes leak from bearings or couplings and cause contamination. Although food grade lubricants do not solve the leakage problems they do minimize risk.

Open top processing systems such as tanks for mixing or storage of products can be a potential area of contamination risk as objects may fall undetected into the tank. If the tank is a mixer the object may be ground down in size and pass through the processing system. If it is metal it may be ground to fine particles which are then not detected by metal detectors further downstream. It is therefore important to protect tanks with lids. The lids or manways can have detectors fitted that indicate if they are open. Some tanks, however, have to be opened as one may be tipping powder from sacks into the tank. In this case pieces of paper sack may pass into the product. There are several ways of preventing this. One is to place a mesh filter over the top of the tank to prevent pieces of sack material entering the system; however, small pieces may still enter and these would be collected by a secondary finer mesh filter. An improved method is to unbag and sieve powders into an intermediate container which is then tipped into the mixer.

3.5.2 *Heating ventilation and air conditioning (HVAC)*

HVAC systems can cause major contamination risks if not designed, managed, maintained and cleaned correctly. The systems normally take the form of ducting, mostly hidden either in the roof void or behind walls. The systems are often forgotten about as one cannot see them. There can be the potential of dust and debris building up in the system or of pests infiltrating. With air flowing through the system and being blown out into the production area this can have quite severe consequences.

The HVAC system needs to be inspected regularly and if necessary cleaned. Some developments have been made to produce automatic inspection 'pigs' which take the form of a robot-type device that can be placed inside the ducting and can inspect by relaying back images from a camera located on the robot. Some companies have designed and installed fully cleanable HVAC systems, even to the extent of cleaning them in place. Care should be taken to ensure any condensation that is collected is piped to suitable drainage system.

There is the use of air socks which are used to distribute air and are placed over a fan unit which forces air into them. This type of system gives a good distribution of air but unless the air is well filtered beforehand dirt and dust can build up within the sock. Similarly, if the sock is not regularly cleaned debris can build up on the outside and can then be deposited onto a food operation below.

3.5.3 *Services and utilities*

Services such as steam pipes or water distribution systems can present a range of potential contamination issues. Dirt and dust can lay on the tops of pipes and lagging can fall off or disintegrate with time. Pipes can collect condensation and begin to rust. Pipes should always be lagged where appropriate, in particular where condensation may occur, and therefore water, contaminated with paint fibres or oxidized metals, may potentially drip on the product below. The lagging should be such that it is non-shedding and sealed to prevent insects entering. The lagging should be carefully cleaned periodically to prevent dust build-up on the top surface.

There has always been a discussion as to the best form of cable protection: cable trays or trunking. Trays give the advantage that one can see any dirt and dust if it collects. Trunking, however, can be tidier and cleaner, and if the trunking is sealed it can be hygienic. However, most trunking is opened, which allows insects and other material to enter and collect. Whether trays or trunking, they require inspecting regularly and cleaning when appropriate to remove any dust build-up.

3.6 Maintenance and repairs

The maintenance of equipment and the building fabric are most important as many contamination issues arise from poor maintenance or as a result of equipment repairs. Planned and preventative maintenance are good methods to adopt as it is the rushed unscheduled jobs which often go wrong, and in which corners are cut and procedures overridden, thus creating additional risks of potential contamination. Although there is an investment required to implement a preventative maintenance or total productive maintenance (TPM) policy, if carried out effectively it can reduce the risk of:

- Wire strands being deposited
- Nuts and bolts being left loose
- Equipment reassembled incorrectly
- Insufficient cleaning

A permit to work system is an excellent method of ensuring that repair or maintenance jobs are carried out according to the required methods. This system also allows one to have an audit trail if things do go wrong so that errors can be put right quickly or batches held for positive release.

The use of any glass associated with tools, instruments, etc., should be very closely monitored within the factory to ensure there is no risk of breakage and potential contamination. Glass thermometers should be not be used.

3.7 Factory hygienic practices

Keeping a factory clean is a difficult task. The main causes of contamination are people, ingredients and air. It is very difficult to eliminate even one of these components and still be able to operate a factory. Some companies with very sensitive foods have either investigated or do use a clean room approach. Clean room technology is obviously used in other industry such as electronics, nuclear, some pharmaceuticals or weapons production. For many food production areas clean room technology is too expensive or does not have a significant impact on improving hygiene.

Many different methods have been used to disinfect production areas. The more traditional method was to spray water using hose pipes or, more recently, high pressure hoses. This can be useful in certain facilities, but it has been proven that hoses can produce very fine spray in the form of aerosols which can be airborne and, after cleaning, settle and foul a cleaned area. Fogging has been used by companies and this actually makes use of the aerosol effect to form a disinfectant fog which then settles on all the areas and equipment, treating the surface and any airborne material.

Foams produced from a mixture of water and cleaning aid are often used. These are sprayed onto equipment and allowed to coat the equipment treating the surface, but they are often good at penetrating where sprays often miss. It is also possible to see what has been coated and ensure no areas are missed.

Smoke bombs are commonly used in the horticultural-based environment. They are also used in food installations but with great care and for specific applications. They are normally used for warehouses and never in areas of direct food contact as residues can occur and odours can cause taints in foods.

3.8 Treatment of raw materials and eradication

3.8.1 *Treatment of raw materials*

Some ingredients have to be treated to kill any contaminating pests. For herbs and spices ethylene oxide was used until its banning. Other processes have now been developed such as steam heating techniques, extrusion, irradiation or microwave technology to sterilize or treat raw ingredients that are potentially contaminated with micro-organisms or spores.

3.8.2 *Social and environmental protection*

There is a growing environmental interest and one has to acknowledge this in the choice of methods that are used for the control of infestations. The use of environmental impact studies can assist in determining whether it is appropriate to use certain chemicals. Many chemicals used have been modified to be ecologically acceptable.

3.9 Tamper evident systems

A growing form of deliberate contamination is that of malicious and deliberate adulteration through tampering. Handling this type of contamination is covered under crisis management in Chapter 2. This marked increase in malicious adulteration has resulted in food manufacturers taking appropriate action to protect the consumer. There are now many forms of tamper proof or tamper evident seals which form an integral part of the food packaging. This ensures that once the food has been processed it is evident or easily seen if anyone has opened the container or package. There are a range of different types of tamper evident systems available, such as:

- Sleeving
- Tabs

- Sticky labels strategically placed over openings
- Overwrapping
- Vacuum sealing
- Breakable seals on tops, lids, etc.

These systems are now widely used and have prevented contamination but have also allowed food companies to ensure a higher integrity of their products. Although this type of system is not 100% foolproof as it does not combat anyone managing to gain access to the factory and contaminate the food prior to it being sealed in the pack.

3.10 Quality systems

Quality systems have been utilized in many industries for many years for component manufacture, precision parts manufacture and materials inspection. It has only been in more recent years that the wider structured approach to quality has been appreciated and utilized. With the implementation of new standards this has promoted the use of documented quality systems. There has been a distinct change in thinking brought about by a 'Total Quality' culture, much of which was talked about and promoted by Crosby, Juran and Deming. The major changes have been away from quality just being about the quality of the product and having quality inspectors, and towards quality being:

- Strategic
- Led from the top of the company
- About the whole organization
- Involves improvement
- Involves everyone

Quality systems are used to lay down procedures and methods to ensure that a product or process is carried out according to that procedure every time. A quality system does not ensure that the quality of a product will be improved. It is a method of making sure that a product is manufactured by the same method and standards every time. The level of detail of the procedures, methods or processes contained in the system documentation can vary significantly.

3.10.1 ISO 9000

Quality control and assurance are a key part of any GMPs. Many companies have now been accredited with an ISO 9000. The first attempt to develop quality standards was in the USA and one of the earliest standards was MIL-I-45208 which was specific for use with inspection system requirements. Other standards were drawn up for use in defence for NATO. These are called the Allied Quality Assurance Publications (AQAP) 1, 4 and 9. AQAP 1 was a quality systems specification and AQAP 4 and 9 were inspection system specifications.

More recently, in 1979, was the first edition of the British standard BS 5750, which was based on the AQAP standard. Following on from BS 5750-1979 was the European equivalent range of ISO 9000 standards which are listed below:

ISO 9000 Quality Management and Quality Assurance Standards – Guidelines for Selection and Use
ISO 9001 Quality Systems – Model for Quality Assurance in Design and Development, Production, Installation and Servicing
ISO 9002 Quality Systems – Model for Quality Assurance in Production and Installation
ISO 9003 Quality Systems – Model for Quality Assurance in Final Inspection and Test
ISO 9004 Quality Management and Quality System Elements – Guidelines

The ISO 9000 standards are now recognized internationally in over 100 countries. The standard means that the company has established written procedures to which it operates. The procedures describe how tasks are performed. The company has an inspection by an accredited inspection company and if it passes is accredited. There are then regular announced and unannounced visits to check on compliance. It is also a requirement to carry out internal audits by trained assessors.

Once the company has been accredited it faces regular inspection to ensure it continues to operate according to its procedures as laid down in its quality manual. The objective of a quality system should be:

- A key company initiative supported by the board
- A means of preventing problems
- Written down adhered to system
- Everyone in the company involved
- All staff trained
- Ensure compliance
- Means of system auditing

Many companies also work to a total quality management system commonly known as TQM.

3.10.2 *Business excellence model and benchmarking*

Many companies have seen it important to improve their methods and processes. One method that has been adopted is that of benchmarking. Benchmarking is a method of comparing one's performance in a quantifiable manner against a set standard. In order to benchmark one has to carry out an assessment. A European model has been established as a way of scoring one's business operations so as to give an overall score. It has been established that over 250 represents a world class manufacturing score. Figure 3.1 shows how the business is divided and what weightings are placed on different parts of the business.

One of the first such systems was that developed for the Buldridge award in the USA. However, the initial assessment did not include a measure of profitability and, therefore, many companies scored very highly but went out of business.

Benchmarking of best practices combined with an organizational enthusiasm for learning, can enable companies to instantly increase their competitiveness through improved management and technical practices by learning from best-in-class companies. The Nabisco Biscuit Company in 1994 benchmarked best-in-class companies with regard to cross-functional team best practices. As a result of the study they changed the way they managed their new product development (NPD) teams. By comparing their practices with other companies and evaluating their performance they were able to make instant major advances without the painful and slow approach. Although this was in the area of NPD, the same approach could be adopted in areas such as GMP, food safety or HACCP. The method of benchmarking can be used at an overall business level or at a manufacturing level and even at an equipment level.

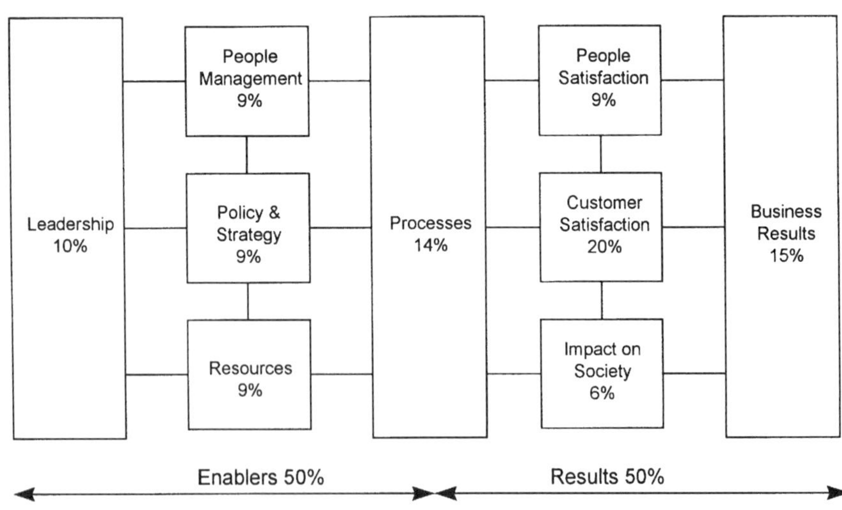

Figure 3.1 The business excellence model.

3.10.3 Self-assessment

The European Quality Forum uses the business excellence model which consists of nine elements which are termed enablers or results. The elements of Leadership; Policy and Strategy; People Management; Resources; and Processes are termed the enablers which enable the organization to harness and release the talents of its people. The elements of People Satisfaction; Customer Satisfaction; Impact on Society; and Business Results are concerned with results the organization has and is achieving. The approach allows one to numerically score a company in each of the areas, thus giving the ability to compare one company's performance against another. An annual award is presented (European Quality Award [EQA]) for the company that scores the highest. A description of each element of the business excellence model is given in Table 3.4.

3.10.4 Quality Function Deployment (QFD) in R & D

QFD allows technical developers to understand what users want and need which the more traditional market research often ignores.

Table 3.4 Description of element in the business excellence model (BEM)

BEM model element	Description
Leadership	A measure of management commitment to its employees, suppliers, customers, stakeholders and the community at large
Policy and strategy	The organization's mission, values, vision and the means by which they will be achieved
People management	The management of all employees and the release of their full potential to improve the organization continuously
Resources	The measure of an organization's ability to manage the preservation and use of resources
Processes	The ability of the organization to identify, and review value adding activities to ensure continuous business improvements
Customer satisfaction	The achieved perception of the organization as judged by its customers
People satisfaction	The organization's ability in achieving in terms of satisfying people needs, aspirations and pride as measured by employees at all levels
Impact on society	How society at large views the organization, its approach to quality of life, the environment and preservation of resources
Business results	The organization's achievements in relation to its planned performance

In addition there are linkages between QFD and a new product development process.

3.10.5 Auditing

Auditing is used in order to assess how good a factory is, whether it relates to hygiene, environmental, ISO 9000, maintenance, HACCP, energy or safety. Most factories are familiar with regular audits from a quality or safety aspect, but few have systems in place to audit other issues such as maintenance, energy or management methods. One can assess a range of issues using an external body to audit the facility. Auditing has grown, although it is not always popular as it can disrupt production when too many audits take place.

Within companies there are usually annual internal audits which should be carried out by trained assessors. It is good for staff from other divisions or other companies in the group to audit each other. Although they are centred around a checklist, audits should be more than this.

Many retailers carry out their own regular audits to assess how well their suppliers are performing and ensure that the required standards are being met. Factories grow complacent and are often insular, so the use of external experts to assess key issues can be most beneficial to a company. The majority of external audits are normally announced (pre-arranged with everyone knowing) but within larger organizations unannounced audits are used and with ISO 9000 are common. The unannounced audit can allow the auditor to get a better, more realistic impression of the way in which the factory normally operates.

References and further reading

Bauer, F. (1982) *Bird Control in Food Plants*. Food Trade Press, Orpington, Kent.

BSI (1991) *ISO 9000 Guidelines for Food*. BSI, London.

CCFRA (1994) *Guidelines for the Design and Construction of Walls, Ceilings and Services for Food Production Areas*. Campden and Chorleywood Food Research Association, Chipping Campden.

CCFRA (1996) *Guidelines on Air Quality Standards for the Food Industry*. Campden and Chorleywood Food Research Association, Chipping Campden.

EHEDG (1993) *Hygienic Equipment Design Criteria*. The European Hygienic Equipment Design Group, Campden and Chorleywood Food Research Association, Chipping Campden.

FDA (1977) *Current Good Manufacturing Practice in Manufacturing, Processing, Packing, or Holding of Human Food*. Federal Food and Drug Administration, Washington, DC.

Hayes, P. R. (ed.) (1985) *Food Microbiology and Hygiene*. Elsevier, Oxford.

HMSO (1991) *Food Safety Act*. HMSO, London.

HMSO (1995) *The Food Hygiene Regulations.* HMSO, London.
IFST (1993) *Guide to Good Manufacturing Practice – GMP Guidelines.* Institute of Food Science and Technology, London.
Imholte, T. J. (1984) *Engineering for Food Safety and Sanitation.* Technical Institute of Food Safety, Crystal, MN.
Jowitt, R. (ed.) (1980) *Hygienic Design and Operation of Food Plant.* Ellis Horwood, Chichester.
Juran, J. M. (1988) *Juran's Quality Control Handbook.* McGraw-Hill, New York.
Juran, J. M. (1992) *On Quality by Design.* Free Press, New York.
Marriott, N. G. (1985) *Principles of Food Sanitation.* AVI, Westport, CT.
Shapton, D. A. and Shapton, N. T. (eds) (1991) *Principles and Practices for Safe Processing of Food.* Butterworth Heinemann, Oxford.
Sprenger, R. A. (1991) *Hygiene for Management*, 5th edn. Highfield, Doncaster.
Stranks, J. (1995) *Occupational Health and Hygiene.* RoSPA/Pitman, London.

4

Legislation

4.1 Introduction

The objective of this chapter is to provide an overview of the law as it applies to foreign bodies in foods. The main emphasis relates to the legal position in the UK which is derived from European Community (EC) directives. The laws concerning the prevention of foreign body contamination in food are, therefore, the same in the rest of the EU and it will be found that similar principles apply everywhere there is food safety legislation. The chapter is written by a layman for the defined purpose only. Whenever advice is required of a legal nature, then the advice of lawyers and other experts specializing in the field should be sought.

In theory the requirements of all the other member states of the EU should be the same or very similar. One of the objectives of the EC is to establish general requirements for food safety and hygiene applicable throughout all the member states as part of the food harmonization programme, thus allowing free trade in food throughout the community. This objective is achieved by the Council of the EEC issuing directives which under the terms of membership of the EC must be implemented in national laws within a specified time period.

Non-EU countries have their own legislation. Advice on what these requirements must be sought from other sources, preferably from within the country in question or by using the resources of research associations such as Leatherhead Food Research Association or Campden and Chorleywood Food Research Association. Legislation world-wide is in a constant state of flux in terms of revision and innovation. Hence, up-to-the-minute statutes must always be determined.

4.2 Summary of the European hygiene directives applicable to food

There are two general directives relating to all food products:

Council Directive 89/397/EEC	General hygiene directive on the official control of foods
Council Directive 93/43/EEC	General rules on the hygiene of foodstuffs.

In addition there are a series of directives relating to specific foodstuffs:

Council Directive 92/116/EEC	Health problems affecting trade in fresh poultry meat.
Council Directive 92/46/EEC	Health rules for the production and sale of milk products
Council Directive 92/5/EEC	Hygiene standards for trade in meat products
Council Directive 91/497/EEC	Health rules for the fresh meat trade
Council Directive 91/433/EEC	Updates 91/497/EEC
Council Directive 91/495/EEC	Health rules for the trade in game and rabbit meat
Council Directive 92/45/EEC	Health rules for the trade in wild game meat
Council Directive 91/493/EEC	Health rules for the trade in fishery products
Council Directive 89/437/EEC	Health rules for the trade in egg products

The directives relating to specific foods have been found to contain some inconsistencies and the EC has committed to rationalizing them. Within the context of this chapter they have little if any relevance as the subject of 'Foreign Bodies' is covered under the general directives.

An EEC document, relating to the review of existing specific product directives, entitled '*Guide to certain rules governing production, marketing and importation of products of animal origin intended for human consumption*' was issued during 1996 by the EC Directorate General for Agriculture. Significantly, the document emphasizes the importance of HACCP systems in establishing hygiene standards. It recognizes that inspectors from enforcement authorities cannot supervise or see all production processes in all establishments all the time and that the responsibility has to be with the manufacturers. For this to be effective manufacturers need to use quality systems based on a HACCP system or something very similar.

4.3 Current UK food hygiene legislation

The major Act of Parliament affecting foreign body legislation as it applies to food is the 1990 Food Safety Act. This is the UK's interpretation of the Council Directive 89/397/EEC which is the General Hygiene directive on the official control of foods. It was introduced into UK law under the Food Safety Act 1990

In addition there are the following regulations made under the act:

- Food premises Registration Regulations 1991
- General Product Safety Regulations 1994
- Food Safety (General Food Hygiene) Regulations 1995
- Food Safety (Temperature Control) Regulations 1995

4.3.1 The Food Safety Act 1990 (SI 1990 No 2484)

The Food Safety Act 1990 is designed to improve the safety of food and food products throughout the complete process from 'field to plate' of food production. Enforcement powers, defence and penalties are specified. When the Act was introduced in 1990 it introduced a new, to the food industry, defence of 'due diligence' (Section 21 of the Act).

The presence of a foreign body in food or the absence or prevention of such an occurrence are the subject of three separate sections of the Act defining the offence:

Section 7 A person commits an offence if he/she renders any food injurious to health by either adding any article or substance to the food, using any article or substance as an ingredient in the preparation of the food abstracting any constituent from the food or subjecting the food to any other process or treatment with intent that it shall be sold for human consumption.

Section 8 A person commits an offence if he/she sells for human consumption, or offers exposes or advertises for sale for such consumption or has in his/her possession for the purposes of such sale or of preparation for sale or deposits with, or consigns to, any other person for the purpose of such sale or of preparation for such sale any food which fails to comply with the food safety requirements.

Section 14 A person commits an offence if he/she sells to the purchaser's prejudice food which is not of the nature or substance or quality demanded by the purchaser.

An offence is deemed to have been committed in the event of a foreign body being found in a food product offered for sale. This is a criminal offence. It is not necessary for the prosecuting authority to prove negligence or carelessness. A defence of 'due diligence' may be offered.

It is the concept of 'due diligence', expressed as having taken all reasonable precautions and exercised all 'due diligence', which is designed to ensure that anyone who is entirely innocent should not be convicted of a criminal offence. As with so much to do with law in the UK the exact definition of 'All Reasonable' and 'All Due Diligence' is open to interpretation by the courts.

4.3.2 The Consumer Protection Act 1987

This Act does not specifically relate to food, it is designed to prevent false or misleading claims or indications of the price of goods, it imposes an obligation to supply goods which comply with a general safety standard. The Act contains provisions for redress for injury and/or damage caused as a result of defective goods.

As with the Food Safety Act it creates an offence of strict liability, which means that the prosecuting body does not need to prove negligence, intention or recklessness. Under both Acts the offences are *criminal offences*. Enforcement of both Acts is the responsibility of either Trading Standards Officers or Environmental Health Officers working for Local Government departments. Prosecutions are initially held in Magistrates Courts or Crown Courts and can be pursued further through the legal process.

4.3.3 Penalties

Magistrates courts have the power to impose penalties up to £20 000 and/or 6 months imprisonment for each offence depending upon its nature. Crown courts have the power to impose unlimited fines but a maximum of 2 years imprisonment. These are penalties imposed by the Crown and are not the same as compensation claims for injury or damages resulting from the presence of a foreign body in food brought under civil proceedings.

Magistrates Courts do have the power to award small amounts of compensation, limited to £1000, while the County Courts are able to award an unlimited amount as compensation.

Civil proceedings can be instituted by the person who suffered from the presence of a foreign body in food in addition to, but not in place of, criminal proceedings brought by a local authority. Indeed, an enforcement authority prosecution may never arise. The type of proceeding and the potential damages will depend on a variety of factors which are beyond the scope of this book. Suffice it to say that any manufacturer is exposed to both criminal and civil proceedings should a foreign body be found in his/her products by a consumer or other interested party.

4.3.4 Responsibility.

In the case of a product manufactured in the UK, then the responsibility rests with the manufacturer if a foreign body is found in a product which either got into it during the manufacturing process or was not removed during the manufacturing process. In the case of prepacked products this is quite easy to define. In the case of product sold 'loose', e.g. cooked meats sold by a delicatessen, the question of responsibility for say an insect found as a foreign body is less clear and will need to be resolved either by mutual agreement between the shop, the manufacturer and the authority or by the courts.

In the case of food products imported into the UK, regardless of their source, the responsibility to ensure they are free from foreign body contamination rests with the importer. The level or amount of quality tests the importer needs to carry out will depend on the source of the product and the relationship of the importer to the manufacturer. Consider the difference between an international manufacturer with manufacturing plants throughout the EEC each specializing in a particular product for distribution throughout the market who has positive control over the quality procedures used in each plant and the importer of a product from a third world country where he/she has no real ability to control quality procedures.

In the case of private label products the position is not clear cut and will to some extent depend on the contractual relationship between the manufacturer and the retailer, and the manner in which the product is manufactured and presented (packed). In some cases the retailer may be able to rely on the quality control procedures used by the manufacturer; in others the retailer may need to carry out his/her own independent quality control checks.

While the various situations described above clearly require different levels of quality control procedures and tests by the person or company ultimately responsible for them, one fact is clear and that is that no one can rely solely on information supplied by the manufacturer or the importer. The person with the ultimate responsibility has to be able to prove that he/she has a continuous process of checking the efficiency and the operation of his/her suppliers' system.

4.3.5 General

The single most important factor that any manufacturer must be able to prove and demonstrate is that the manufacturer has considered the potential causes and sources of foreign body contamination in the product, and that a system is in place to ensure foreign bodies are not present in the finished product. To do nothing or to have no systems in place is absolutely unacceptable for any business. This does not necessarily mean that a small establishment has to have the same complexity and cost involved in its system as a multinational company. The small company may also be able to rely on the systems used by suppliers who are many times larger than they are, particularly where the suppliers are using systems such as BS EN ISO 9000. A larger company may be expected to use their experts to check their suppliers' systems.

The Acts described above in practice are only invoked when a consumer makes a complaint to the local authority. If the consumer decides to make a complaint to the manufacturer or the shop from where the product was purchased then, providing the complaint is dealt with in a manner which satisfies the consumer, most probably the matter will end there. It is, therefore, important that the manufacturers and distributors have an effective method of handling and investigating complaints which provides a prompt response to the consumer generating goodwill rather than frustration which may lead to the complaint being referred to the authorities. This subject is dealt with in Chapter 16.

4.4 The 'due diligence' defence with specific reference to foreign body contamination

4.4.1 Introduction

There is no clear single definition of what constitutes 'due diligence' and all reasonable precautions in UK law. This would be impossible to define as no two businesses use exactly the same raw materials and process them in exactly the same way using identical methods of control and inspection. There are three principles which must be met regardless of the detail of the system.

The first principle must be to do something. Any business that does nothing to consider the possibility of its product being contaminated by foreign matter is clearly negligent. It is accepted that the amount of consideration and investment put into the matter will not be the same for a large organization as a small one.

The second principle is that whatever system the business adopts it must be within the control of the business. This does not mean that specialist advice from outside cannot be used. Indeed there are occasions when this is strongly recommended. What must not be done under any circumstances is to rely entirely on outside organizations to ensure foreign body contamination does not occur.

The third principle is that whatever actions, decisions, plans, etc., that are developed by the business must be recorded. The records, whether electronic or hard copy, must be kept available and stored for a reasonable length of time.

The use of quality control systems is becoming increasingly common as witnessed by the increasing number of companies who obtain certification to EN BS ISO 9000 Part 1 or 2. To achieve this certification the business will have adopted a written system of risk assessment, identification of critical points within the process, the establishment of controls and provision for a continuous review of the effectiveness of the system, and a system of continuous improvement, all of which is recorded. This may be in a formal HACCP analysis of the process or a less formal procedure in the case of the smaller enterprise. It is clear that even the smallest food producer must give consideration to these factors as they apply to his/her product. Failure to do so will be seen as totally unacceptable.

There is not a strict definition of what is a small company and what is a large company. Campden and Chorleywood Food Research Association, Guideline No. 5, identifies the size of the enterprise and the impact the cost will have on the commercial viability of the enterprise as factors which must be considered when evaluating alternative measures.

These components of a quality control system can be identified as either 'due diligence' or 'reasonable precautions'

'Due diligence' items are:

- Adoption of a formal plan
- The keeping of records

Reasonable precaution items are:

- Assessment of risk
- Establishment of control points and methods of control
- Continuous review of effectiveness
- Continuous improvement to correct system failures of the system

It has been said that any business that does not have a metal detector on the end of the line cannot be seen as 'due diligence'. This is not necessarily true as in many cases a detector either could not be used because of the form of the final pack, e.g. a metal can, or because the presence of foreign bodies can be better controlled at another stage in the process or because a metal detector is not the appropriate inspection device to use. The analysis of risk and the definition of a control point are the proper techniques to be used in deciding what equipment should be used where.

4.4.2 *Food Safety Act 1990. Code of Practice No. 1: Paragraph 16*

Codes of practice are a concept that saves the lengthy process of making regulations. They give guidance to local authorities on the enforcement of the law. Because they can be quoted in court they effectively have the force of law and are generally respected and adhered to. A number of codes of practice have been issued under Section 40 of the Food Safety Act of which code number 1 is particularly relevant to foreign body questions. This code, reproduced by courtesy of LACOTS from their document *Guidance on Food Complaints*, states the following:

> *District Councils should investigate and take legal proceedings, in all cases of mould or foreign matter (such as glass or metal shavings) found on or in food. The district council may seek the opinion of experts such as the public analyst or food examiner in handling cases.*

This is a clear instruction to apply whenever a complaint is made which appears to the District Council to be valid. LACOTS (Local Authorities Co-ordinating Body on Food and Trading Standards) has issued a document on 'guidance for dealing with food complaints made to local authority environmental health departments'. In practice, the situation should not be so draconian as the introduction states that it 'encourages EHDs [enforcement authorities] to take a common sense approach to complaints choosing sensible action appropriate to risk and the minimum necessary in order to protect the general public'.

4.4.3 *The 'due diligence' defence: what is it, what does it mean*

In any manufacturing process it is impossible to guarantee the production to be free of defects all the time. This fact is gradually becoming recognized by the food industry, although it has long been recognized by the engineering industry. Engineers are trained to work with safety factors to cover the potential for error in product quality by building in a 'safety margin' or a little extra. Unfortunately this approach cannot be applied to food products. Secondly, engineers have analysed failures, and used the lessons learned to develop additional controls and preventative measures for a long time. One of the most public faces of this work is the results of the investigations that go on when an aircraft is lost or a 'near miss' occurs. The term 'due diligence' applies equally to engineering products and to food. One of its meanings encompasses recognizing that errors will occur and making strenuous efforts to prevent their occurrence.

4.4.4 *All reasonable precautions in the context of foreign body contamination*

The nature of the product and the process needs to be considered in developing a quality control process that can claim to include 'all reasonable precautions' to prevent the occurrence of foreign bodies in the final product. There is no single set of rules applicable to all processes.

The definition of what will constitute all reasonable precautions will also vary from company to company and be proportional to the potential risks. Some products are much more likely to be contaminated by foreign bodies than others. For example, any process removing meat from a carcass has a built in potential for bone slivers being carried over in the product, while a company producing confectionery by boiling sugar is unlikely to suffer from bone contamination, it is at risk of metal contamination coming into the process in the raw material.

The processes used also have an influence on the potential for contamination. For example, slicer blades used in bread slicing are liable to break, any process using glass containers is always at risk from glass shards generated by container breakage, any product packed in pre-made containers, e.g. cans, is at risk from contamination getting into the packages during transport and storage, etc.

The risk of contamination at all stages of the process from the receipt and unpacking of the raw material through to the finished product and the packaging of the product as well as the safety of the packaging must be considered. A large organization will carry out a fully documented hazard analysis of all stages of the production, identifying potential hazards and planning control methods and checks.

A smaller organization may not have the resources to develop such detailed records but it must be able to demonstrate it understands what it is doing and how it sets about producing a product free from foreign body contamination. A record should be available to show that the organization has given careful consideration to what it does. It is not sufficient for an owner manager to say to the enforcement authorities, or indeed a major supermarket if it supplies such, after a complaint that 'I didn't know that can happen'. The manager needs at least to be able to show records of the consideration of the process for the prevention of foreign body contamination and that the manager has considered what may happen based on knowledge and experience and actions taken to prevent contamination occurring.

In completing the review of the potential causes of contamination the manufacturer will also establish control methods to prevent the foreign bodies being carried over into the finished product. This may be achieved by the use of cleaning processes, the use of manual inspection or the introduction of detection equipment. The types and functions of these are described elsewhere in the book, as are the controls and records to be used with them. Where the potential hazard cannot be removed or detected by normal methods it may be essential to implement alternative procedures. An example of this would be where a machine component could break during the process and where the component is manufactured from a material that is undetectable by any of the available methods. In this case a procedure would be implemented to inspect that component at predetermined intervals, to ensure it is not becoming weak through wear or indeed broken. This will require the establishment of the procedure and the training of the operatives to carry out the inspection properly. It will also require a product quarantine process to be implemented, in the event of a breakage being found during the regular inspection, to ensure the contaminant does not leave the factory.

There is no clear definition of what is reasonable for a company to be required to use for the removal of contaminants from a product or indeed in the selection of equipment to perform a task. A multinational company could be reasonably expected to have a knowledge of whatever is state of the art at any particular time. There is no doubt that they will be made aware of the latest developments by the equipment manufacturers who will naturally target them whenever there is a new product – indeed they will probably be involved in the early development stages. Further, because of their size they will have departments charged with engineering development. On the other hand, a small company will not be such an immediate target for the equipment manufacturers, and will not have engineers reading all the latest literature and working on development, so it is unlikely the small company could be reasonably expected to have the same knowledge.

Equally, when the decision to invest in a new piece of equipment is made the cost effectiveness of the investment will be proportional to the size of the enterprise and may not be practical when measured in terms of value to the business or in terms of availability of capital.

To summarize, the enterprise must use its resources in proportion to its size to analyse all potential sources of foreign body contamination no matter where they arise and to use this information to establish procedures to remove the foreign bodies should they occur.

4.4.5 *'Due diligence' in the context of foreign body contamination*

Before anything else can happen the business must formulate its policy towards quality and state the principles it will adopt. In the case of a very small enterprise this may only amount to a clear recognition of the need to produce a product free from contamination, while in the largest organizations it will be the adoption of a prescribed system of quality control and the allocation of resources to operate the system.

The effectiveness of the 'due diligence' system depends on records being kept which demonstrate the system has worked, or if it has not, identifies the failure and records the corrective action taken to prevent repeat occurrences and to ensure any product at risk of foreign body contamination is prevented from reaching the consumer.

In the case of a large organization the records will cover every factor affecting the process including the training provided to the personnel involved in the production process. Where the system is operated to BS EN ISO 9000 then the regular external auditing of the process and the records should identify any failures of the system. However, this should not be relied upon as the sole check of the system – regular in-house auditing of the process, with the requisite records, is essential. In designing a system it is important that records show a regular pattern of supervision and checking. It is not sufficient to set up a system which only records failures, the system must be capable of demonstrating continuous monitoring of the process. The records must show where checks were made and that everything was correct as well as when it was not. Records which only show exceptions are insufficient – they must record the normal condition as well. Records of any remedial actions should be kept as well as any decisions not to implement a remedial action or to defer implementation.

An example of this is where a sensor with an air-operated reject system is in use. If the record does not show that the reject system was tested and operated properly at each test it is impossible to prove that it did not miss rejecting a contamination should a complaint of a detectable piece of metal be received. If the record only shows times when it failed to operate and there is no record at the relevant time it is impossible to be sure of the operational condition of the reject. Whereas if the record confirms the system did operate properly before, after and even during the period the item, subject of the complaint, was made then a stronger proof exists.

The frequency of checks of the system will be established empirically. This frequency must be constantly monitored and records must be available to confirm that the frequency of check is the optimum for the particular item.

A few example of the records to be kept are:

- *Manual inspection.* Manual inspection it is necessary to be able to demonstrate that the personnel have been trained to perform the given task and that their activity in carrying it out is recorded.
- *Machinery damage.* Where a machine may suffer damage which could lead to foreign body contamination, e.g. being belt damage. Belt condition needs to be monitored at regular intervals. Perhaps at the start of a run when a written form should record that a specified individual actually inspected the machine to ensure damage had not occurred. If damage is detected then remedial

action should be recorded and quarantine or disposal of the potentially contaminated batch recorded.

- *Detection devices.* Where detection devices are used which supply data records these must be made to be meaningful in light of the identified hazard. Where the equipment does not provide data the regular checks by specified methods must be undertaken and recorded, with action and records made where the equipment is found to be at fault.
- *Contamination norms.* Where the process includes manual or automatic devices to detect and remove foreign bodies then the volume of detected contamination should be compared to a norm. Where this norm is exceeded then action should be implemented to reduce the excess. This could mean changing a source of supply or alterations to the process or the machinery.

In summary, a control system has to be implemented to ensure the precautions and preventative methods built into the process work. Great emphasis must be placed on ensuring the record system is complete and continuous. Where any fault in the system is detected then the corrective action implemented is to be recorded. It is no use relying on outside agencies to check the system is working all the time, the best they can do is to provide a snapshot of the system at one point in time, it is only the continuous in-house effort which will ensure the system works.

The small enterprise has the same objectives but will have a much less complex manufacturing procedure. Records still need to be kept that will demonstrate the business is aware of its responsibilities and how it goes about meeting them. What these are will depend on individual circumstances. The small business should utilize any resources available for advice and assistance including those of the Environmental Health Officer.

4.5 Enforcement of the law in the UK

As previously stated the law is enforced in the UK by the appropriate enforcement authority usually either Trading Standards Officers or Environmental Health Officers employed by Local Government.

Any business premise will have a local authority to work with. This is referred to as the home authority. The home authority plays an important role on behalf of the manufacturer because it is to them that any initial contact should be made by another authority in the event of a complaint being made.

Any food manufacturer should strive to establish a good working relationship with their local enforcement authority. The objective being to ensure that local officers know the manufacturer's business and understand how it operates. The manufacturer will take notice of and co-operate with officers and listen to advice. It should be remembered that the manufacturer is the expert in a particular process and where there is a good relationship he, the manufacturer, has the opportunity to establish with the officer the efficiency of the control systems and the safety of the process. The advantages to this are considerable to both parties, in particular when the local authority is referred to as the home authority by another part of the country, simple questions can be answered and resolved quickly and amicably to everyone's satisfaction.

The Act itself gives powers to enforcement officers which include the power to detain food where it is seen as unsafe and to serve improvement notices where regulations have been contravened. It also defines who may enter premises and what the limits are to their authority once they have entered the premises.

These entry provisions are quite draconian. Section 32 of the Food Safety Act 1990 states that an authorized officer has, upon production of an identification document showing their authority, the right to enter premises within their authorities area, at any reasonable hour, for the purpose of establishing if there is a contravention of the Food Safety Act or any regulations made under the Act. Section 32 also gives the enforcement officer the right to enter any premises at any reasonable time for the purpose of obtaining samples, inspecting or seizing food which may be likely to cause food poisoning. Section 32 of the Act also gives enforcement officers the right to enter any business premises within or outside their area to ascertain if there is evidence of a contravention of the Act within their area.

As far as admission to private premises, a house, admittance can only be gained by the authority giving the occupier 24 hours notice or on presentation of a search warrant.

The manufacturer is not totally powerless in the face of these provisions. Enforcement authorities using them have to do so strictly within the law and where necessary within the requirements of the Police and Criminal Evidence Act (PACE).

Any manufacturer when presented with a situation where an officer demands to inspect the premises should first of all ascertain whether this officer is from the local authority or from outside the area as this has a significant effect on how far the officer can go and what the manufacturer is required to tell the officer. However, as in any situation confrontation should be minimized as much as possible, and by both the officer and the manufacturer being aware of what they can and cannot do it should be possible for the visit to remain amicable and professional.

There is a distinct difference between the powers the local officer have and those of an officer from outside the area. The officer from outside the area does not have right to carry out a general inspection of the premises, and must restrict questions to those relevant to seeking evidence of a contravention of the Act. In the case of a foreign body complaint the prosecution does not have to prove intent on the part of the manufacturer – the fact the foreign body has been found is enough. Therefore, there should not be any reason for an outside authority to visit the manufacturer. He should be able to obtain information about the manufacturer from the local authority. However, the outside authority may want to see what action the company is taking to prevent foreign bodies entering the product and if the company has a 'due diligence' defence. The company is not required by law to cooperate in this, although in practice it may be preferable for the company and the authority to be open with each other so that providing the company can show it has a good system, preferably supported by the view of the local officers, the authority does not waste money on a prosecution doomed to failure from the start.

In the event that entry is refused then the authority can apply for a warrant to the local Justice of the Peace. Providing the JP can satisfy them of the need to enter the premises, a warrant will be issued which then gives the officer power to enter the premises using reasonable force. If the premises are unoccupied at the time of entry the officer is required to leave the premises secure when leaving.

On entering the premises an officer has certain powers and the business is required to provide certain information. Failure to do so can result in contravening Section 33 of the Act which deals with obstructing officers carrying out their duties.

The Act specifically gives the officer the right to inspect any records, whether these are in hard copy or on computer. The manufacture must cooperate in making these available or accessible to the officers. The officers have the authority to seize records which may be required as evidence in the event of a prosecution. These powers are subject to PACE. This means in simple terms that when an officer visits a manufacturer the officer must explain the reason for the visit. If the manufacturer is not suspected of an offence the officer must state the reason for making the visit and obtain permission to enter the premises. If, on the other hand, the manufacturer is suspected of committing an offence, not only must the officer obtain permission to enter the premises and explain that the manufacturer is not required by law to consent to the visit, but the officer must also explain that anything taken may be used in evidence against the manufacturer.

4.6 Conclusions

There are few golden rules which apply to all organizations in ensuring they are taking all reasonable precautions and exercising 'due diligence' to prevent foreign body contaminants finding their way to the consumer.

Those that are of a general nature:

- All companies must consider how to prevent foreign bodies in their product
- All risks must be identified with an estimate of their likely frequency and the potential danger to the consumer
- The considerations must be written down
- A system must be implemented and the result of its application recorded
- The system must be checked and records of the checks kept
- A philosophy of continuous improvement must be applied
- All personnel must be properly trained in their duties and understand the importance of them

The details of these rules will depend on the type and the size of the company. What is reasonable for a small operation may not be reasonable for a large multi-national. A full HACCP system may be expected of a company whose sales are measured in millions of pounds, while a company with sales of £100 000 may only be expected to record consideration of the process and action to be taken to be recorded in the form of a simple note. Equally, the larger company could be expected to purchase items of equipment costing £100 000 while the smaller company could rely on manual inspection.

There are no clear rules – in the end the only bodies with the power to rule on an individual cases are the courts. Without documentation demonstrating thought and effort there is no hope of the courts accepting a 'defence of due diligence'. They are the final arbiters of whether the system does constitute 'due diligence' and this will depend on how they view the efforts made.

Training is an essential item to the defence of 'due diligence'. Manufacturers must be able to demonstrate that the people they rely on to carry out part or all of a process both understand what they are doing and the importance of carrying out their duties correctly. They must be aware of what to do in the event of a failure in the system and who to report it to. Where their work involves the keeping of records, they must understand what they are doing and why. In developing a training programme the requirements of the prevention of foreign bodies must be included. Everyone must be aware what the term means and, while not expected to see everything that goes through the system, they must be aware of the benefits of monitoring the process in any way they can.

These comments apply to everyone involved in production regardless of department or job. For example, maintenance teams will be taught to work in a clean and tidy manner and to dispose of scrap materials in a controlled manner, but it is just as important that the operator or cleaner who returns to the line after a repair automatically makes a check to make sure the maintenance team have not forgotten something.

Where training depends on a learner watching an experienced operator there should be an overall description of their job available for reference to ensure all eventualities are covered. With more formalized training reference to a job description should be an automatic part of the training.

Finally, all manufacturers will have a local authority under whose jurisdiction they are located. Establishing a sound, amicable and professional relationship with the authority should be an objective of all. This will not prevent the law taking its course when required, but will play a part in ensuring that where the manufacturer is operating correctly this is recognized and less time is wasted on pointless arguments and more is spent on constructive developments.

5

Equipment purchasing and costs

5.1 Introduction

A decision to purchase a particular type and brand of foreign body detection and removal equipment has two effects on the future of the business. One is the economic effect and the second is the effect on quality. This chapter is primarily concerned with economic factors; quality factors are discussed elsewhere.

In evaluating the advantages and disadvantages of various equipment the rationale behind the decision in terms of 'due diligence' must be considered during the evaluation process. The original specification in terms of detection capability must be satisfied by the item purchased and where this is not achieved then a record must be available supporting the basis of the purchase decision.

There does not appear to be any dramatic new technology imminent which will make current systems obsolete (Chapter 18). When any of the new technologies do mature into practical solutions the time taken for them to be refined to a level suitable for normal industrial use is likely to be 3–5 years. X-ray systems are a case in point: the first of the in-line scanning systems was launched in 1984/85 and it took a further 6–7 years before the latest generation of machines were developed.

The decision to carry out specific process will be based on the analysis of risk. Where a potential risk is identified that can be reduced by the introduction of an expensive device, the justification to purchase, or not as the case may be, will be affected by the costs which will be incurred in relation to the economic viability of the organization. The factors considered in the decision-making process need to be recorded.

For example, the potential lifetime of the equipment will have obvious cost implications. Potential lifetime will depend partly on how a piece of equipment compares to 'state of the art' at the time of acquisition and partly on its predicted working life.

The analysis of what is the 'state of the art' today and what will it be in the future is a complex task which will require taking outside advice and questioning manufacturers. The meaning of the term 'state of the art' will depend on the type of equipment. The newer, the technology the faster significant developments take place and the contrary. In the context of foreign body detection and the food industry the term 'state of the art' will also have a relationship to the size of the enterprise. While a digital metal detector system with a centralized data collection system and every conceivable automatic feature could be described as 'state of the art' for a multi-national operation, for a small family operation a stand-alone metal detector with relatively simple automatic monitoring and control of its settings and reject system would represent the 'state of the art' for them.

Having made the decision, as well as recording the basis for the decision, of the specification of the equipment, the total cost is calculated. A common mistake in the decision-making process is to limit consideration of costs to the obvious purchase price and not to fully consider the other factors involved. The information obtained will not only provide a basis for cost comparisons between suppliers, but also help to establish the test calibration and maintenance programme.

5.2 Costs

5.2.1 *Capital cost*

The major component of the total price for the equipment is the 'ex factory' (or depot) cost from the supplier. Depending on the location of the supplier, the costs of delivery, and in some cases customs clearance and importation, can be significant. Companies in the EU must ensure that any machinery they purchase meets the requirements of the directives on safety, EMC and hygiene, and be certified to conform. The cost of this certification will be significant if the user tries to obtain the certification himself; manufacturers and manufacturers distributors and agents must provide the certification within their quoted prices.

5.2.2 *Installation costs*

Before a machine can be put to use it has to be installed in-line, which can incur significant costs. These include the cost of unloading the machine at the user's premises, which may require hiring lifting equipment, the placing of the machine in-line and any modifications to the existing line in order to accommodate it. Power and other services need to be supplied; not only do these need to be available, but they must be connected to the new machine. Satisfying this requirement can involve the purchase of additional equipment, e.g. air compressors, and the purchasing of specialist services such as electricians.

5.2.3 *Compatibility with existing systems*

When the equipment has to fit in to existing systems, for example feed back loops to other machines, the purchaser must ensure the new machine will be compatible with the existing systems or factor-in the cost of modifications to make everything work as a unit.

5.2.4 *Spare parts*

Where the company policy is to hold spare parts then the cost of the spares recommended by the manufacturer to ensure continuous operation has to be included in the acquisition cost.

5.2.5 *Obsolescence and replacement*

The decision on when a machine becomes obsolete will depend on many factors including the size of the operation, the application, and service and spare parts availability. With the rapid changes in technology discrete electronic components are often made obsolete by the component manufacturers. While they will normally have an alternative available this may not suit a particular circuit and thus a complete system can be made obsolete for the lack of a single component. In the purchasing decision process the length of time the equipment manufacturer will guarantee to support his/her equipment is important. The equipment manufacturer's policy on product 'life time' needs to be defined and considered, as must the length of time the particular machine has been on the market and what the manufacturer's replacement plans are. Some manufacturers only guarantee to support equipment for 5 years from the date they declare it obsolete and replace it by a new model. In calculating the total cost of the equipment a forecast of the life of the machine must be made bearing in mind the likely causes of obsolescence as well as the anticipated life the machine has before wearing out.

5.2.6 *Upgrades*

Given that all equipment will be modified and improved by the manufacturer, the company policy on upgrading existing equipment is a factor to be considered in making a purchasing decision.

5.2.7 *Operating costs*

Any machine used in a production process will require some supervision and examination during the course of its operation. No machine can be installed and forgotten. The costs involved in the support, monitoring, maintenance, calibration and recording of a machine can vary significantly.

(a) Repair and maintenance

The cost of repairs and maintenance need to be estimated. The items subject to wear in normal use need to be identified and their anticipated usage considered, e.g. belts, motors, pneumatics, sensors, etc. Then the risk of accidental damage has to be evaluated where the application has built-in hazards. Routine maintenance needs have to be identified including lubrication and adjustments.

(b) Cleaning

All machinery has to be kept clean. Ease of cleaning, requirement for special resources, need to disassemble or cleaning-in-place (CIP) need to be examined and costed, and compared between equipment designs.

(c) Supervision

Does the machine have automatic compensation systems to account for drift and wear or does it require manual monitoring and adjustment. In the event of machine failure (minor or catastrophic) are there 'fail-to-safe' and alarm systems fitted.

(d) Testing and calibration

The frequency and complexity of routine calibration and maintenance are very important with inspection equipment. Costs and cost comparisons between systems are very important as these processes will be demanded by the quality control system and will have to be carried out thoroughly and recorded. These are fully discussed in Chapter 13. The availability of traceable test standards needs to be specified and their cost included. Manufacturer's service and calibration support, and the availability and cost of contracts to carry this out are to be included. Of significance will be the level of approval the manufacturer's service department carries and its capability of providing a satisfactory support service (ISO 9000, etc.).

(e) Supplies

Where the machine requires supplies, e.g. paper for printers or compressed air for pneumatic systems, the potential cost liability needs to be specified and compared between options.

(f) Training

When new equipment is installed staff need to be trained in its use and application, and this training needs to be refreshed from time to time. The manufacturer's support in terms of documentation and personnel need to be costed and evaluated.

5.3 Supplier classification

Having carried out an analysis of the various options and suppliers it is recommended that the supplier be audited to ascertain their financial stability and history. Where there is no history of working with a supplier, it is recommended that a reference list of existing customers should be obtained and references taken from existing customers. Where the supplier is an agent or distributor, the length of the relationship and contractual terms should be investigated, and references sought on performance against promise. From this a rating of the supplier should be established as a comparison against the options available.

5.4 Supplier standards

The supplier will almost certainly be required to enter the food manufacturer's premises to carry out installation or maintenance work. It is essential that the supplier be aware of the specific hygiene and safety requirements of the food industry, and that his/her personnel are trained to work to the GMP requirements of the industry.

5.5 Questionnaire

An example of a questionnaire is given to demonstrate a method of evaluation (Figure 5.1). The precise details will vary but the principle will hold of comparing the stability of the supplier, his/her costs and

XYZ Speciality Foods ltd

Equipment & Supplier Evaluation		Form No 1200 Issue 0002 Date 25.7.1997
Project analysis		Project leader
		Approval
	Brand A	**Brand B**
Basic machine ex factory		
Tooling & ancillaries		
Options		
CE Marking and customs clearance		
Delivery to site		
Total cost equipment delivered		
Lifting		
Foundations		
Services (Air/Gas/Water/Power)		
Line modifications		
Installation		
Initial training		
Spare parts stock		
Total installation costs		
Estimated annual maintenance Parts		
Estimated annual maintenance Labour		
Annual support contract		
Annual test and calibration		
Total annual service costs		
Supplies		
Cleaning		
Services		
Training		
Total estimated running costs per year		
Depreciation		
Estimated costs over 3 years		
Guarantee period		
Exceptions to guarantee		
Age of machine design		
New model expected		
Spare part availability guaranteed for (years)		

Figure 5.1 Equipment and supplier evaluation form.

the cost of owning the machine, with the intangibles which go toward making a decision. A format of this nature will also provide a useful record for the future and should be part of the overall quality system employed by the organization. The form is referenced and shows the date of any changes. Provision is made to summarize the project analysis and to continue to relate the purchasing decision to the project requirements.

6

Physical separation methods

6.1 Introduction

Although physical separation processes are not as technologically sophisticated or as glamorous as some of the other inspection technologies, they can provide an effective means of detection and separation of contaminants. Most companies who manufacture foods will use screens or sieves in some shape or form. A simple screen or filter may be used for a liquid feed to ensure that there are no components from the machinery or processing equipment upstream trapped before it enters the next stage of the process. This type of filter or trap assists in ensuring safe food production, but can also protect items of equipment that could be easily damaged, such as an homogenizer, if large, hard materials were to enter it. Screens and sieves are often an effective means of removing foreign bodies from ingredients that are to be used in a process. They are effective in many cases because the shape or particle size of the contaminant is different to that of the ingredient. This method is particularly effective when there is a very regular ingredient or product which has a very characteristic shape and size. They can also be used to grade the materials according to their size and shape.

Dry materials are often used in the food industry as dehydration or moisture control is an effective means of preservation, in addition to the reduced costs of transportation because one is not transporting large quantities of water. Many key and major food ingredients are supplied dry such as:

- Flours
- Sugars
- Herbs and spices
- Soup and sauce mixes

Most of the above list are food materials which are grown in an agricultural environment and are harvested from the field. In order to optimize the use of physical separation methods one has to also understand the effect of ingredients on the process and on the final quality of the food being manufactured. Potentially, a physical process may cause damage to the surface or structure of certain produce such as bruising or marking. This damage may then result in the ingredient or final product being downgraded or having a reduced shelf life.

6.2 Representative samples

Many of the techniques and systems described below depend on obtaining a representative sample of the materials to be analysed in order to be sure that the results from the analysis are representative of the larger mass of material, whether it be a large sack, tanker or ship load. For solids there are a number of established techniques which enable one to take a representative sample and reduce it to a smaller sample size which is still representative of the larger sample amount.

For large samples the technique of cone and quartering is used; this is where sample quantities of material may be up to 1 ton. The technique involves mixing the sample thoroughly, this can be achieved using a spade, fork or mechanical digger, and then heaping it into a uniform cone. The pile is then divided into four equal fractions by splitting from the tip of the cone. One of the quarters can then be heaped into a cone again and the operation repeated until a sample of a reasonable size is obtained, usually 20–30 kg. To reduce smaller quantities of materials to obtain samples, a sample splitter or divider can be used. The splitter will consist of a hopper at the top with a grid inset into the base. The grid has channels from the base with are directed in alternative lateral directions so that collection pots can be placed either side. The material is tipped into the top hopper, left to flow through the grid and split into the two sample pots. This process can be repeated by tipping one of the pots through again until the required sample size is achieved.

A spinning riffle is similar to the splitter, but rather than having two sample pots it can have many sometimes 50 or more. Material is placed in a hopper mounted above a static cone. Around the base of the cone are a number of sample pots that rotate around the axis of the cone at approximately 1 r.p.m. Any material falling onto the cone will have an equal probability of falling into any one of the rotating pots. This type of system is used where a large number of representative samples are needed for comparative testing. Another system design operates by pouring the sample into the top of the system and allowing it to fall onto a spinning disc which distributes the material evenly into the receptacles placed around the disc.

Two other common laboratory types of dividers are the rotary cascade and the centrifugal. Another type of divider is the rotary whole stream, which uses a set of revolving chambers to take samples from a falling stream of material.

Where samples are required from a large consignment or batch of materials, such as a road tanker or ship, then it is usual to take a sample stream by splitting the main product stream as it flows. One can either continue sampling throughout the transfer of the whole batch or sample intermittently. Another approach is to use an in-line sampler which takes grab samples at set intervals that can then be combined as a representative sample. There are many different designs for grab samplers. Most project a sample chamber into the stream using a drive mechanism (hydraulic or compressed air driven). For lorries with open access from the top, such as grain lorries, one can use spear sampling systems that automatically plunge into pre-set or operator guided positions within the lorries load and use a vacuum to withdraw a sample.

6.3 Particle characterization

In order to select and use the most appropriate form of separation technology for separating solids from mixtures one has to understand something about the particles that one is attempting to separate. A common approach is to characterize the particles and this can be carried out using a number of different techniques. The physical attributes and properties are quite varied and include the following as shown in Table 6.1.

6.3.1 Shape characterization

The shape of the particles is important if they are to be separated. Often scientific research is based on spherical particles; however, it is

Table 6.1 Physical attributes and properties of materials

Category	Attribute
Thermal Properties	Boiling point, drying characteristics, freezing point
Appearance	Shape, size, size distribution, colour, reflectance, texture
Solubility	Concentration
Electrical	Surface charge, conductor
Surface properties	Adsorption, hydroscopic, hydrophilic
Rheology	Viscosity, flow behaviour
Material Properties	Density, hardness, magnetic

Table 6.2 Measures of particle shape

Measure	Description
Volume diameter	sphere of same volume
Area	sphere of same surface area
Sphericity	particle shape see equation
Settling velocity	sphere with the same settling velocity
Feret's diameter	mean length between two parallel lines drawn tangentially to the particle

most uncommon to have spherical shaped particles, most particles are of an irregular shape. Shape characterization, therefore, has to be expressed in some recognizable terms. The most common forms of quantifying shape are shown in Table 6.2.

A good measure of a particles shape is its sphericity.This is calculated as:

$$\phi = \text{surface area of a sphere of same volume as particle}/\text{surface area of particle}$$

6.3.2 *Sieve analysis*

Sieves can be bought in various different forms, sizes and to various standards. The technology of sieving dates back many years. A laboratory nest of sieves can be used to carry out a sieve analysis. This analysis allows one to characterize a material by its distribution in particle size. Figure 6.1 shows a typical distribution of particles.

A statistically representative sample of the material has to be obtained in order to determine this distribution. This sample is then separated into its different size fractions by passing through a series of sieves. This series or nest of sieves comprises a number of sieves which have different aperture sizes – the largest aperture size is

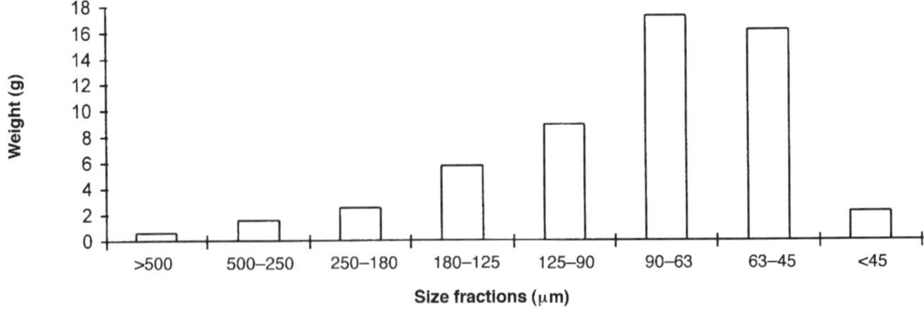

Figure 6.1 Typical particle size distribution.

located at the top of the nest and the sizes reduce down through the nest until one locates a base collection tray. The sieve consists of a metal rim which is slightly tapered to the base of the rim and locates into the top of the sieve below. The smaller diameter end of the sieve has a mesh of wire attached to it, usually this is welded. The mesh material can be made of stainless steel for larger sizes and nylon for smaller aperture sizes Figure 6.2 shows some typical mesh designs for different sized sieves.

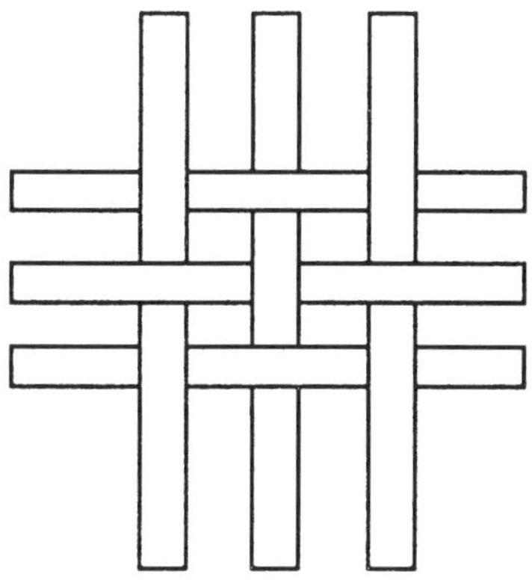

a) Plain weave

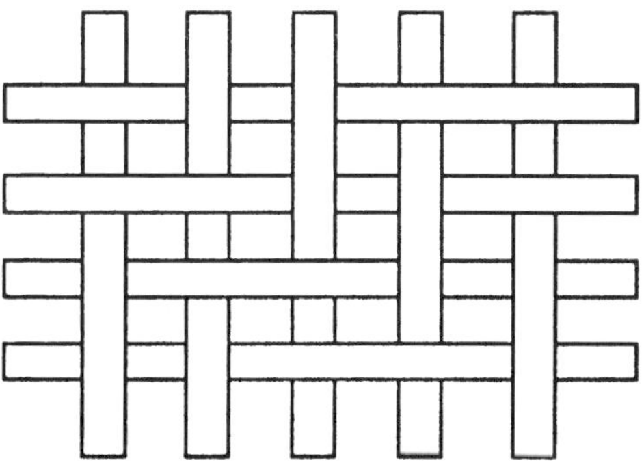

b) Twilled weave

Figure 6.2 Typical mesh designs for different sized sieves.

The weight of each clean sieve is noted and amount of material placed on the top sieve weighed. The sieves are then clamped together on the shaking machine with the sample placed in the top sieve. The sieves are then shaken for a set period of time and then the sieves are weighed again the difference noted which is the weight of material retained on that sieve. These weights of material can then be expressed as a percentage of the original weight of the sample. The weights can be accumulated either as a percentage of material that is over that screen size (oversize) or as a cumulative total under that screen size (undersize). Table 6.3 shows a typical sieve analysis.

The weight measured in grams is the weight of material which has been retained on that sieve except for the last size which is the weight of material which has passed through the smallest sieve. The percentage oversize or undersize can then be calculated and plotted against particle size and used to obtain the mean particle size and the standard deviation as illustrated in Figure 6.3. These measures can then be used to mathematically characterize the particle size distribution.

There are a number of standards for sieving and these include the British Standard, BS4 10: 1996, ISO R 565 and ISO 3310, and ASTM E11:81 and E11:95. In the USA there is an alternative called the Tyler series. The general procedures for sieving are detailed in BS 1796 (1976).

For the series of sieves to be used to characterize the particle size distribution it is important that the correctly sized apertures are selected. A commonly used series is one such that the aperture widths of the adjacent sieves is the square root of 2, i.e. 1.414. The reason for selecting this difference is that it then means that the aperture area doubles for each sieve. Other sieve series are based on fourth root of 2 (i.e. 1.189) or on the 10th root of 10 (i.e. 1.259). A rule of thumb guide to selecting how many sieves to put in a series is to

Table 6.3 Typical particle size analysis

Sieve size range (μm)	Weight (g)	Weight (%)	Cumulative % undersize	Cumulative % oversize
>500	0.62	1.13	98.87	1.13
500–250	1.57	2.86	96.01	3.99
250–180	2.56	4.66	91.35	8.65
180–125	5.73	10.44	80.91	19.09
125–90	8.91	16.23	64.67	35.33
90–63	17.21	31.35	33.32	66.68
63–45	16.12	29.37	33.95	96.05
>45	2.17	3.95		

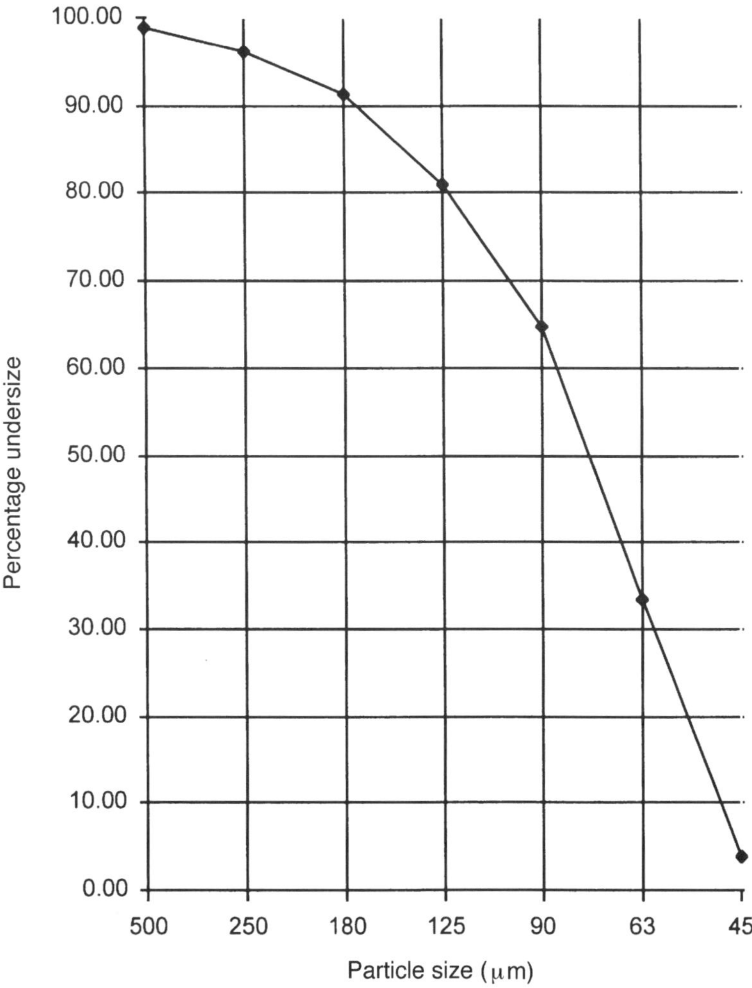

Figure 6.3 Sieve analysis plot.

ensure there is 5–10% of material retained on the largest aperture sieve and that there is 5–10% that passes through the finest sieve.

6.3.3 *Elutriation or sedimentation methods*

These techniques can be used to characterize particles and depend on the fact that the terminal falling velocity of the particles increases with their size. Elutriation in some ways is the reverse of sedimentation and it utilizes the fact that if particles enter into a stream of liquid being pumped vertically upwards they will be carried in the stream if their terminal falling velocity is less than the velocity of the upward liquid stream. This technique has been used as a standard measure and a British Standard for this method is BS 893. Analysis of the data can be carried out similar to that described for sieving above.

6.3.4 *Microscopy*

It is possible to examine particles under a microscope from which measurements can be made to characterize the particle shape and size. Very small sub-micron particles can be examined using an electron microscope. With the advancements in image analysis systems it is now possible to semi-automate this analysis. Some early systems such as quantimet were used to investigate particle shape. Normally statistically representative samples of product are obtained very carefully as this technique requires a small sample size. The technique does have the advantage of being one that can be used for very small particle size down to 0.001 μm using electron microscopy. Systems now allow one to carry out rapid analysis and apply various algorithms to the image analysis, providing such parameters as:

- Surface area
- Circumference
- Voidage
- Mean diameter
- Shape factor

The technique is predominately used as a two-dimensional system but advances in stereo microscopy are now providing three-dimensional systems.

6.3.5 *Other methods of particle size analysis*

There are other methods for particle size analysis and one popular method is a specialist particle size analyser. These systems utilize a laser beam which is directed at the particles which are entrained in a liquid of gaseous phase. One of the earliest systems to use this effect was Malvern. The light from the laser beam is diffracted by the particles, and the level of diffraction is measured and analysed to give a measure of the particle size distribution. Another more traditional method is the Coulter counter method.

Image analysis techniques can be used to measure the shape and size of the particles usually in two dimensions, although the particles could be reoriented and re-measured. A typical image analysis system can measure a range of features such as the average diameter or radius circumference, area, etc. Early systems were used for inspecting grain to assess quality attributes and looking for foreign objects, in particular stones. The systems were rather time consuming to use as an operator had to examine every particle. With the development of more sophisticated image processing systems it is now possible to automate the imaging technique and provide a rapid method of two-dimensional particle size analysis. Other more recent methods include light and X-ray scatter and electro-sensing.

6.4 Separation by shape and size

The separation of materials by using their physical attributes, such as size and shape, is nothing new. Many of the technologies used today have been around for many years and some since early man. However, the understanding of the properties of the material and the optimization of the design of such equipment has developed and continues to develop. Some of the technologies currently used to separate foreign materials from a final product or from ingredients are briefly described in the following sections.

6.4.1 Sieving

The process of sieving is used to separate any material which is not of the required particle shape. The process is primarily selective on shape as the sieve is contracted from a mesh of regularly sized apertures. The use of sieving in the food industry is widespread and is used for foreign body detection in dry food ingredients. In addition, many retailers or manufacturers of food products specify that all dry ingredients should be sieved prior to use.

There are a range of different sieves that are used. The sieve itself is usually metal and circular. The design is such as to ensure that all the material will pass over the mesh and be allowed to move freely. One important aspect of sieving is to ensure that the sieve does not blind. Blinding is a symptom of when the mesh of the sieve becomes blocked with either particles agglomerating or by too much oversize material being caught in the mesh. The sieve is vibrated in order to increase the throughput of the sieve and make it more efficient through preventing blinding. The vibration is controlled by oscillating the sieve. The vibration causes the particles to move and cover the surface of the sieve, thus utilizing all the mesh rather than just a portion. In order to size a sieve correctly one requires the following key parameters:

- Particle size distribution
- Size fraction required
- Throughput required

From these parameters it is then possible to size the sieve, i.e.:

- Sieve area required
- Sieve mesh size required

Sieves used in a manufacturing environment will be used to produce two or three fractions. Normally it will be to separate out oversize material and, therefore, all material that passes through the sieve mesh is used and that retained is either reground or discarded as it contains foreign matter. The sieve may also be used to remove fines (material with a small diameter of the order of microns) and in this case there could be two meshes.

Sieves are often operated in a batch mode. They need to be correctly sized to match the amount of material to be sieved in order to achieve the best performance. Most sieving systems can also be operated continuously, in which case material will exit the sieve system once it has passed through the mesh. In a continuous mode the sieves need to be checked regularly for build-up of retained material, blinding and to analyse what material has been retained. Sieves can be easily damaged and it is important to inspect them regularly because if the wires start to break up it is very difficult to detect them further on in the process. Some materials which clump or are difficult to feed can be assisted by a rotating paddle. It is also advisable to have a grating above the sieve in many instances, otherwise a sudden large mass of material falling onto a sieve can damage it.

In order to prevent blocking of the apertures, i.e. 'blinding', anti-blinding devices such as brush-type sweepers are often used. Another common approach is to use balls on the surface of the screen; the balls are made from an elastic material such that as the screen vibrates the balls bounce against the underside of the screen or sieve above, helping to dislodge any trapped material. A more recent development has been that of using ultrasound to cause finer oscillations and assist in the break-up of agglomerates or clumping of materials. The discharge, particularly of fine material, can often require assistance and there are a number of different mechanisms such as rotating paddles, vibrating cones, etc., that can be utilized. Figure 6.4 shows a typical design of a multi-deck sieve indicating some of the additional features.

Sieves are widely utilized in the food industry, and they require regular inspection and cleaning. The sieve mesh can be eroded and break, and often because of the fineness of the wire it cannot be detected downstream.

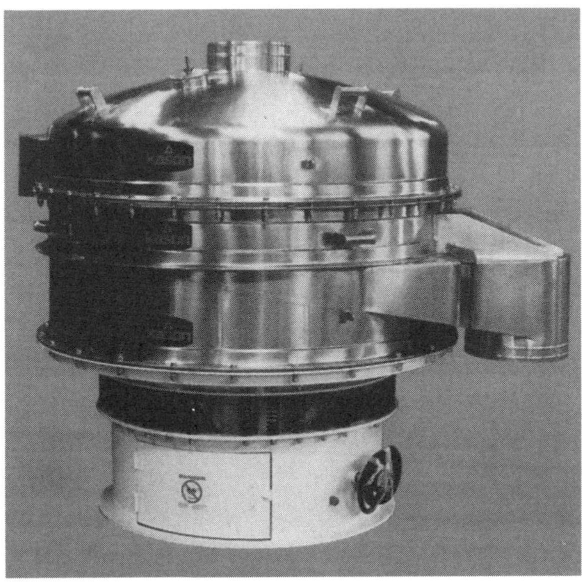

Figure 6.4 Multi-deck sieve (Kason).

6.4.2 Screens

Screens are similar to sieves but are usually continuous and are extensively used in the food industry. Screens are used for particles that are free flowing and have particle sizes of above 250 μm. There are a wide range of different types of screens and some of the more common include:

- Rotary
- Vibrating
- Trommel
- Sieve bend

For vegetable harvesting in the fields and on the farms, products are passed over very coarse gently vibrating screens which convey the vegetables but at the same time remove the earth and sticks and stones that have been picked up or attached. A screen is similar to a sieve in that it consists of a metal mesh or fabric which is attached to a frame. The frame may then be housed in a casing.

The construction of the mesh or fabric is very important as it has to be robust but also designed to a strict tolerance so that it has a specific aperture size and, therefore, will allow only a certain size fraction to pass through it and will retain material above that size. Some meshes are constructed to allow specific shapes through, and the apertures are checked for size and shape. The shape allows the screen to be more selective and is often used for materials that are of a regular shape but may contain some misshapen.

Screens suffer from similar operational problems to sieves in that they suffer from blinding that affects the capacity and efficiency of the screen. As with sieves, balls can be places between the decks to assist in reducing blinding. The efficiency of a screen can be determined by the following equation:

$$E = (c - f)/[c(1 - f)] \times 100$$

where E is the overall efficiency (%), c is the fraction of material above the cut point size in the overflow and f is the fraction of material above the cut point size in the feed. The fraction of materials can be measured by obtaining representative samples from the feed and overflow and sieving them. Obviously one requires a system which has a high efficiency. A usual method of selection is to trial a screen under the expected operating conditions and to measure the performance before the screen is purchased. Most screen manufacturers will provide trials facilities for this purpose.

6.4.3 *Rotary, gyratory and reciprocating screens*

Reciprocating screens consist of a rectangular shell which contains frames with different grades of cloth attached to each of the tiers or decks. These are placed inside the shell with the coarsest grade screen on the top and finest at the bottom. The screen is inclined along its length with the inlet being located on the top at the highest end and the outlet on the base at the lowest end. Figure 6.5 shows a typical design of a reciprocating screen. The outlet is at the lower end of the inclined screen.

Material passes over the screen and out via a chute either to be collected or to provide a direct feed for the next stage of the process. The lower end of the screens/frame is attached to a fixed point via a bearing. The higher end is attached to a reciprocating arm and a motor. The reciprocating arm causes a rotational movement to the whole screening machine which is extenuated at the higher end. This type of motion creates a circular whirling path for the material as it passes over the screen, therefore exposing the material to a larger surface of the screen and thus providing a reasonable opportunity for undersize material to fall through the mesh.

Reciprocating screens can be used for a variety of functions as they can be fitted with screens with specific aperture shapes and sized to allow products of certain shapes to pass through. Their use is, therefore, varied, but includes confectionery applications, animal feeds, etc. Like other screens, they have to be inspected regularly to

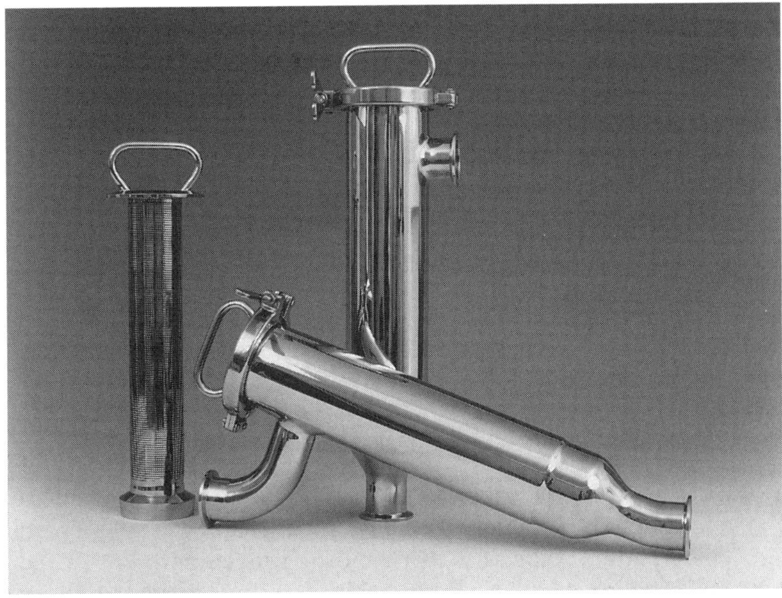

Figure 6.5 Typical rotary screen (Rotex).

ensure that the screens are not damaged as they can snag or tear if abrasive or sharp objects pass over them.

The reciprocating screen can provide, for a single and multiple pass system, the benefit of utilizing less floor space than a conventional screen. This reduction is due to the fact that the screen is inclined thus reducing the floor space. From a safety point of view care has to be taken to ensure that no-one is close to the moving parts of the screen as it can deliver quite a sharp blow.

The gyratory type of screen is similar to the reciprocating screen, but the type of motion generated is that which is gyratory. A system normally comprises a nest of screens or sieves which are supported on a table or base plate. The motion is generated from underneath by a motor with shaft which drives a weighted system. The weights are placed so as to create the required motion profile. The screens are often circular in design.

6.4.4 *Vibrating screens*

Vibrating screens are similar to rotary but differ in the type of movement that is applied to the screen. The motion of vibrating screens is different from rotary in that it is a more random high frequency motion. The vibration is induced vertically and this can be carried out in a number of different ways, the most common being either by rotation of a mechanical reciprocating device applied to the casing or by an electrical device operating directing on the screen. Electrically produced vibrations are generated by applying an alternating current to a moving magnet. They usually produce a high frequency with a low level of movement.

There are a variety of different types of vibrating screens which can come in different shapes, designs and sizes. Vibrating screens are very similar to sieves except they are continuous and have a higher throughput.

6.4.5 *Trommel screen*

The trommel screen, rather than shaking or vibrating, rotates around its horizontal lengthways axis. The wall of the cylindrical conveyor is made usually of a strong mesh or metal grid. The cylinder can be inclined so as to aid the discharge and create a flow of material through it. The material to be separated is fed in at one end of the cylinder and the unwanted material falls through the mesh, and the product which will be larger than the mesh aperture will pass along the inside of the cylinder and be discharged at the other end. The cylinder is normally rotated at a moderate speed of a few revolutions per minute. The rotation of the cylinder causes the material to be dispersed and, therefore, exposes it to the mesh surface.

The speed of the rotation should be such as to prevent the product or particles being carried too far around the internal circumference of the cylinder otherwise they will fall down and cause damage to other particles or cause attrition. The angular velocity ω at which the particles would be carried all the way around is:

$$\omega = \sqrt{(g/r)}$$

where g is the acceleration due to gravity and r is the radius of the cylinder minus the radius of the particles. It is best to keep the velocity of the cylinder at a fraction of this velocity to allow optimum performance and reduce any potential product damage.

This type of separation system can be quite harsh on the product and is, therefore, only suitable when operated dry for quite robust products such as nuts or foods with a hard outer shell or coating. However, when this type of screen is operated wet it has a much gentler action on the product as the water cushions it. As a wet system it can, therefore, be utilized as part of a vegetable preparation line. If fine delicate meshes are used with trommel screens and dense large material passes through, the mesh will deteriorate rapidly and become damaged. It is, therefore, recommended to use coarse strong meshes.

6.4.6 Filters and strainers

For liquid processing there is usually a requirement to remove any foreign objects prior to filling and this is achieved by the use of in-line filters or strainers. This will prevent foreign objects damaging the filling machine or being blocked in the system as well as to ensure that foreign objects are not filled into containers. The main function of the filter/strainer is to entrap solid material on one side, which is material to be removed, from the liquid. The strainer can be used to entrap foreign bodies such as metallic objects or other non-soluble materials such as fibres and plastics.

The strainer or filter is normally housed in a special purpose surround and this is then connected in-line as part of the pipework system. The strainer should be located in an accessible position so it can be regularly inspected for wear, and to remove and inspect objects that have been trapped. The inspection of materials caught by the strainer can be indicative of any processing problems, in particular non-dissolved or suspended ingredients.

There is a limit to the fineness of filter as a fine filter will reduce the flow of liquid through it because of the increase in pressure drop across the filter. If a filter collects a lot of material it will blocked or blinded. The amount of blocking or clogging of the filter can be automatically detected by using pressure sensors – these detect any increase in pressure across the filter and can alert the operator to clean the filter. If too much material is being caught in the filter it may be that too fine a filter is being used or it could be there is a process-related problem or there is a need to introduce another separation technology to remove the solids.

Most filters or strainers should be cleaned daily or more frequently and inspected for damage, and the material that has been collected should be inspected. Filter cloths or meshes can wear and break, and any inspection should include such a check. Filters can remove much finer material than screens.

6.4.7 Plate-and-frame filters

Although the purpose of many filters is not primarily as a preventative measure for foreign body contamination, many of them are very effective at entrapping foreign objects. For many food processes it is necessary to clarify a liquid by separating any solids or particulates which may affect the quality and cloudiness. These types of filters have been used in the brewing and drinks industry in order to separate out yeast cells or impurities. The particle sizes are usually quite small (less than 50 μm).

A plate-and-frame filter is one that is constructed in the form of a press. Metal frames, now mostly stainless steel, are covered with a filter cloth, and are positioned horizontally and located into the frame. The filter is sized for the throughput and the amount of solids to be removed. Once all the filter frames have been located into the frame the end plates are placed at either end and the filter is tightened, normally by hydraulic means, to ensure a seal between each of the plates. On the end plates are ports for the liquid/slurry entering the press and the filter liquor leaving. The filtrate flows out such that it can be seen – this enables any damage to the filter cloth to be immediately visible.

The solids are collected on the cloth and are referred to as a cake. The thickness of the cake grows over time as more solids are deposited. The pressure drop across the cake also increases, which makes it more difficult for the filtrate to pass through. One of the major variables is the thickness of cake that is allowed to form before removal. The thickness will depend on the permeability of the solids being removed.

Many of these types of filters have traditionally been used in the brewing, wine and drinks industry, but are now less popular as other more continuous filters offer reduced downtime for cleaning and some require less floor space.

6.4.8 *Cartridge filters*

Another type of filter system used to remove suspended fine (small particle diameter) solids from liquids or gases is the cartridge filter. The cartridge filter is often used for air supplies in order to filter out dust, insects and other non-desirable matter.

The cartridges can be made from a variety of materials and are housed in a shell which is made of a robust construction, normally stainless steel. The filters themselves are often quite fragile, particularly fine mesh, and therefore they are strengthened by a supporting cylindrical frame.

6.4.9 *Membrane filters*

Membrane filters are a very selective form of filter for very fine particles or are more commonly used to separate liquids which have different molecular sizes. There are several types of filter, i.e. ultra-filtration (UF), reverse osmosis (RO) and microfiltration (MF).

Although these type of filters are not usually installed to separate and filter out foreign bodies as such, they are very effective at doing so. This type of filter is more commonly used to concentrate fruit juices by selectively filtering the water out and for clarifying. Water can be filtered to provide a cleaner or de-mineralized supply for special requirements. In the dairy industry membranes are used from milk processing streams. Therefore, they are commonly used as a solids concentration system prior to drying.

The membranes are very carefully constructed from materials such as ceramics. The pore structures do get blocked but they can be cleaned out by 'back-flushing' the system, which forces trapped particles or molecules out of the filter. Figure 6.6 shows a typical membrane filtration system

One benefit from this type of system is that it provides a means to also re-use water that would commonly be evaporated and lost.

6.5 Air classification and separation systems

Systems based on air separation have been used in farming for many centuries for processes such as the separation of wheat from chaff ('winnowing'). Many more systems have developed for separation

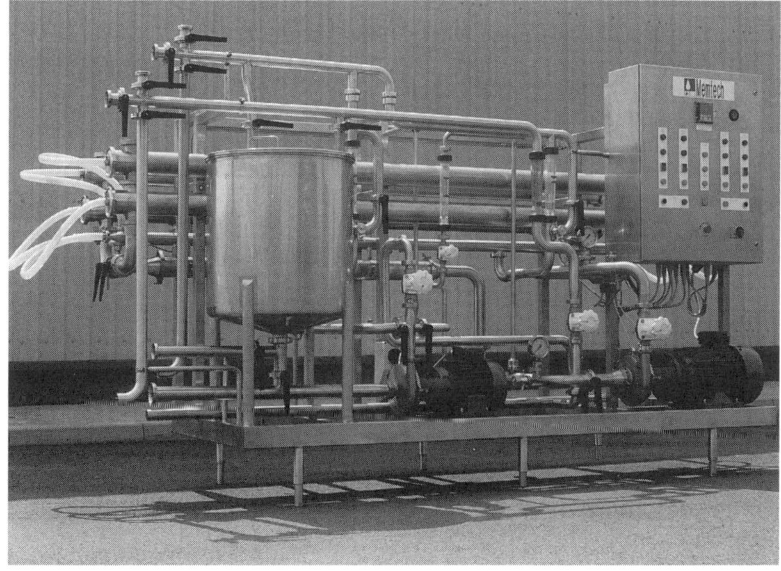

Figure 6.6 A typical membrane filter system (Memtech).

using air as a classifying medium. These are described in the following sections.

6.5.1 Cyclones and hydrocyclones

Cyclones and hydrocyclones are used to separate particles at the fine end of the range. Some processes produce dense, hard fines which are undesirable. The cyclone is used to remove fines or concentrate fines. The fine material is usually less than 1 mm in diameter.

The principle of the cyclone is that the geometry and flow of the carrying gas, usually air, causes a vortex which has sufficient upward velocity to carry the finer particles within it and thus carry them out through the upper outlet. Outside of the vortex the pressure is lower, which allows the larger, denser particles to fall downwards under gravity as they are too heavy to be carried upwards by the vortex and, therefore, pass through the lower outlet. An illustration of a typical cyclone is shown in Figure 6.7.

In order to function well they require a vortex finder to be positioned between the inlet and the overflow. This prevents material short circuiting and passing straight into the vortex and out through the overflow stream.

This separation technology is commonly associated with dryers and other similar equipment so as to remove fine material, thus ensuring that the product is of the correct particle size. The cyclones can be used to either extract fines which require removing from the process or waste stream or to remove aggregates or oversize particles which require further processing. Although this separation is primarily used for grading and quality purposes, it does allow foreign bodies to be detected and removed.

Hydrocyclones have always been of a low cost but this has reduced further by the construction of cyclones from plastics. In the food industry this can cause cleaning problems if wet cleaning-in-place is necessary. Larger cyclones are constructed from metal and can be made from food grade materials.

6.5.2 Air filters

Air supplies to food factories are important as air is used for a number of activities such as:

- Compressed air supplies to equipment including air actuated valves
- Transportation of materials – pneumatic
- General positive pressure air supply

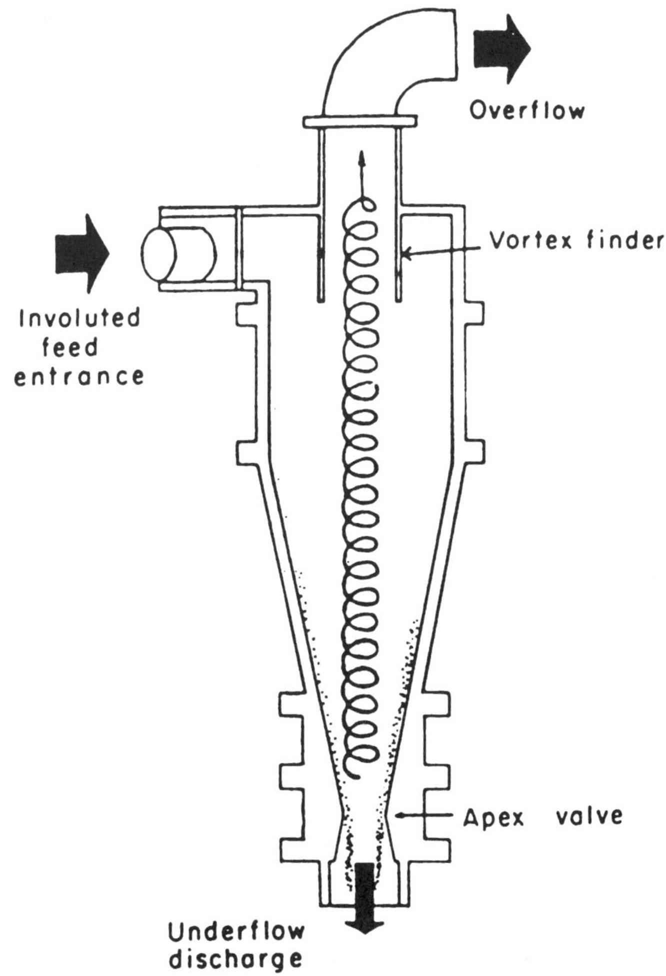

Figure 6.7 Diagram of a cyclone.

- Cleaning and purging of pipe systems
- Drying systems
- Cooling systems

The air supplying the above processes or services often comes into direct contact with foodstuffs, it is, therefore, essential that the correct quality and filtering systems are utilized so that contaminants are not introduced into the food manufacturing systems. It is often assumed that the air is clean as the human eye cannot see any microparticles or gaseous materials that the air is transporting. The air supply can be tested using standard environmental techniques to analyse what is present. It is important to carry out this exercise prior to deciding which industrial system is to be most suitable for the factory air supply.

There are a number of different methods of treating air, and the method is dependent on the use of the air and whether it has to be sterilized. The quality of air is quantified by a number of factors such as:

- Particulate matter – fibres, dust, spores, etc.
- Gaseous – volatile content

Air contains many potential contaminants, most of which are unseen by human eye. These contaminants can be categorized as shown in Table 6.4.

Within factories air is an important medium for many purposes. It is most important that when air is used in the process it is of the appropriate quality for its use.

6.5.3 Air intake filters

Air intake systems are to be found in all factories and there are some basic design principles that are important such as:

- Siting the intake point upwind and some distance from the air exhaust
- Protecting the air intake with louvres or suitable protection to prevent vermin and birds entering
- Making sure that there is no flaking or roofing material that is likely to shed

Table 6.4 Classification of contaminants in air

Contaminant	Size range (μm)	Characteristics
Dust	0.1–75	generated by fragmentation of materials
Fumes	0.001–1	small solid particles of condensed vapour, especially metals
Smoke	0.01–1.0	aerosol foaming from incomplete combustion of organic matter
Mist	0.01–10	very fine spray or aerosol as droplets
Vapour	0.005	gaseous state of substances which are liquid or solid at room temperature
Gas	0.0005	substances which normally gases at room temperature

- Ensuring that the air supplied and the prevailing wind direction does not carry dust or other contaminants from adjacent or upwind sites.

These need to be considered before looking at methods of filtering or treating incoming air. The incoming air will always carry some dust and particulates. One needs to assess what air requirements are necessary for the particular factory or process. The use of HACCP and HAZOP are useful tools to ensure that the risks have been evaluated and assessed correctly. Following the assessment one then has to design the required system.

6.5.4 *Sterile air filters*

For certain uses of air it will be necessary to use a sterile air intake. This type of system can be similar to that used for clean room environments.

In order to achieve a clean room environment one has to filter and treat the air to remove dust particulates. The main method of doing this is to use ultrafine filters such as HEPA filters these are filters made from a special fabric.

6.5.5 *Aspirators*

An aspirator is a system which uses air to flow as a separation medium. The air entrains one of the materials to be separated and carried it in its stream. The remainder of the material is too dense or large to be entrained in the air stream, and, therefore, falls into a receptacle or chute where it is collected.

6.5.6 *Air classifier*

An air classifier operates on the basis of entraining particles in a gaseous (usually air) stream. The system is constructed as a large cylindrical chamber with a perforated sloping base. About a quarter the way up is an entry point where the feed material enters. Air is blown in through the base and through the perforated plate. The perforations are of such a size that air will pass through them but the material to be separated will not. The fine material is entrained in the air stream and raised to the outlet at the top of the column where it exits via a discharge port. The coarse material will pass directly over the perforated plate and out through the base in the coarse discharge chute. Although not terribly sophisticated, the technique is effective.

6.5.7 *Zig-zag classifier*

The zig-zag classifier is very similar in principle to the conventional air classifier. It works on a principle of entraining particles in an air stream which passes up through a series of zig-zag profiles. This has the effect of impacting on the rising particles such that they are knocked back – if there is insufficient air velocity to carry them they will fall back down to the base and be carried out through the coarse discharge at the base. Particles that make it up through the zig-zag profiles to the top are discharged as the fines stream. Within this type of system the particle size range is normally between 2 and 50 μm

6.6 Gravity systems

Another physical property that can be utilized as a means of separation is that of density. The difference in density between materials can be quite marked and the densities of some typical materials and foods are given in Table 6.5.

As one can observe, most metals, stones, bricks, glass, etc., have specific gravities much greater than that of water and, therefore, will sink. Therefore, water can be used as an effective separation media for separating such contaminants from food such as fruit and vegetables which float in water.

6.6.1 *Float–sink*

The use of a controlled density to separate materials has been used for many years, particularly in the mineral processing industry. It has been developed to a fine art by using liquids with controlled densities to allow a fine separation using the float–sink properties determined by the density of materials.

The principle of the technology is very simple. The heterogeneous material to be separated is tipped into a tank of liquid – usually water. The material more dense than water will sink and that which is less will float. What this means in practice as applied to the food industry is that produce such as most fruits and vegetables will float whilst contaminants such as soil, glass, and stones will sink. These products are also usually conveyed by water allowing the water to wash the products at the same time as separating and conveying them. The process is normally continuous and products flow over a series of weirs into increasingly cleaner tanks.

Table 6.5 Densities of materials

Material	Specific gravity (water at 4°C=1.0)	Density (kg/m³)
Lead	11.34	11340
Stainless steel	7.80	7800
Tin	7.2–7.5	7200–7500
Cast iron	7.2	7200
Stones – granite	2.6–2.7	2600–2700
Glass	2.4–2.8	2400–2800
Brick	2 (approx.)	2000
Soil	1.12	1120
Hard woods	0.50–0.80	500–800
Cereal	0.5–0.8	500–800
Soft woods	0.40–0.55	400–550

6.6.2 *Shaking tables*

A shaking table is a wet separation system used in the mineral processing industry, but does have some application in food particulate separation and could potentially play more of a role. The system is used to separate different materials that have varying densities.

The principle behind the technology is that if one uses a table, inclines it, allows a liquid to flow over it and particles are suspended in the liquid, smaller particles will not move as fast as larger particles as they will be submerged in the film of liquid. Denser particles will move more slowly than less dense materials and this causes a lateral movement of the material.

6.6.3 *Sedimentation*

Sedimentation is a means of separating fine particles from a liquid. The slurry or liquid with suspended solids in is pumped into a large tank or lagoon. Over time, the solids settle and fall to the bottom. Those that are more dense will settle immediately, whereas lighter, less dense materials will be carried further in the liquid stream before settling. By the inlet there is usually a baffle plate to prevent material entering. In order for the particles to settle they must have a higher density than the liquid medium, usually water, as indicated in the equation below.

The liquid with the very fine suspended solids flows out from the top where it can be pumped away and filtered to be reused or it can be pumped to further processing or other forms of purification. The solids can be discharged from the base by using a selection of cavities where the solids collect and flow down towards the discharge. The cavities nearest the inlet will house the coarser material and those nearer the liquid outlet will contain the finer material. The rate of sedimentation is a function of the particle size and density, and the density and viscosity of the fluid the particle is settling in. The relationship is shown by the equation:

$$V_g = [d^2(\rho_p - \rho_l)]/18\eta \times g$$

where V_g is the sedimentation rate, d is the is the particle diameter, ρ_p is the particle density, ρ_l is the density of the continuous (liquid) phase, η is the viscosity of the continuous phase and g is the gravitational acceleration (9.81 m/second^2), For a continuous sedimentation system the throughput Q is a simple function of the surface area and the limiting settling velocity ν_{lim} such that:

$$Q = \nu_{lim}A$$

From the discharge the solids can be removed either by pumping or screw conveyors. One way in which the throughput can be increased is by fixing plates in the settling tank so as to increase the effective area. Figure 6.8 shows a typical sedimentation tank with inlet and outlets.

6.6.4 *Centrifuge systems*

Centrifuges are common to the food industry and are primarily used as processing systems for operations such as the separation of cream from milk or solids from fermentation broths. There are a number of different designs of centrifuges but they all rely on the same principle. The feed material can consist of two or more types of materials with different densities. One of the phases is continuous and a liquid, whilst the other can be another liquid or solids. The phases can-

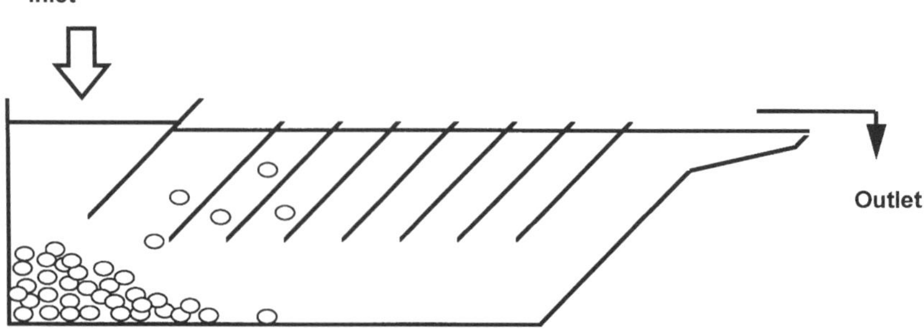

Figure 6.8 Sedimentation system.

not be completely soluble in each other. When the composite material is subjected to a high gravitation force through spinning the materials can be separated.

With sedimentation one of the limiting factors is the acceleration due to gravity. Because a centrifuge spins the acceleration can be greater than that of the earth. Centrifugal acceleration is shown by the equation:

$$a = r\omega^2$$

where r is the radius and ω is the angular velocity. The sedimentation velocity now becomes:

$$V = (d^2\Delta\rho/18\eta)r\omega^2$$

Using an electric motor to drive a shaft which has metal discs welded to it one can create a spinning sedimentation vessel with a large surface area. The discs can be rotated at very high velocities usually several thousand to over 10 000 r.p.m. The system works by forcing the denser material in a radial direction whilst the less dense material or liquid phase moves less and, therefore, the two can be separated on this basis. The design of centrifuges allows them to be operated continuously and also to be cleaned quickly *in situ*. Figure 6.9 shows a typical configuration of a centrifuge.

The primary function of a centrifuge is not usually as a foreign object removal system, but this may be its secondary purpose. One of the main reasons for this is that the cost of a centrifuge just to remove foreign objects is too high.

6.7 Other classifiers and separators

There are a wide range of other types of separators some of the more common types are briefly described in this section.

6.7.1 General classifier

There are a number of different types of classifiers used, all of which are based on a similar basic principle. The classifier is a machine which is inclined, the suspension of solids is added to the classifier part way along, the dense material will sink quickly whilst the less dense will stay suspended and be carried in the liquid phase back down the incline and over a weir. At the top of the classifier the coarse material which has sunk has been mechanically transported up the incline and out of the machine. Figure 6.10 shows a simplified diagram of a solid–liquid classifier.

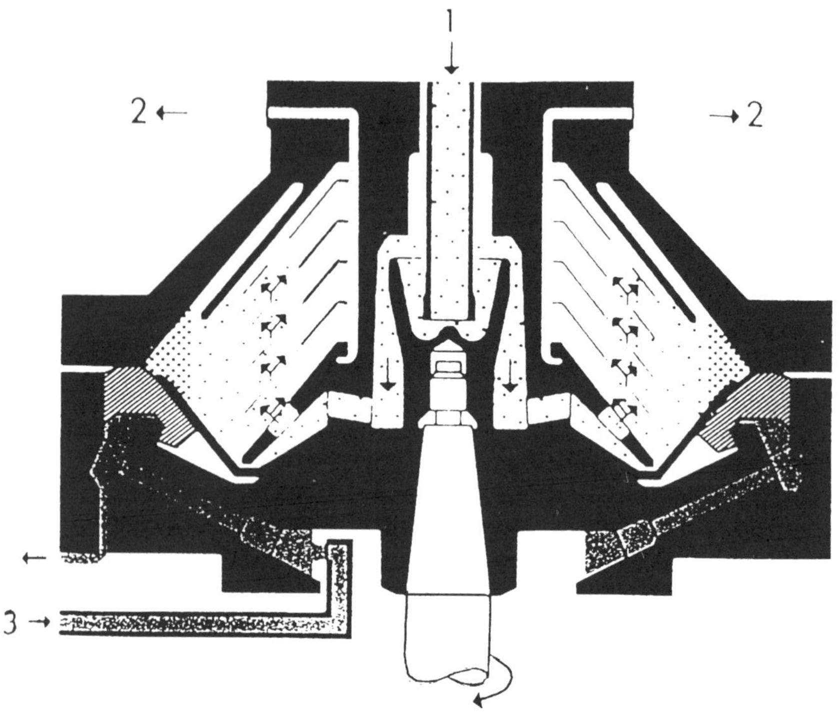

Figure 6.9 A typical centrifugal separator. (Courtesy of Alfa-Laval.)

6.7.2 Electrostatic separator

An electrostatic separator functions by using the different electrical properties of the materials to be separated. The system is designed so that material is fed from above and flows either down through a chute or over a drum. An electrode is placed near to the drum on the side where the material is falling. The charge on the electrode will attract an opposite charged particle sufficiently that its path can be deflected as it is drawn closer to the electrode. In being deflected as it falls under gravity it will land in a different location to that material which does not have a charge and, therefore, its flight has not been deflected. This type of separation system is used to separate materials which are usually fine dry particles or powders.

6.8 Selection of separation equipment

There is a wide range of different equipment available that can be used to separate and classify solids and slurries. Table 6.6 summa-

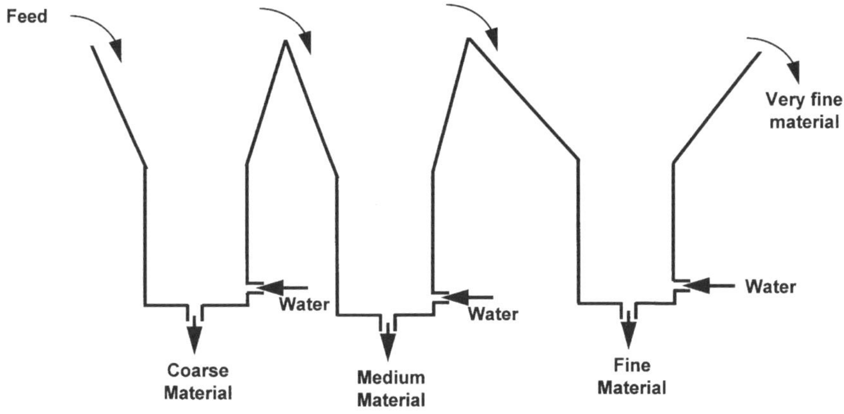

Figure 6.10 Simplified diagram of a solid–liquid classifier.

rizes the major types food separation technologies. The basic cost categories are given although more precise costs will be dependent on the specific applications. The general uses of each technology are also indicated.

Although there is a wide range of technologies, few are actually used solely to remove foreign object or contaminants. It is important for the food manufacturer to be aware of the wide range of equipment there is available and the potential for its application.

Table 6.6 Summary table of physical separation technologies

Separator classes	Types within class	Typical particle size	Typical field of use	cost
Sieves	metal molecular	10 μm–2 mm	flour, grain, powders	low
Screens	rotary vibrating trommel	250 μm–25 cm	confectionery, fruit and vegetables	low
Filters	plate and frame candle membrane cartridge	< 1–250 μm	beer, wine, fruit juices and drinks dairy and fruit juices air and dust	medium
Cyclones	hydrocyclone cyclone	~ 1 μm–2 mm	slurries and dust	low–medium
Centrifuge	centrifuge decanter	0.5–500 μm	diary, drinks, biotechnology	high
Classifiers	zig-zag	2–50 μm		
float sink	water dense media	~ 50 μm–50 mm	fruit and vegetables	low
sedimentation	lagoon tanks	~ 1 μm–2 mm	water re-use	medium–high

References and further reading

Brennan, J. G., Butters, J. R., Cowell, N. D. and Lilly, A. E. V. (1990) *Food Engineering Operations*, 3rd edn. Elsevier Applied Science, London.

Fedoc, P. (1993) Air classification. In *Encyclopaedia of Food Science and Technology*. Academic Press, London.

Fellows, P. J. (1996) *Food Processing Technology, Principles and Practice*. Woodhead, Cambridge.

Grandison, A. S. and Lewis, M. J. (1996) *Separation Processes in the Food and Biotechnology Industries*. Woodhead, Cambridge.

King, C. J. (1982) *Separation Processes*, 2nd edn. McGraw-Hill, New Dehli.

Address

British Standards Institute, 389 Chiswick High Road, London W4 4AL.

7

Machinery design and hygiene

7.1 Introduction

This chapter is aimed at assisting the equipment design by presenting some of the key design issues as well as allowing the user a greater appreciation of the issues involved in the design of food inspection machines. The design criteria for foreign body inspection systems or machines is as important as any other food processing equipment. The equipment has to comply with all the necessary regulations and has to be fit to meet the requirements of its use. Generally, the regulations are uniform across most countries although there are some countries that have differing requirements. In the majority of cases there are no specific regulations as to the exact design of an inspection machine but there are however general guidelines. New UK and European standards are being written for specific machines used in the food industry, and this may well cover inspection machines in the future.

It is worth considering some principles that can be applied to all food processing equipment and these have been listed according to three categories in Table 7.1.

The cleanable category must be adhered to as any build-up of dirt or debris will potentially pose a contamination threat and also the dirt could harbour bacteria. Safety is important both for employees but also for food safety regarding the consumer and the third category is that of general issues relating to the construction of an inspection machine.

Equipment that comes into direct contact with food has to be easy to clean, smooth with no cracks, seams, chips, pits or internal corners. It is vital that the contact surfaces with the food are non-toxic, non-absorbent and corrosion resistant. In some countries it is necessary that the contact material is approved by a regulatory authority.

Table 7.1 General equipment design categories

Category	Design guide
Cleanable	smooth surfaces – crevice free and non-porous
	materials of construction – preferably stainless steel
	no recesses or dead spaces where dirt and material can harbour
	all components securely fixed with locking fittings such that no parts may fall off
	welded parts and joints are continuous with no pitting
Safety	appropriate emergency stop
	electrical connections to required IP rating
	safety guarding where necessary
	appropriate interlocks
	ports and windows made of shatter proof material
	food grade lubricants
General	surface finish – non-flaking
	selection of appropriate materials of construction
	food contact surfaces – non-toxic
	floor attachments – designed hygienically
	gear boxes, pumps, etc. located away from food

7.2 Machine design

The design of the machine is important and a number of key design issues have been reviewed in the following sections. It is obvious to most food experts by just looking at a machine whether it is a hygienic design.

7.2.1 Machine inspection

It is important that all food contact surfaces are easily accessible for inspection and they will also need to be convenient for cleaning. Many machines have protective panels that have to be removed for inspection or cleaning. These panels should be designed to allow safe removal – preferably they should not too heavy for one person to remove. It is preferable that fittings are of the quick release type and that fittings remain attached to the panels or the equipment frame/assembly. This will prevent them being lost or falling into the machine and it also aids the speed of removal and reassembly.

If there are any specific requirements for inspection of a particular item of equipment these should be detailed by the equipment manufacturer and complied with by the operator. Many foreign body detection or inspection machines are enclosed and, therefore, need to be designed such that inspection can be made easy either through an inspection window, a port or by the quick and easy removal of a panel.

7.2.2 *Maintenance*

Often machines are not designed with maintenance in mind. However, the ease of maintenance is an integral part of equipment design. Once the machine has been installed in a factory the operator and engineers will have to live with the design for many years. Machines should be designed such that they are easy to dismantle to replace or repair parts. Easy opening mechanisms enable parts to be inspected and worn parts easily replaced or repairs carried out, thus allowing the operators and engineers to look after the equipment. Hidden or difficult to reach access will only encourage poor maintenance.

Regarding inspection, removable panels are useful for quick and easy access but care must be taken with fasteners to make sure they are easy to open but robust enough for engineers working under pressure, in addition to being hygienic such that they do not allow dirt to accumulate and can be easily cleaned. On a practical level it is helpful to be able to utilize the same tool on a wide range of machines, so where possible the use of industry standard fittings assists maintenance staff.

Another useful design issue to aid maintenance is the use of common components, whether this is bearings, fasteners, seals, etc. It allows the maintenance staff to keep fewer spares and to be more familiar with the components.

Self-diagnostic systems are being employed and incorporated into many machines now, and these allow the machine itself to monitor key components or variables and report if there is any deterioration in their performance. This type of system can be used to check the life of components such as X-ray generators, lights used in illumination, holes in screens, etc. This self-checking aids in ensuring that the equipment is operating at peak performance at all times, which is essential in the case of inspection machinery.

7.2.3 *The machinery directive, CE marking and other standards*

Any new food equipment supplied to Europe now has to be CE marked. This was a new regulation introduced into the UK in 1996. CE marking was developed as a means of knowing that an item of equipment had been designed by the supplier to conform with the regulations. The regulations focus on a number of factors, in particular that of safety. The European Machinery Directive (EMD) was started about 1987 when the first EC discussions began. This then developed and it became law from the 1 January 1995 that no machinery could be sold in the EC, including domestic markets, which did not legitimately bear the CE mark. Failure to comply with this EC law is now a criminal offence on the part of the manufacturer or his/her representative in Europe and may also result in the removal of the machinery from the market. In the most severe instances, penalties of up to 3 months' jail and a £5000 fine could be imposed. The main directives are:

- The EMC directive – enforceable January 1996 – 89/336/EEC
- The Low Voltage directive – enforceable January 1997 – 73/23/EEC
- Both of these have now been revised by the council directive – 93/68/EEC

CE marking is not an approval like UL or CSA, which always involve independent testing, it simply indicates the product complies with the directives and applicable standards. The primary objective of the directive was to promote free trade and the main purpose of the common safety requirements set down in the directive was to remove trade barriers. The EMC directive is also one of many pieces of European legislation bringing uniformity to the technical regulations for equipment throughout Europe. The standards have been selected mostly from existing international standards so as to have a neutral effect with the rest of the World. European member states are no longer able to impede the import of machinery, as long it is designed and built to conform with certain essential safety requirements and certificated to do so, by carrying the so-called CE mark.

The regulations do not cover second-hand machinery, unless such machinery is imported from outside the EC or European Free Trade Area (EFTA). However, machinery which has been overhauled and/or modified will be required to be rebuilt or modified to comply with the EMD. A further directive, the Second Amendment to the Machinery Directive, has been agreed in Brussels. This covers hoists and work platforms for lifting people, but not classic lifts and building site hoists, which will be covered by other legislation. It also covers safety devices.

Products for outside the EC/EFTA do not have to be CE marked, but it could be a sales advantage. For most equipment companies the Act means they need to ensure that the machinery they supply meets the safety requirements set down and that they have adequate documentation to demonstrate conformity. A Technical Construction File (TCF) is one of the key requirements of conformity which then allows a declaration that the machinery complies and affixes the CE marking. This is covered by the Work Equipment Regulations, which are divided into two parts:

- General Regulations 1–10 became law on 1 January 1993 and includes a requirement for risk assessments
- Specific Regulations 1–10 had to be met by 1 January 1997

If a machine is modified it has to comply only if its performance or function is altered. If there is no alteration of performance, it is classed as a repair and does not have to be CE marked. If a machine is used as part of a production line, it only has to comply if it is capable of being operated as a stand-alone machine.

One of the key requirements of the Act is to produce a TCF. This does not have to be a major task – the objective of the TCF is to make it possible to draw some kind of conclusion about whether a product complies with relevant directives, without it having to undergo conformance testing. The TCF is used in the same way as a laboratory test report – to show that the product meets legislative requirements and can carry a CE mark. Basically, a TCF is a product file of information from a number of technical sources. It comprises:

- An overall drawing of the machinery, including control circuits
- Full detailed drawings, accompanied by any calculation notes and/or test results required to check the conformity of the machinery with the essential health and safety requirements
- Lists of the essential health and safety requirements, transposed harmonized standards, and other standards and technical specifications which were used when the machinery was designed
- Description of the methods adopted to eliminate hazards presented by the machinery
- Optionally, any technical report or certificate obtained from a competent body or laboratory; if declaring conformity with a transposed harmonized standard, any technical report giving results of tests carried out at the manufacturer's choice either by themselves or by a competent body or laboratory
- A copy of the instructions for the machinery

(a) The electromagnetic compatibility (EMC) directive

The EMC directive requires products to generate no harmful electromagnetic emissions and be immune to defined electromagnetic disturbances and phenomena. EMC is the ability of an electrical/electronic device or system to function reliably in a typical electromagnetic environment (such as an industrial shop floor or a domestic home) whilst not unduly affecting that environment. It is not measurable as such, but it is possible to test equipment by monitoring its emissions or subjecting it to simulated emissions to establish EMC against internationally recognized standards.

According to a formal advice document from the EC, the EMC directive is applicable to 'electrical and electronic apparatus, as well as to the equipment and installations which contain electrical and/or electronic components'. The term, 'apparatus' has been further defined by the commission as being a finished product delivering an 'intrinsic function' and 'directly usable by the end user', and which can be sold as a single commercial unit.

(b) The low voltage directive

The low voltage directive (73/23/EEC) directs developers to implement safety standards which apply to the products and environment they operate in. It applies to all electrical equipment, designed to operate (normally) in the voltage range 50–1000 V(a.c.) or 75–1500 V(d.c.). Areas covered are product labelling and marking, i.e. working voltages and frequency, the design of product enclosures must ensure that users cannot gain access to hazardous areas and service people must be warned of hazardous areas.

The design must minimize the risk of ignition using materials that can withstand fault conditions. Cabling and insulation should be able to carry the power in the environment it is intended. Mains driven equipment sold as 'ready to use' must be fitted with a suitable mains plug with a correct fuse. PCB layout is defined in terms of track spacing (creepage distance) and component spacing. Operator areas are also defined in terms of handles, knobs, grips, etc.; the specification defines the temperature rise for these items, it will not allow these to exceed a certain value as the operator would find it hazardous to touch them for fear of being burnt. External surfaces are also considered for temperature rises. It specifies maximum earth leakage current for a mains connected device, generally 3.5 mA, if devices exceed this, then they must carry a warning label. If lithium batteries are fitted then warning labels must show how to dispose of them.

Panel instruments have been classified as components but it has become common practice to CE mark them for EMC compliance. This makes the panel builders job a lot easier, as the CE mark must be applied to complete installations not just individual products.

One needs to provide evidence that one took all the necessary steps to ensure the system supplied meets the directive. It is beneficial if the subsystems are CE marked from reputable suppliers and the installation instructions are followed correctly. Compliance with the EMC directive is normally demonstrated in one of two ways:

- *Self-certification* – this may involve having the tests done at a specialist test house or in-house testing.
- *Technical construction file* – this requires detailing the design, specifications, drawings and all information which will allow the approval authorities to technically vet that your product was tested and, if re-tested independently, it would comply. These

details are submitted to a competent body (normally a NAMAS accredited laboratory) for approval.

(c) Other tests

The following tests should be carried out with the product running a typical application with appropriate cables attached and varying its position to identify maximum emissions.

- Radiated emissions are tested by typically scanning from 30 to 1000 MHz at a distance of 10 or 30 m, depending on the class.
- For conducted emissions a scan from 0.15 to 30 MHz is performed using a line impedance stabilization network (LISN), the limits are defined using two different techniques, quasi peak and average.
- Radiofrequency electromagnetic field (susceptibility) tests are carried out to ensure the product performs to its intended functionality when subjected to a field with a strength of 3 or 10 V/m through the frequency range of 27–500 MHz.
- Electrostatic discharge (ESD) is tested to simulate static discharge from the human body, it incorporates an 8 kV dual polarity air discharge and 4 kV contact discharge, the unit under test must not fail under either condition.
- Fast transients are tested by inducing the mains and data cables connected to the equipment under test.

An EU declaration of conformity must be made once the testing is complete and reports are produced. Copies must then be available for the authorities such as trading standards officers to review in cases of 'due diligence'. The form of the declaration is laid down in Annex 1 of the EMC directive and it must:

- Identify the manufacturer or the authorized representative within the EU
- Describe the equipment to which it relates
- Define the standards to which conformity is declared
- Identify the signatory who is empowered to enter in to commitments on behalf of the manufacturer or its representative

These agencies will test equipment thought not to comply and if they fail can prohibit sales in the UK and Europe. They can even seize products or entire systems.

In the USA there are a number of different regulatory authorities that relate to food processing equipment depending on the food sector the equipment is to be utilized in. Most regulations are standardized. The main authorities are the Food and Drug Administration (FDA), US Department of Agriculture (USDA) and the 3-A. For these agencies it is usual to submit a particular item of equipment for their examination along with any pertinent data or samples.

There is also the US National Testing and Certification. It is usual that products are tested by a laboratory which is accredited by the Occupational Safety and Health Administration (OSHA), US Department of Labour. The testing laboratory will test and evaluate equipment and materials for the workplace to determine conformance with US national regulatory standards. Accreditation of testing laboratories is carried out under the Federal OSHA Regulations, 29 CFR, 1910.7. This federal law establishes OSHA as the agency that determines which laboratories have the legal authority to certify products used or installed in the office workplace.

Certification for Japan and other countries can often be carried out by companies that specialize in providing a certification service. Due to the deregulation efforts of many governments, third-party certification is often possible. In Japan one of the main laws is the DENTORI law (Electrical Appliances and Materials Control Law). Category B products and products not listed in the DENTORI law can be tested and certified to both international and Japanese safety standards by independent testing agencies. The Japanese S-Mark license is for products that pass the compliance test for the DENTORI or IEC standard and Japanese deviations. The S-Mark can also be obtained when testing to IEC standards for international approvals, such as the GS mark, CB scheme, CE marking, NRTL (ANSI/UL 1950), GOST Certification and Nordic.

7.2.4 Materials of construction

The choice of materials from which food processing equipment, separation and inspection systems are manufactured is generally governed by how the equipment is to be cleaned and the type of products that will be processed or inspected. The materials used have to meet the hygiene requirements as laid down according to the particular country the machine is to be used in. Materials need to be stable, non-toxic, durable, non-tainting, non-reactive with the product, inert to cleaning chemicals and sanitizers, non-corrosive, non-absorbent, and non-shedding (flaking, chipping and eroding).

Generally stainless steel is seen as being one of the most suitable materials for construction and one that meets the above requirements. This is because of its strength, non-rusting, and resilience to acid and caustic cleaning. There are different grades of stainless steel. The main food grades that can be used are shown in Table 7.2 and their use is selected based on the use of the contact material.

Table 7.2 Main types of food grade stainless steel

Grade BS 1449 pt2	Grade AISI	Grade DIN	Formed	Maximum carbon content (%)	Molybdenum content (%)
304 S15	304	1.4301	Annealed/cold drawn	0.08	–
304 S11	304L		Annealed/cold drawn	0.03	–
316 S13	316	1.4401	Annealed/cold drawn	0.10	2.5
316 S11	316L		Annealed/cold drawn	0.03	2.0
317 S15	317			0.06	3–4
410	410	1.4006	Annealed/heat treated	0.15	–

Stainless steels such as austenitic are more workable and less brittle than chromium stainless steel and is also corrosion resistant. Generally 304 or 304L grade are commonly used unless the food is low pH, such as some dairy products, or if the cleaning requirements also demand low pHs, in which case 316 is preferable. If the food product is extremely corrosive or requires special cleaning then it may be necessary to construct the machine or apparatus for a special alloy such as titanium. Coated metals such as chromium plating are unsuitable and should be avoided as wear and flaking can occur which will lead to contamination.

Welding of metal section, pipework and tubing is important, and there are a number of different methods for welding. It is important that the welders are qualified to weld the selected materials using the most appropriate method. There is a considerable amount of skill involved to provide first class quality welds. Inexperience can often produce welds that look attractive from the outside but are poor on the inside – this is particularly relevant when welding pipes. Many food companies specify that non-destructive testing is carried out on a number of selected welds to check the integrity. X-ray radiography or die penetration is often used to ensure that the weld is sound and there are no cracks, pin holes or crevices in the weld. Where a foreign body detection device is to be fitted into a pipe system, the inspection device, usually a magnet or metal detector, can be directly welded to the adjoining pipes. However, for inspection and maintenance purposes it is usually preferable to weld on hygienic fittings. There are a number of different types of fittings that can be used. The most common are Tri-clover IDF or RJT. Seals to be placed between the fittings will require selection according to the materials to be processed, cleaning chemicals and temperature. Common materials utilized for seals are nitrile rubber, silicon rubber, viton and ethylene propylene diene monomer.

Other materials that may be utilized for certain parts are various plastics. The plastics used have to be non-degrading. Those which are commonly used are polycarbonate, high density polyethylene, polypropylene and unplasticized polyvinyl chloride. The use of these materials is in items such as conveyors belts, spigots, etc.

The selection of different materials which are in contact with each other should be selected so that there is no electrolysis that may occur that will destroy the bonding or weld used to hold the materials together. There are some rules of thumb on the selection of materials. Any material which is used for moving parts and that is likely to break up such as certain plastics, wire mesh belts or certain rubber used for belts to convey materials should either not be used or be readily identifiable either by a foreign body inspection device or clearly visible. Other than in most explicit situations, glass and wood should be avoided as they can present a contamination risk. Glass can crack or shatter, presenting a major risk. Wood can easily splinter or can create a contamination risk.

Metals such as copper, although an excellent conductor, are unsuitable in most cases as they will react with many food products. Aluminium may be used as a food contact surface, but aluminium alloys need to be checked. Aluminium has the advantage of being easily worked and light, and it is resistant to some cleaning chemicals but not with regular use of low acid or high alkalis chemicals. Iron and steel are used for structural purposes although some companies have preferred to utilize stainless steel for structures as iron and mild steels are susceptible to corrosion.

7.3 Hygiene

The hygiene within most food factories is very important and in some factories it is more important than others. Where a product is to be sold directly to the consumer and consumed without heating or further processing, such as chilled products, there is an increased level of risk regarding food safety. It is these worst case scenarios that equipment has to be designed for. Traditionally, food processing equipment has been designed for its processing function rather than its hygiene. With changes in eating habits and increased concern over food safety it is essential that the hygiene of equipment is kept as high as possible.

Much equipment presently used for the separation of products, i.e. screens, sieves, etc., is difficult to clean due to the nature of the equipment. The small holes and non-smooth surfaces create problems. Items such as sieves and screens also have to be dismantled regularly to be cleaned. It is not suitable for many dry processes to clean equipment with liquids and, therefore, dry cleaning techniques are required such as brushing, wiping, etc. Although elementary, these techniques do require attention as they can be a source of contamination from microbes, fibres shedding or other loose material.

Usually food products have a final inspection post-packaging. In this case the level of cleaning required is minimal and hygiene less of an issue as the product is protected from the machinery. Many companies will allow alternative materials of construction to stainless steel such as plastics or mild steel.

Moving parts have to be lubricated and whatever joints, gaskets, bushes or seals are used they normally leak at some point in their life. The lubricants used should be 'food grade' such that if they contaminate the food they are non-toxic and edible. Many companies now insist that all oils and lubricants are food grade, and these are normally made from vegetable matter such as rape seed or similar.

7.4 Methods of cleaning

Cleaning is an important element of any food manufacturing system. There are a number of different methods of cleaning. The ideal from a manufacturer's perspective is to be able to clean quickly and effectively so as to maximize machine availability for production. In order to clean quickly, cleaning-in-place (CIP) is ideal. However, most inspection machines do not lend themselves readily to being cleaned-in-place except for those in pipe systems. For CIP it is important that the velocity of the cleaning fluid is sufficient to cause turbulent flow so as to create eddies currents which increase the cleaning action. For the average 50–76 mm diameter pipe the velocity of the cleaning fluid should be above 2 m/second. No cleaning system should be introduced without assessing whether it adds to the risk of foreign matter incursion.

In order to clean most inspection machines, one has to carry out a manual or semi-manual clean. The cleaning can still be carried out using a range of different methods such as:

- Scrubbing brush and bucket of suitable cleaning solution
- Jet spray system of water or water/cleaning agent
- Foaming system where the cleaning chemical and water are physically foam prior to application
- Wipe clean with clean non-shedding material
- Soaking in a tank of cleaning fluid
- Air jet for dry product
- Vacuum system for dry products

In order to clean a machine, the method is important in order to ensure the machine is properly cleaned. The following general steps are a guide to effective cleaning:

- Remove by hand all solid waste or debris from the machine and place in receptacle
- Rinse the machine to remove smaller solids
- Apply diluted cleaning chemical – detergent selected and applied according to the manufacturer's recommendations
- Rinse off cleaning agents
- Apply disinfectant

Some other general points to bear in mind are:

- Work from the top of the machine down otherwise one may recontaminate or dirty a part of the machine that has already cleaned
- Ensure material is removed from any recesses or concealed places

For an individual item of equipment a specific cleaning schedule should be developed. This schedule is documented such that it includes:

- How the equipment should be cleaned – dismantling, where to clean, etc.
- Frequency of cleaning
- Cleaning regime
- Chemicals to be used
- Level of cleaning required (e.g. micro count, visual, etc.)

A record should be kept of when the equipment was cleaned and by whom and a note of any problems. For the cleaning and hygiene of in-line equipment which is to undergo CIP, a European working group formed as part of a European funded project has developed a standard by which to test equipment that is to be cleaning in-line. It is planned that the standard is called after the project/group name of the European Hygienic Engineering Design Group (EHEDG).

Equipment will be certified to comply with the standard by subjecting it to trials using a specifically designed rig which allows a controlled soil to be applied and then the item is cleaned *in situ* using a set cleaning regime. The equipment or components are then swabbed to determine how clean they are.

7.4.1 *Power – jet cleaning*

This type of cleaning method is based on using a pressurized jet of water which is usually hand held and directed onto the surface that requires cleaning. The type of system can be either a mobile high pressure system, from a fixed point or via a ring main system. The system works by pumping water/detergent through a pipe/hose and then at the end of the pipe through a nozzle. The nozzle is usually located on the end of a lance and creates a restriction, thus creating a pressure in the system and a high velocity as the liquid passes through the restriction. The pressure created can be up to 100 bar.

This type of cleaning is usually more suitable to large, open areas rather than equipment. The high pressure of the jet directed at some equipment can damage it either from the impact pressure, by the ingress of water and by affecting the calibration of sensitive equipment. The pressure of the jet can be used to remove more stubborn soil that is difficult to remove.

The high pressure jet systems are effective at removing soil but can present a secondary problem through creating large amounts of aerosols (airborne fine droplets). The aerosols can spread contamination and soil.

7.4.2 *Foaming*

A foam clean allows the detergent to be applied to the soiled surface and remain in contact with the surface for long enough to breakdown the soil and make it easier to wash off. The foam can be generated from a number of different types of systems. A mobile high pressure system can be utilized where detergent is injected into the water stream. The foam is produced by using a specially designed nozzle that draws in air. A ring main system can also be used. The ring main may have two rings, one for detergent and one for water, or there may just be a high pressure water ring main and the detergent is supplied locally at the application point. It is important that the foam has the appropriate bubble size and miscell level so as to have the right stability, therefore ensuring that it does not collapse too quickly but also is not so stable as to be difficult to break down.

Foam cleaning is effective for large pieces of equipment or equipment which has an intricate design as the stable foam blanket that is created clings to the equipment and reaches all parts of the machine.

7.4.3 *Misting or fogging*

This method of cleaning is one that uses a low energy jet to spray a detergent solution onto a surface. This type of cleaning is more appropriate to open surfaces and areas as the spray hangs in the air and disinfects the airborne particulates and organisms. One has to be careful where the mist lands so as not to contaminate already clean surfaces.

This type of system works by pumping water through an injector usually using compressed air to atomize the cleaning fluid. The centralized system is similar to the foaming system but the nozzle/applicator design is different so as to create a mist.

7.4.4 Dry cleaning

Many food processes are dry and using water or liquid chemicals to clean would cause major problems, and lead to potential contamination and growth of micro-organisms. It is, therefore, necessary to use dry cleaning techniques and methods such as vacuum systems, compressed air, wiping, brushing or sweeping.

(a) Vacuum

One of the most common methods of dry cleaning is that of vacuuming. Vacuum cleaning systems can either be both mobile or part of a central system with suction points located at different points around the factory. Vacuum systems can be most effective as they can be used to reduce the level of dust as well as picking up and removing waste materials.

The system has to be effectively designed to allow sufficient vacuum to remove the size and density of materials. More critical is the method by which the vacuum system can be cleaned such as to avoid internal build-up of waste inside the vacuuming system which could harbour and grow bacteria. In most cases sufficient air velocity, used only to remove dry materials, and routine internal inspection and cleaning will be adequate to ensure the system performs well. It is also possible to use an air-jet vacuum system so the air jet can be utilized to dislodge any material and the vacuum to remove the soil.

(b) Other methods of dry cleaning

There are other methods of dry cleaning. Air jets are used to remove material from difficult to reach locations. The use of compressed air jets should be limited because it can lead to increasing the distribution of materials over a wide area and the fluidization of the dust which may take sometime to settle.

Sweeping and brushing are commonly used cleaning methods. They can be effective but do require a reasonable labour input. Brushes and brooms can add a contamination risk as the bristles will often be lost and could enter into the food production system. One way of minimizing the risk of contamination from bristle is to use brightly coloured bristle (even fluorescent bristle) such that they can be easily spotted and removed – colour coding can also assist in locating where the bristle originated so as to increase vigilance.

Where material has solidified onto equipment surfaces it may be necessary to use specialist cleaning techniques. It is possible to hire cryogenic cleaning systems which use carbon dioxide to shot blast the surface by generating carbon dioxide pellets using a special gun attachment connected to a carbon dioxide cylinder. The cleaning works by attrition and lowering the temperature of the soil so it hardens further and can be removed.

7.5 Microbial contamination

Micro-organisms exist all around us and are present in many foods. Most food processes have a processing step to reduce microbial levels of contamination. Within all food processes the level of active micro-organisms has to be controlled. The control is through heat processing, sterilization, pasteurization, pH control, temperature control (chilled or frozen) and packaging. Some micro-organisms are deliberately introduced as part of the process or final product such as in yoghurt, beer, cheeses and other fermented products. However, many micro-organisms cause spoilage of foods such as moulds, yeasts, and some bacterias. There are also dangerous organisms which include mycotoxins, some bacterias and viruses.

The level of microbial contamination that an inspection system may be subjected to will depend on the environment where it is housed and the type and nature of the product to be inspected. A lot of inspection is carried out at end of line when the product is in its final packaging and protected. This will reduce the likelihood of contamination either of the product or of the machine.

Where an inspection process is carried out on a raw product or one where there is no subsequent sterilization or heat processing step one has to take considerably more care. If any food passing through an inspection system has a high microbiological count, micro-organisms could be transferred onto other products passing through the same inspection machine, and at certain conditions of temperature, pH and moisture this could lead to other food becoming contaminated.

7.6 Chemicals used for cleaning

There are a variety of chemicals that can be used to clean equipment. Some of the most common are detergents such as acids, alkalis, surfactants, phosphates or other similar chemicals. Detergents act by reducing the surface tension and enabling oils/grease to be penetrated and dispersed into globules which can then be freed and flow in the liquid cleaning media. The choice of chemical will depend on the type of soil which is to be removed. Types of soil include:

- Product residues
- Solids deposited from product
- Scale deposited from water
- Calcium salts

Detergents need to be environmentally friendly. Often detergents are alkaline and this is through the addition of chemicals such as caustic soda (sodium hydroxide), sodium carbonate or sodium metasilicate. The selection of an acid or alkaline detergent will depend on the soil to be removed. Polyphosphates are often used to soften water as they act as good dispersion agents and they also possess good anti-corrosion properties.

7.7 Disinfectants

After the soil has been removed from a machine by cleaning there may still be micro-organisms present which have survived the cleaning processes. Disinfectants are used to kill micro-organisms by altering the metabolism or structure of the micro-organism. Some of the common chemicals used as disinfectants are:

- Aldehydes
- Hydrogen peroxide
- Peracetic acid
- Chlorine-based chemicals
- Amphoterics
- Phenolics
- Quaternary ammonium compounds

7.7.1 Choice of disinfectant

The choice of disinfectant will depend upon its use such as the particular food process, type of food and the microbiological requirement. Probably the most important factors to the food manufacturer are the cost of the disinfectant, its ease of use and application, and its microbiological effectiveness. Some disinfectants are toxic and, therefore, their use is restricted. Some compounds have health and safety implications, and, therefore, their use needs to be closely monitored and the appropriate protective clothing has to be worn. Certain chemicals will require special conditions to be most effective such as

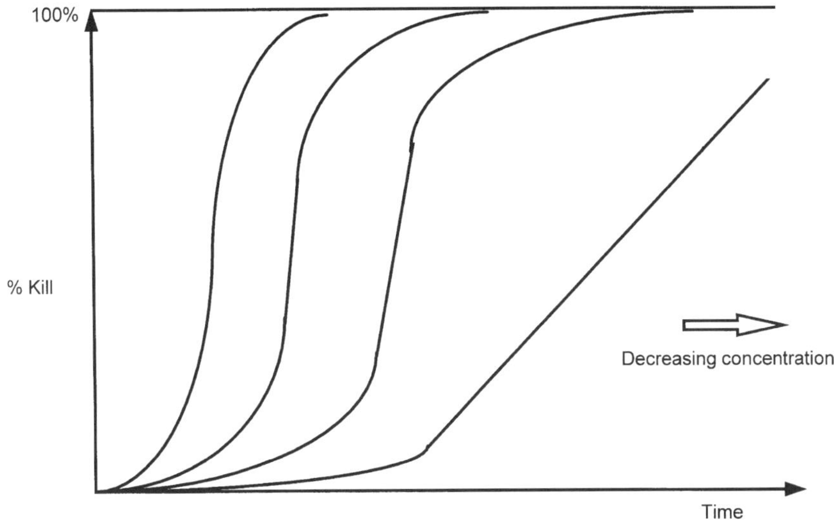

Figure 7.1 Effect of time on degree of kill through disinfection.

concentration and temperature. The physical and chemical properties may affect effective use such as level of foaming, pH, water hardness, reactions with seals or other equipment components.

The application of disinfectants is important and in particular the contact time. Figure 7.1 shows how the degree of kill of organisms increases with increasing contact time.

Disinfectants such as hypochlorite and peracetic acid can be used specifically to oxidize enzymes. Table 7.3 shows some of the advantages and disadvantages of specific types of disinfectants.

Another method of disinfecting is the use of heat. This method is effective but it is often the case that machine components cannot withstand the temperatures required to sterilize a machine by this method. It can also be potentially quite expensive in terms of heating and the time taken to cool the machine down again ready for use.

7.7.2 *Environmental issues associated with disinfectants*

As with cleaning chemicals, disinfectants are usually disposed of by washing them down the drain into the sewage system. They therefore then make their way to the municipal sewage treatment plant. The environmental impact that this has on society is becoming of increasing concern. A number of countries have developed models to assess the environmental impact of disinfectants in terms of

Table 7.3 Major types of disinfectants

Disinfectant	Advantage	Disadvantage
Chlorine based	low cost, organic material, breaks down, can be used with hard water	corrosive, strong odour, volatile, deactivated by soil, acid risk, non-environmental; efficiency is dependent on pH and initial oxidative load in the system
Quaternary	low corrosion, toxicity and volatility, biodegradable, safe to skin	high cost, resistance, restrictive spectrum of use, deactivated by soil, foams
Peracid	low taint, environmentally friendly, effective with hard water, wide range of use	corrosive, volatile, not low cost, requires specialist handling has restricted shelf-life
Amphoterics	low corrosion, toxicity and volatility, safe to skin	high cost, resistance, restrictive spectrum of use, deactivated by soil, foams

assessing the risk. Most local authorities set maximum consent levels over which the discharge must not exceed, otherwise a penalty or prosecution will take place.

7.8 Machine hygiene regulations

Over recent years there has been a move in Europe and other countries to ensure that equipment is better designed for use in the food industry. The EU initiated a harmonization programme for food safety and hygiene. This resulted in a Council directive on the hygiene of foodstuffs which is entitled the EC Food Hygiene Directive (93/43/EEC) 1993.

Hygiene rules have also been developed for a number of specific food product groups and these are given in Table 7.4.

The Food Safety (General Food Hygiene) Regulations, 1995, states that all articles, fittings and equipment with which food comes into contact shall be kept clean and:

> *... be so constructed, be of such materials, and be kept in such good order, repair and condition, as to minimize any risk of contamination of the food.*
>
> *With the exception of non-returnable containers and packaging, be so constructed, be of such materials, and be kept in such good order, repair and condition, as to enable them to be kept thoroughly cleaned and, where necessary, disinfected, sufficient for the purposes intended;*
>
> *... be installed in such a manner as to allow adequate cleaning of the surrounding area.*

There are a large number of new standards for specific types of food machines which have either been written or in progress (Appendix I).

Table 7.4 Guidelines for specific food product groups

Directive	Specific products
92/46/EEC	Milk and milk-based products
92/5/EEC	Trade in meat products
91/497/EEC	Fresh meat
91/493/EEC	Fishery products
89/437/EEC	Egg products
94/65/EEC	Minced meat and meat preparations

References and further reading

AISI (1974) *Steel Products Manual: Stainless and Heat Resisting Steels*. American Iron and Steel Institute, Washington, DC.

ASTM *Alloy Designations for Cast Stainless Steels, ASTM Standard A781/A781M,* Appendix X1. Steel Founder's Society of America, Chicago, IL.

Deutches Institut fur Normung (1985) *DIN 17 440*. Beuth Verlag, Berlin.

EC (1993) *Food Hygiene Directive (93/43/EEC)*. Brussels, Belgium

EHEDG (1993) *Hygienic Equipment Design Criteria*. The European Hygienic Equipment Design Group, Campden and Chorleywood Food Research Association, Chipping Campden.

FDA (1997) *Food Drug Cosmetic Law Reports, Section 178.3570*. Food and Drug Administration, Washington, DC.

HMSO (1995) *The Food Safety (General Food Hygiene) Regulations*. HMSO, London, UK

8

Magnets

8.1 Introduction

It is a common misconception that only sizeable pieces of mild steel can be picked out by the use of magnets. In fact with the advent of advanced materials technology magnets can be used to pick out extremely fine metallic dust and some grades of stainless steel, particularly fasteners which have developed some magnetic properties as a result of the processes used in their manufacture.

Ferrous contamination can enter the process at almost any stage from 'the field to the plate'. It can occur during harvesting, transport or storage of crops. It can occur as ingested material in some animals or enter the material during slaughter and processing. During processing it can arise during transfer, thermal processing, size reduction, mashing, blending, slicing and packing.

Magnets are one of the oldest methods available to the food industry to remove metal contamination from food, having been around since the 1890s. They also tend to be an under-utilized resource. Modern magnets benefit from the latest developments of materials science. They now have the capability to remove metal contaminants far smaller than anything currently detectable by metal detectors or X-ray machines.

Before the introduction of modern magnet materials, electromagnets were used where maximum field strength was required. This is no longer the case. Electromagnets required a d.c. power supply which made them not only relatively costly but also unsuitable for use in wet conditions.

While a magnet only has the capability to remove magnetic materials, i.e. ferrous metals, they can be used under the extremes of temperature found in the food industry and in wet or dry processes. Their great advantage is that they only remove the metal, not the process material, therefore they do not generate product waste.

Incorporating them into the line, ahead of conventional metal detectors, X-ray machines or optical sorters have the advantage of ensuring even the smallest magnetic particles are removed while reducing the amount of rejection from the inspection devices, reducing product waste and making monitoring of the process simpler.

8.2 Materials used in magnet construction

Permanent magnets were made originally from steel alloys, a typical alloy contained 5–10% cobalt, 0.9% carbon and was of little or no use in the removal of metallic contamination from a process line. By the 1940s alloys were introduced with greater magnetic properties which were almost unmachinable and were used in the form of sintered materials. These 'ceramic' or 'ferrite' materials as they are known were principally barium or strontium ferrite. Other materials had also become available, examples being 'Alnico', an alloy containing 10% aluminium (Al), 20% nickel (Ni) and 13% cobalt (Co), and 'Reco 2A', an alloy containing 20% nickel, 7% aluminium, 20% cobalt, 7% copper and 6.5% titanium. Ferrite, Alnico or Reco magnets had similar magnetic properties, which are given in Table 8.1

During the 1970s rare earth magnets started to appear for industrial purposes with far greater magnetic properties. The introduction of samarium–cobalt rare earth magnets increased the magnetic strength available by a factor of two to three times the strength of the earlier materials.

By the 1980s material technology had advanced again, and new neodyium–iron–boron rare earth materials have been introduced with even greater magnetic properties.

8.3 Performance

The performance of a permanent magnet is evaluated in terms of its energy product which is expressed as BH_{max}. Gauss and oersted are

Table 8.1 Comparative magnetic properties of permanent magnet materials

Material	Energy Product BH_{max}	Remanence magnetism *Br* (Gauss)	Coercive force *BH* (Oersted)
Ferrite, Alnico, Reco	3–6	3700	3000
Samarium–cobalt (rare earth)	25–30	11000	9000
Neodymium–iron–boron (rare earth)	30–40	12000	10000

units of the centimetre–gram system (cgs) This has been superseded by the SI units Tesla and ampere/metre (1 A/m), respectively.

Gauss (tesla) is a measurement of the flux density and oersted (A/m) is a measurement of field strength. The figures shown in the Table 8.1 demonstrate the dramatic difference in magnetic properties of rare earth materials. Samarium–cobalt or neodymium–iron–boron rare earth material makes permanent magnets an important tool for the removal of ferrous metal contamination from process materials

8.4 Operation

A magnet operates by attracting a metallic particle then holding it on its surface. To achieve this the magnet must generate a magnetic field of sufficient strength to magnetize any magnetic metal particle that passes through its field. It must also generate a magnetic gradient of sufficient strength to draw the particle to it against the physical resistance of the product through which the particle must pass as it moves to the magnet surface. The magnetic force acting on the particle is the product of the magnetic field strength and the gradient.

The selection of the material the magnet is made from will depend on the application. Moving relatively large particles of easily magnetized materials, such as steel nuts and bolts, from a product with low resistance to the movement of the particle, e.g. grain flowing under gravity in a tube, requires a relatively low intensity field. This will be satisfied by the use of a ceramic (or ferrite) magnet. On the other hand, where small, difficult to magnetize particles must be drawn from a product which will resist their passage, e.g. fine metal shards in liquid chocolate, a high intensity field will be required. This will be satisfied by the use of a rare earth magnet. Where the application exceeds 80°C then the samarium–cobalt material is required.

In application the magnet material is protected from the environment by a case completely surrounding the magnet. In many cases the magnet is not a single block of material but an assembly of several individual magnetic components built up to provide the characteristics required by the application. The case is manufactured from stainless steel.

8.5 Types of magnets

There are four main ways magnets are used in the processing of food. These are:

- Plate magnets

- Rod magnets
- Pipeline magnets
- Magnetic drum systems

8.5.1 Plate magnets

A plate magnet is simply a box containing permanent magnets. Its size, or working face, will be made to suit the particular application. The normal application of these magnets is to remove relatively large pieces of metal and generally they are manufactured from ceramic magnets.

They are commonly placed above conveyors carrying product, particularly at the reception of harvested crops. They are also found at the base of chutes, or in ducts carrying material between process stages or storage and usage. Where the application calls for the removal of fine particles, rare earth magnets may be used but it may be preferable to investigate the use of an alternative style to achieve the best result.

Plate magnets are installed above conveyors at a height sufficient to just clear the product and it may be necessary to install a product levelling device in front of the magnet to prevent blockage or spillage. The depth of the material on the belt should be minimized – this can be achieved in a variety of ways, including increasing belt speed or spreading the burden evenly across the full working width of the belt. The shallower the product burden, the more effective the magnet will be.

Were the magnet is to be installed in a duct, then similar actions should be taken including the introduction of weirs and product guides to achieve a minimum product depth across the magnet without interfering with product flow or capacity. A typical system is illustrated in Figure 8.3.

Provision needs to be made to access the magnet for cleaning. This may be by swinging the magnet clear of the conveyor to give access to it or dropping the magnet on a hinge so that it forms a door when used on chutes. It is important that the magnet face can be easily accessed and observed for regular cleaning purposes. Plate magnets can be heavy and their weight must be considered when designing access.

8.5.2 Rod magnets (grids)

Rod magnets are stainless steel tubes containing cylindrical permanent magnets built up to achieve the length required by the application. The rods are then arranged in single or multiple rows to form

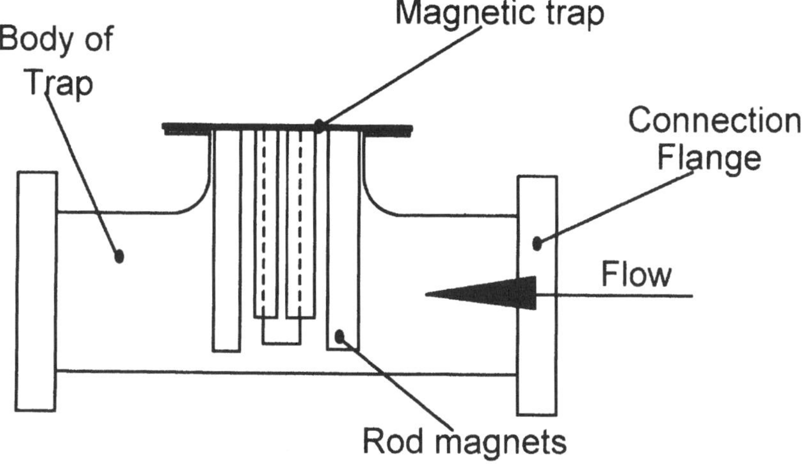

Figure 8.1 Magnetic pipeline trap. (Courtesy Boxmag Rapid Ltd.)

grids. The spacing of the rods within the grids is optimized to ensure the maximum magnetic effect is exerted on any metal particle passing through the grid.

The grid may be arranged in a drawer to allow it to be extracted for cleaning. This can be a manual or pneumatic operation.

The product, typically a powder or granular product, flows through the grid where metal particles are removed by powerful magnets, typically 9000–10 000 gauss, and held on the tube until it is cleaned manually. Careful design of the grids ensures that flow rates are not compromised and in those cases where the product has a tendency to form a bridge, the grid can be vibrated electromechanically or air used to ensure blockage does not occur.

The use of the high power rare earth magnets ensures the removal of very fine particles of iron or rust. Where the objective is to trap larger contaminants the ceramic magnets may be sufficient. See Figure 8.4.

8.5.3 Rod magnets (pipeline traps)

The use of metal detectors or X-ray machines on liquids flowing in pipes leads to quite large volumes of reject material for the reasons discussed in the relevant chapters. The use of a magnet pipeline trap results in all magnetic metal contaminants being removed without the loss or wastage of the product. Viscosity, temperature and pH of the material have little or no effect on the efficiency of the system. They are an improvement on the use of filters. However, when the

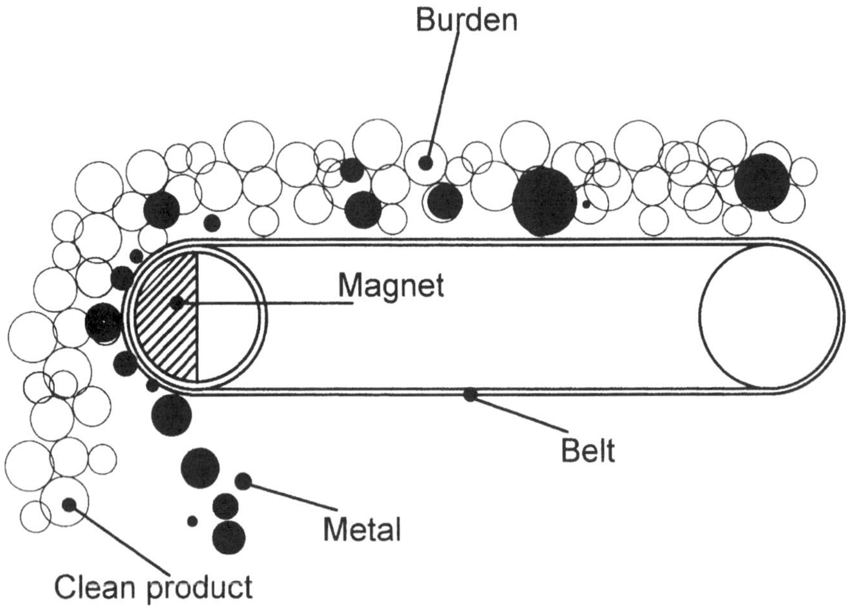

Figure 8.2 Magnetic drum separator. (Courtesy Boxmag Rapid Ltd.)

product is 'lumpy', e.g. meat products, plate magnets may have to be used which may require modification to the system to accommodate them.

The same type of rare earth rod magnets are used as in the grid system. In this case they are arranged as shown in Figure 8.1 and placed in the product flow. Any magnetic material passing over them is held, allowing the clean product to continue without any interference.

The rod assembly is simply lifted out of the pipe for cleaning.

The system is supplied as a complete unit to fit a specific pipe size, e.g. 50, 75 and 100 mm. It can be obtained with a heated jacket for use on applications such as liquid chocolate.

8.5.4 Magnetic rods (plain)

A single magnetic rod is a useful tool for incoming quality control or indeed in process quality inspection for bulk products such as powders or granules. Simply inserted into a container of product and 'stirred' round it will perform a very rapid assay of the level of metallic contamination present.

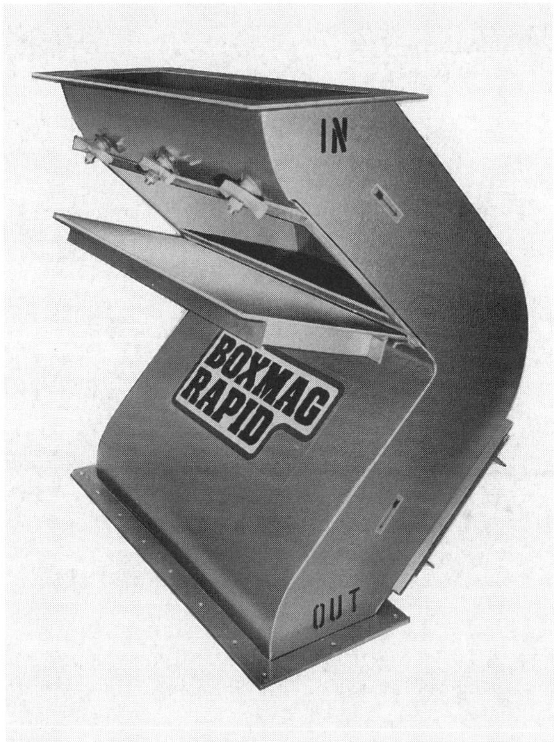

Figure 8.3 Magnetic plate separator incorporated in a section of ductwork. The plate is hinged to allow easy cleaning. (Courtesy Boxmag Rapid Ltd.)

8.5.5 Magnetic drums

A magnetic drum separator comprises a rotating drum which contains a fixed permanent magnet extending through approximately 180° around the periphery. Material to be treated is fed onto the top of the drum, magnetic metals are attracted to the magnet unit and held onto the drum as it rotates. Non-magnetic material is thrown from the drum by centrifugal action from the rotation. The magnetic particles are held until the drum surface leaves the magnet at which point the magnetic particles are thrown from the drum or cleaned off by a scraper system.

These systems are used to extract magnetic contaminants from free-flowing materials such as tea, sugar or grain. Where the objective is to remove large particles, then ceramic materials are used. Where the objective is smaller particles, then higher intensity rare earth magnets are used. See Figure 8.2.

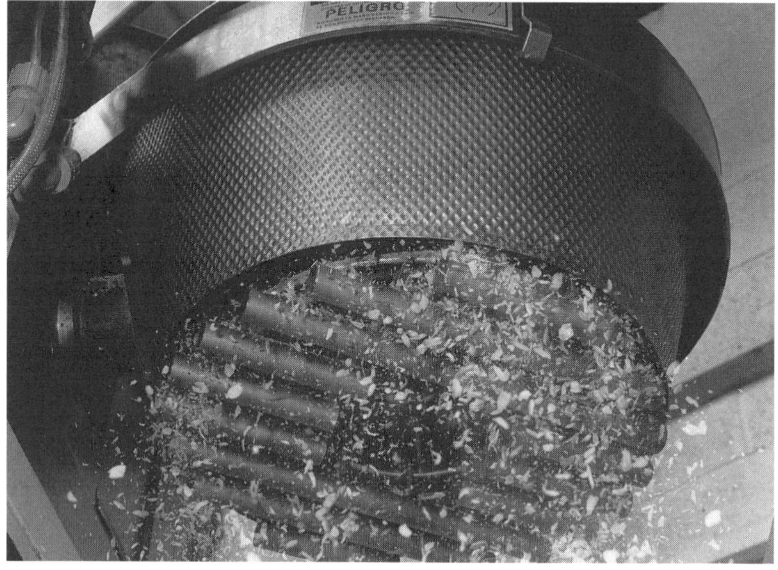

Figure 8.4 A rare earth magnetic grill detects and removes pieces of broken cutting blades during nut chopping. (Courtesy Boxmag Rapid Ltd.)

The capacity of drum magnets is based on the volumetric capacity per unit width of the drum. To extract larger particles, nuts and bolts, etc., the calculation is based on 100 m^3/hour/m drum width, with the capacity dropping to 15 m^3/hour/m of drum width for fine particles.

8.6 Safety precautions

Magnets are not dangerous to human beings as far as is known. They can, however, present dangers to other pieces of equipment which is why they carry warning labels. They will disturb magnetically recorded information, tapes, discs, credit cards, both mechanical and electronic watches, and pacemakers. All magnetic separators have to comply with the EC directive on EMC which is embodied in the UK's machinery safety Act.

The performance of permanent magnets is affected by temperature. Ceramic magnets can be used at temperatures up to 350°C. However, there is a significant loss of field strength at temperatures above 180°C. Rare earth magnets have a maximum working temperature of 150°C.

8.7 Limitations

Magnets will only remove magnetic materials, they will not remove any of the non-ferrous metals such as bronze, copper or brass, they will not remove any non-metallic impurities such as plastic or paper, and in general terms they will not remove stainless steels except in certain instances.

The sensitivity or ability to remove a specific particle size depends upon the following criteria

8.7.1 Material bulk

The bulk of the material through which the contaminant has to be dragged. The process of attracting a particle to the magnet surface will be proportional to the thickness of the burden through which it has to pass. All the time it is travelling through the product it is travelling with the product past the magnet itself. If the time taken to travel through the product exceeds that to travel past the magnet, then a particle initially lying at the furthest edge of the product to the magnet may not be removed.

8.7.2 Product speed

The time available to attract a metal particle will be inversely proportional to the product speed. Therefore, product speed and distance to be travelled to the magnet surface must be optimized to ensure maximum sensitivity. In practice this can be achieved by selection of the site for the magnet and its design and selection.

8.7.3 Contaminant susceptibility to magnetic force

The susceptibility of materials differs in descending order. It is:

Iron
Mild steel
Magnetic stainless steel
Rust
Scale
Abraded non-magnetic stainless steel

8.7.4 Contaminant size

As already stated, magnetic susceptibility is also proportional to particle size.

8.8 The application of magnets in a quality control system

8.8.1 General

The choice of location, style and type of magnet will be derived from the risk and hazard analysis applicable to the operation. This is discussed in more detail in Chapter 2. Having made these decisions, the magnet has to be managed within the system, and its performance monitored and recorded. The performance of a magnet, providing it is not subject to mechanical shock or extremes of temperature, will remain constant. However, this does not mean that it can be taken for granted and ignored – it must be checked at regular intervals. In operation, metal contamination will build up on the magnet surface, which must be removed at regular intervals. Examination of the contamination removed can also provide invaluable information about the process.

8.8.2 Performance measurement and tests

The field strength of a magnet can be measured quite simply by using a commercial gaussmeter fitted with a Hall effect probe. As with any measuring equipment, the traceability of calibration needs to be recorded, when the meter is calibrated against a reference magnet. While the user can carry out this test, reputable magnet manufacturers will carry out the work if required and in most cases calibration by an outside source is preferable.

The calibration process is not required to be carried out frequently – in practice an annual calibration should prove sufficient, unless the magnet is known to have been subject to mechanical shock, e.g. dropped or subject of extremes of temperature. Under these circumstances the calibration process should be carried out before production continues.

8.8.3 Cleaning the magnet

As previously stated, magnets must be cleaned at regular intervals. The frequency of cleaning will depend upon the particular application on a particular line. The question of establishing the frequency of monitoring equipment performance is discussed in Chapter 13.

The cleaning process needs to be clearly specified. It is not enough to say clean the magnet – the manner of cleaning and the way it is to be carried out to prevent metal contamination falling back into the product must be stated. Some magnets are provided with mesh sleeves which are withdrawn, removing the metal contamination and leaving the surface clean. Some magnets utilize mechanical or pneumatic assistance in opening them for cleaning and it is essential that the magnets are correctly re-positioned after cleaning.

It is recommended that the operators responsible for this work be trained, and that the training be recorded and repeated.

Drum magnets are an exception to the general rule as these by definition are both self-cleaning and powered. While the magnet will not need cleaning, the extracted contamination will need to be removed and the system checked to ensure it is operating correctly. As with manual cleaning, the work and inspection process must be clearly specified and the operators trained in the necessary work to be carried out.

8.9 Analysis of metallic contamination

Every time the magnet is cleaned some metallic contamination should be found and removed. Depending on the application, a description of the expected contamination should be drawn up so that a comparison can be made between what is expected and what is found. Where the magnet has been installed for a specific purpose, e.g. to catch pieces of a knife which is known to break occasionally, then a description of the material expected to be discovered is required.

When contamination removed exceeds the limits set out in the description of the anticipated contamination, a procedure should be implemented to evaluate the cause and introduce corrective action. Where the overall quality system calls for inspection of the magnet in the event of an equipment breakdown, e.g. when a knife fails, then the metal contamination removed needs to be examined to ensure the complete broken component has been retained in the system. Where this is not the case then product quarantine is implemented.

8.10 Records

Records need to be kept of the risk and hazard analysis on which the decision was based to introduce a magnet. This will include the descriptions of expected findings – when these are exceeded the product quarantine procedure is introduced.

Records need to be available of the checks and cleaning process as they are carried out and confirmation the material removed is within expected limits. The record needs to be simple but designed to record both when the system is operating as expected and when there is a potential problem (Figure 8.5).

To ensure the system is capable of operating properly all the relevant factors are specified in a written training manual, and person-

XYZ Speciality Foods ltd

Magnet Performance Record				Form No 1201 Issue 0005 Date 25.7.1997
Line reference			Magnet reference	
Date	**Time**	**Classification of Material removed**	**Operator**	**Comments**

Figure 8.5 Magnet performance record. *Line reference* identifies the line. *Magnet reference* identifies the specific magnet. *Date, Time* and *Operator* identify who carried out the cleaning and when. *Classification of removed material* allows for a record to be made which will normally show the system is performing as expected. Within specified limits = OK. Exceeds specified limits = X. *Comments and Action* allow for a record to be made when the expected levels are exceeded. It provides space for details of action taken to be entered, e.g. Informed line manager.

nel who have been trained and achieved a satisfactory level of competence identified.

8.11 Economic considerations

Magnets are the cheapest, automatic means of removing ferrous metal contamination from a food process line. Once they are installed, except in one or two specific instances, they are self-contained and do not consume any utilities. Their predicted life is in excess of 10 years. In operation, a minimum of expertise is required to supervise them and providing they are in position they will continue to operate.

By removing only the contamination they reduce the wastage that occurs from other detection devices; further, the material removed is readily available for immediate examination and it does not require any costly separation procedures, thus providing a cost-effective instant picture of the condition of the product or the line.

Maintenance of the magnet, except for a regular test of efficiency, is not required. It is only where it is built in with a mechanical system for opening/closing or operation that maintenance is required to ensure continuation of performance.

9

Metal detection

9.1 Introduction

Metal detectors are the most common type of foreign body detector in use throughout the world (Figure 9.1). The technology has been known for many years. A patent was registered in the USA during the last century covering the principles of the balanced coil design. The first industrial metal detector incorporating this technology was developed by Bruce Kerr in 1948. The application was to sort a batch of confectionery known to be contaminated following a machine failure.

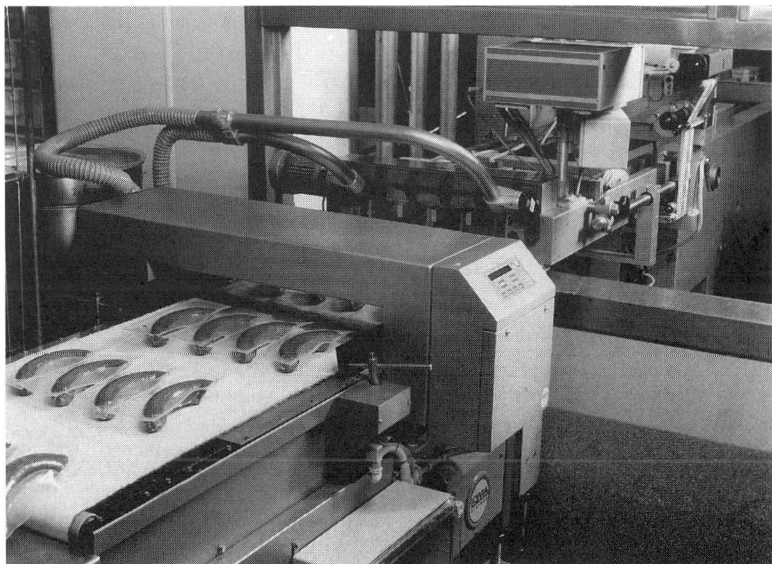

Figure 9.1 Typical metal detector installation. (Courtesy Loma Engineering Ltd.)

Since that time several types of metal detector have been developed for various applications. The type known as 'balanced coil' systems (section 9.2), in principle capable of detecting all metals, is the type normally used in the food industry, with the 'ferrous-in-foil' type (section 9.3) being of secondary importance – they are only capable of detecting ferrous metals. The use of balanced coil metal detectors for use with metallized film has been developed in response to the growth of the use of this material for packaging (section 9.4). There is a further type commonly used in the plastic industry which is discussed in section 9.5

Over the years the method of construction has more or less standardized to the wrap round, closed-coil type. Applications for the separated-coil type are limited and these are mainly found in non-food applications.

While 'open-end section' metal detectors were used by the food industry, their use is now restricted to heavy industrial, non-food, applications because of the deterioration in stability/sensitivity caused by the demands of the construction. (Open-end section metal detectors are constructed so that the side section of the aperture can be removed to facilitate installation over a belt. Breaking the coils degrades performance and stability is reduced.) The types of metal detector sold for use in the quarry industry are totally unsuitable for the detection of foreign bodies in food products. Treasure hunter metal detectors and security, hand held, metal detectors are equally unsuitable for food applications.

The development of the microprocessor and other modern solid-state devices has had a dramatic impact on the performance of metal detectors – not so much in terms of the minimum size of particle that can be detected under ideal conditions but in the improvement in stability and reliability in real-life applications where the environment is hostile to the use of extremely sensitive equipment. Only a few years ago setting a metal detector up was a lengthy and tricky operation. The adjustments were made manually and in many cases the detector had to be built differently depending on whether the application was on a wet or dry product. The detectors required frequent manual correction and adjustment, with in many cases the sensitivity having to be reduced because of environmental considerations. The latest detectors are able to set themselves up to optimize detection automatically. They can recognize wet or dry products and make the necessary adjustments to optimize performance. Once they have set themselves they continuously monitor their settings, compensating where necessary to allow for changes in the product or drift in their electronics. Digital technology allows settings to be stored for recall and information on performance to be sent to central computers. The traditional methods of testing functionality have been replaced by the metal detector automatically demanding a function test, which if not carried out according to a predetermined specification will generate an alarm signal in the same way as any other failure.

Coupled with the advances in the design of the metal detectors, the mechanical handling systems have also been improved. Reject operation control has benefited from the introduction of solid-state devices to control the timing of operation signals. The operation of reject devices, the condition of reject bins and various other features can now be monitored by electronic sensors connected to the metal detector self-monitoring circuits and the information utilized by the metal detector electronics as part of its self-check system.

Most manufacturers are now able to offer a range of systems to suit almost any application in the food industry.

As with any of the available detection or removal equipment, no metal detector is capable of detecting every piece of metal which passes through it. There is always a limit to its sensitivity. This limitation is subject to a variety of causes which may be product related, application related or contaminant related. An understanding of what these are and the reasons for them is necessary if metal detectors are to be used to their maximum efficiency within a process. As already discussed, metal is a major source of complaints – it can come from a variety of sources, but in many cases it can be prevented or removed.

9.2 Balanced coil metal detectors: construction

9.2.1 General

All metal detectors comprise a search head housing the sensing coils and a control unit.

The control unit contains the electronics driving the system and operating the detection circuits. With the advent of digital electronics it may also contain the circuits providing and storing the data. To house the additional power supplies needed to operate all the latest features and to provide terminals for input and output signals there may be a second box, in addition to the control unit, containing power supplies and connections for input and output signals. The details of construction will vary from manufacturer to manufacturer.

At first glance a metal detector appears to be a box with a passage through it. Manufacturers strive to make the external design as smooth as possible for hygiene purposes. The box is correctly described as the case of the metal detector – an essential component of the system. A metal detector signal is triggered by the system detecting voltage changes as small as 1 millionth part of a volt

(0.000001 V). To construct a system with this sensitivity, that will operate reliably under production conditions, is one of the major challenges a metal detector manufacturer has to overcome.

The case itself being made of metal has an effect on the coils. Any movement of the case relative to the coils can cause a false detection signal – the amount of physical deflection that will cause this is measured in microns. The total assembly of the case and coil has to be totally rigid, and able to tolerate the mechanical effects of vibration from motors, reject systems, passing traffic within the plant and other machinery. It also has to be able to tolerate temperature changes both ambient and from radiated heat sources, e.g. ovens. A metal detector placed at the outlet of a biscuit oven is a difficult application that has been satisfactorily solved by the metal detector industry. Not only does the case have to perform those functions, it also has to provide an electrical screen to shield the assembly from interference by radiated electrical signals such as those generated by motors, switch-gear and other electrical equipment.

To achieve these properties manufacturers have adopted various construction techniques. The case may have flat sides and top and bottom surfaces or it may have the top and/or the bottom crowned in some way. A benefit of constructing the case with crowned surfaces is that it increases the mechanical rigidity of the case. An additional advantage of having the top of the search head domed or crowned is that it prevents it being used as a convenient place to leave tools, pens, pencils, etc., which could then fall into the product. To maximize physical strength and minimize the effects of humidity, water and dust, the case may be completely filled with a 'potting' compound, the constituents of which vary depending on the manufacturer.

The control unit may be built into or bolted onto the search head, in which case it is generally referred to as an integrated system, or it may be connected to the search head by a cable either so that it can be mounted separately to make access to the control unit more convenient or because the search head is too small to accommodate it.

Construction techniques using painted steel, aluminium or plain stainless steel for the case and the control unit are selected depending upon the application. Models are available that are designed to withstand high pressure and steam cleaning up to IP 66 and even IP 67.

9.2.2 *Closed coil (Figure 9.2)*

- *The case.* This is usually constructed from aluminium but now more and more are in stainless steel to meet the needs of industry.

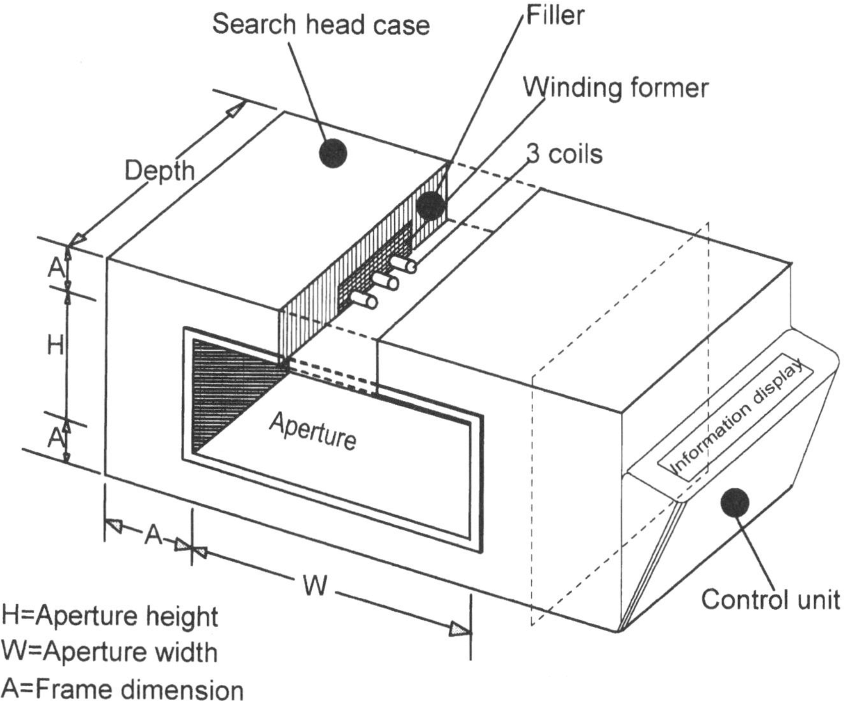

Figure 9.2 Closed coil metal detector.

The purpose of the case is to provide the mechanical enclosure for the assembly but most importantly it has to act as an electrical screen to prevent outside electrical interference disturbing the electrical field generated in the assembly.

- *The coils.* A centre coil and two outer coils, wound on a former. These are carefully constructed to make the three coils as near as possible the same and equally spaced on the former. The coils themselves are made from a single turn of a very thick copper wire.
- *The filler.* The coils and former are supported by a filling compound so that the coils are geometrically equi-spaced inside the case. The filling compound gives mechanical rigidity to the assembly and plays an important part in the stability of the system.
- *The aperture.* The hole in the case surrounded by the coils and being the passage through which the product will pass. This is normally lined with a hygienic, non-metallic, plastic material to allow the field to fill the aperture. The quality of the construction and the seal achieved for the aperture lining is important particularly where the application is wet.

9.2.3 *Separate coil (Figure 9.3)*

- *The upper case* encloses a drive or oscillator coil. This is manufactured from aluminium, mild steel or stainless steel depending on the manufacturer and the application.
- *Spacers*. These are metal components, manufactured from the same material as the rest of the case which are bolted to the upper and lower cases creating the aperture through which the product will pass. Their size controls the height of the aperture.
- *The lower case* encloses the two receiver coils, manufactured from the same material as the upper case.
- *The coils* are supported on formers in a similar manner to the closed loop system.
- *The filler* is a material supporting the coil assemblies as in the closed loop system
- *The aperture* is defined by the size of the upper and lower cases and the size of the spacer between them. Unlike the closed coil system, it is only sealed on its upper and lower surfaces.

9.2.4 *Comparison of closed coil and separate coil construction*

- *Mechanical rigidity*. Because the closed coil system is manufactured from a welded box style of construction it has an inherently greater mechanical rigidity and stability than the bolt-together construction of the separate coil construction.

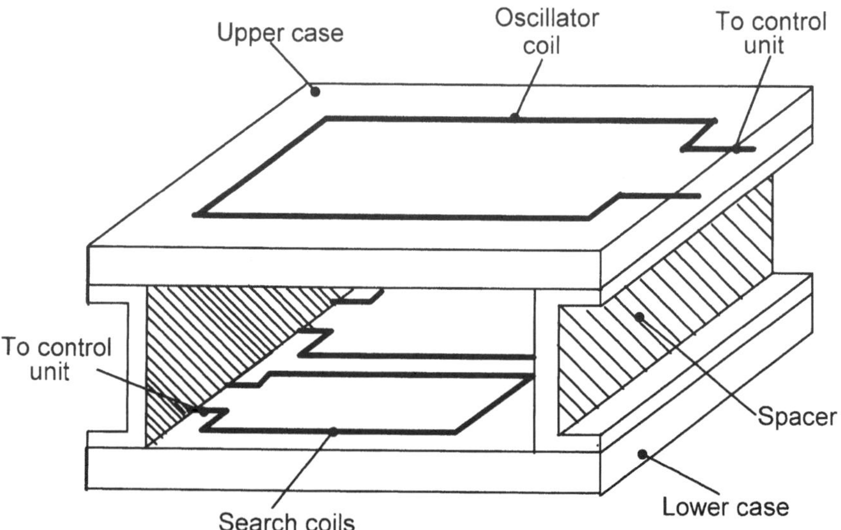

Figure 9.3 Separate coil metal detector construction.

- *Stability*. The optimum dimensions for the size of the case is calculated in proportion to the size of the aperture for closed coil systems. The separate coil system tends to utilize standard components so that the 'depth' and the 'frame size' dimensions are common irrespective of height. This results in lesser stability.
- *Sensitivity*. The coil is wrapped around the aperture in the closed coil system giving a more constant field strength. Constructional difficulties result in less accuracy in the coil alignment of separate coil search heads. These factors have the effect of reducing sensitivity in the separate coil system.

9.2.5 Search head dimensions

The size of the search head is proportional to the size of the aperture, and manufacturers calculate an optimum size for the 'frame' and 'depth' dimensions to suit their construction. Although there is a degree of similarity between the search head sizes adopted by the various manufacturers, there is not a recognized standard for this feature. Manufacturers offer varying styles of search heads to suit particular applications. This is particularly noticeable where the size of the aperture is small and for which the control unit is shown as a separate item. This may result from the calculation for optimum dimensions resulting in the search head dimension working out to be less than the dimension of the control unit. It may result from the need to fit the search head in a restricted space, e.g. in a typical drop-through application between a multi-head weigher and a bag maker. The manufacturer's advice should be sought on the most suitable search head for a given application giving due regard to any loss in sensitivity resulting from the use of small search heads.

9.3 Balanced coil metal detectors: principles of operation.

9.3.1 General

The systems (Figure 9.4) have been described as 'balanced coil' systems. This describes an ideal electrical state that exists only under certain conditions and from which the name is derived. The detection principle applies to both methods of construction.

The centre coil of the assembly is connected to a source of an oscillating current which generates an electrical field around the coil. This is radiated in all directions rather like radio waves which are emitted by a transmitter.

Continuing the analogy, the radiated waves or signal are picked up by the balance coils located at either side of the centre coil (simi-

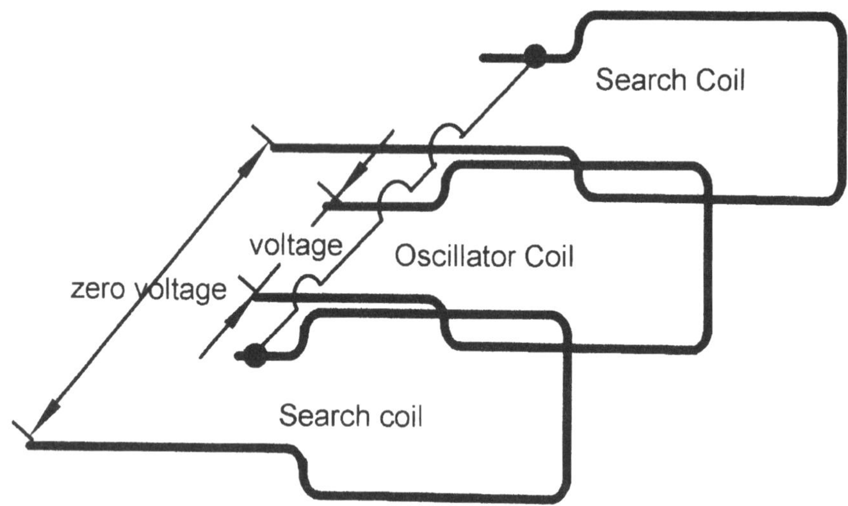

Figure 9.4 Schematic diagram of three-coil arrangement.

lar to an aerial on a radio). This has the effect of generating a voltage in the coil which is used by the detection circuits.

The balance coils are connected to each other in such a way that the signal received by one coil is equal and opposite to the signal received by the other coil, which therefore cancel each other out leaving 0 V across the circuit. In an ideal, theoretical, situation the three coils would be of exactly the same size and be exactly spaced, parallel, etc., so that the signal value picked up by each balance coil would be exactly the same as the other. Unfortunately, this is a theoretical position – in practice the accuracy cannot be achieved and other means are used to achieve the balance state. This adjustment is carried out during the manufacturing process so that when construction is complete any further adjustments due to drift, whatever the cause, are within the capacity of the automatic balance system.

The introduction of a piece of metal into the assembly will have an effect on the field (Figure 9.5). Depending on the type of metal it will either attract the field or repel it, in either case it will change the balance state; however, it has been achieved by causing the signal received by one coil to be different to that received by the other, resulting in a voltage in the circuit. This is the detection signal which may be as low as 1 millionth part of a volt (0.000001 V).

The principle is simple. It is the execution that is complicated by the effects of interference, the electrical properties of various metals, the shape of the metal contaminant and the electrical properties of some food materials.

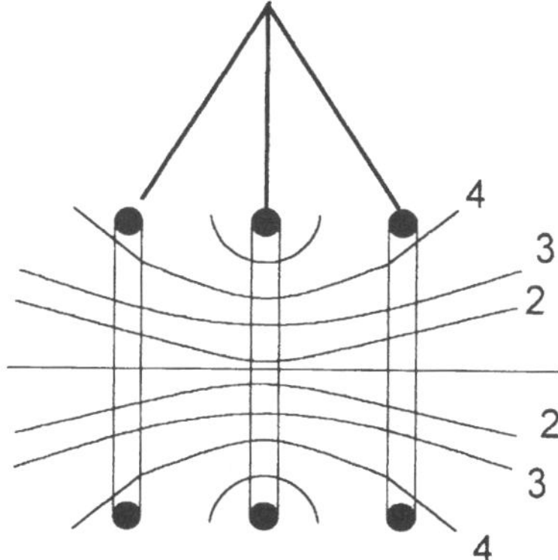

A. Balanced condition.

No metal present.

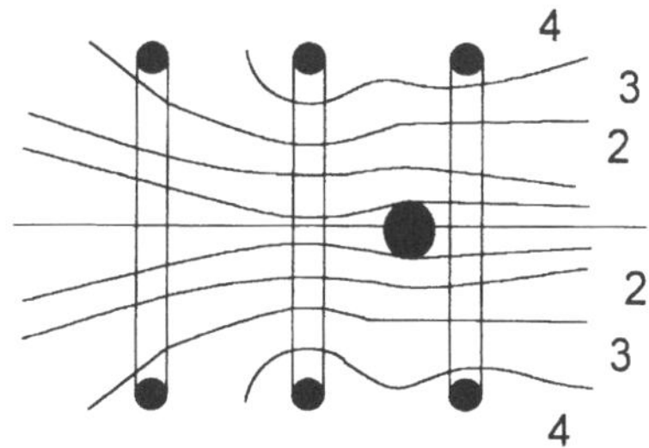

B. Unbalanced condition.

Fe metal present.

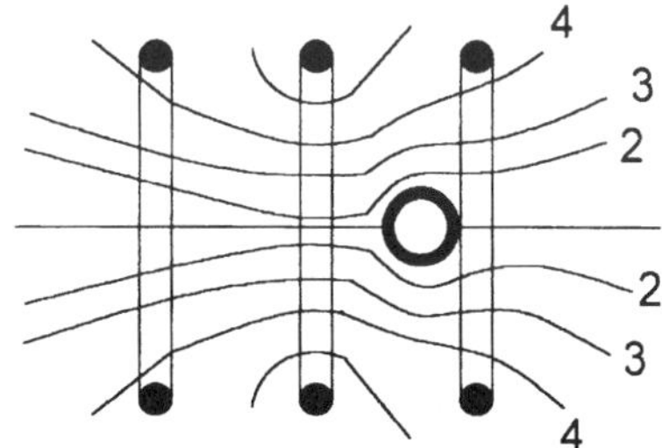

C. Unbalanced condition.

Non ferrous metal present.

Figure 9.5 The effect of metal in a three-coil system.

9.3.2 *Limiting factors*

(a) General

As previously stated, the sensitivity of metal detectors is limited. This section deals with the factors which affect sensitivity:

- Uniformity of sensitivity in the aperture
- The type of metal
- The type of product (includes metallized film detectors)
- Metallized film (included as a limiting factor even though answered by special purpose metal detectors)
- The size and shape of the metal
- The size of the product
- The environment
- The product speed

Magnetic metals are the easiest to detect under all circumstances. Non-ferrous metals, copper, brass, etc., are as easy to detect as magnetic materials when the product is small and dry, e.g. packs of plain biscuits, although in the same conditions stainless steel will be about 1.5 times more difficult to detect. When the product is very large, non-ferrous sensitivity will reduce by up to half of that of ferrous but at the same time stainless steel sensitivity may be reduced by a factor of 2 or even more. When the product is wet, then size for size the ferrous sensitivity will remain fairly constant while the non-ferrous and stainless steel sensitivity will reduce by a significant factor – the value of which will vary from application to application.

(b) Uniformity of sensitivity in the aperture

The maximum sensitivity of any closed coil metal detector will be found at the edges of the aperture, i.e. the plane closest to the coils. The least sensitive point will be at the geometric centre of the aperture, i.e. the point furthest away from the coils. When detector sensitivity is specified without product it should always be specified at the geometric centre of the aperture. Similar rules apply to separate coil construction except that it is only the two sides which are active.

(c) The type of metal

In terms of metal detection there are three types of metals. The first two types are magnetic (ferrous) metals and non-magnetic (non-ferrous) metals. In practice, while pure non-ferrous metals do occur, e.g. copper and aluminium, most metal contaminants are alloys of iron and carbon with additional elements, non-ferrous metals, or alloys such as brass. The third and most difficult type to detect is stainless steel.

The term stainless steel describes a range of special steels with varying mechanical properties and resistance to corrosion. There are two main subdivisions: non-heat-treatable types (SAE 301, 304, etc.) and heat-treatable types (SAE 414, 415, etc.). Because of their characteristics the first types are much more difficult to detect while some grades of the second type are as easy to detect as ferrous metals. Therefore, when specifying stainless steel detection levels reference should be made to the grade of material.

Stated simply, ferrous metals, e.g. iron, are detected because of their permeability. Non-ferrous metals are detected because their low permeability generates eddy current losses. Permeability and eddy current loss both generate signals which are detectable and distinguishable by metal detector electronics. Because most metals are alloys of one type or the other, their effect on the field generated by a metal detector is frequently a combination of both effects.

The measure of detectability is not a constant for a given material. It will vary depending upon the frequency of the current applied to the centre coil of the three-coil assembly. Normal metal detectors operate within the range 10–1000 kHz. Figure 9.6 shows the relationship, in principle, between frequency and signal strength for the effects of permeability (*P*) and eddy current (*E*) loss for magnetic and non-magnetic materials. (P and E are sometimes referred to as *X* and *R* or resistive and reactive signals.)

Figure 9.6 shows how the two effects, i.e. *P* and *E*, apply to the two types of metals and that while there is a preferable frequency for one material this may have an opposite effect for the other. The selection of frequency, therefore, is a compromise in most cases.

The differences can be exploited in the selection of the frequency and setting of a metal detector for a specific application. Where the product is a dry, electrically non-conductive material, the highest possible frequency is selected to optimize detection. Where the product is wet, then the frequency is often reduced to optimize sen-

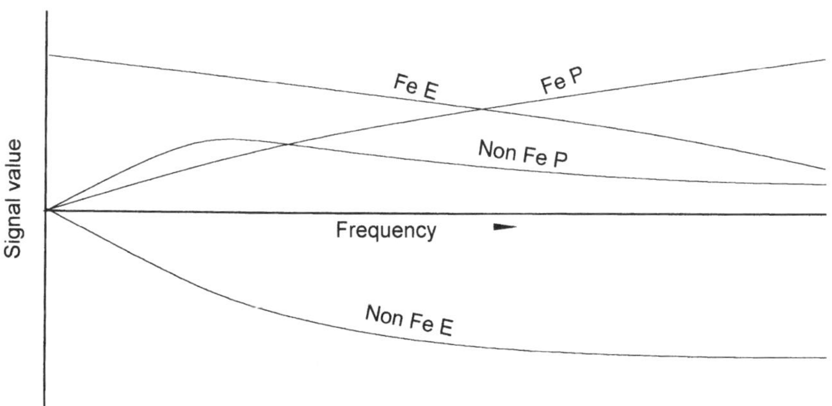

Figure 9.6 Effect of frequency on field strength.

sitivity which limits the extent by which sensitivity can be maximized by the operating frequency.

(d) The size of the product

The size of the metal detector aperture will be proportional to the size of the largest product which has to pass through it. Therefore, the larger the product, the larger the aperture. As previously stated, the least sensitive point in a metal detector aperture lies at the geometric centre; therefore, as the aperture increases in size, the further this centre point is from the coils and the lower the sensitivity becomes. This change is on a logarithmic scale and there is a noticeable increase in sensitivity when approaching a side of the aperture

In selecting the aperture size for the metal detector allowance must be made for the product in its 'worst' condition to pass without causing an obstruction, e.g. if the product lid can be open, this has to be allowed for, as failure to do so cannot only cause false rejects through mechanical interference but cause blockages on the line. In all cases there must be an air gap between the product and the aperture liner. When dealing with conductive products or packs wrapped in metallized film it is preferable to allow a minimum of approximately 25 mm clearance between the product and any side of the aperture.

There is a secondary effect sometimes referred to as bulk effect. This is a monopolar signal which can only be prevented from causing false reject signals by reducing the sensitivity. The cause of this monopolar signal is unclear, although it appears mainly with larger, denser products. Digital technology (discussed in section 9.6.2) is able to minimize this effect.

(e) The type of product: product effect or the electrical properties of products

Some products, particularly wet products, are electrically conductive. This includes obvious examples such as raw meat or bacon, but other products such as bread, jam and cheese are also electrically conductive. The electrical properties of the product interfere with the operation of the metal detector. The measured electrical property in unit terms of the product may be lower than that of metal. The product size will normally be very large in comparison to a potential contaminant. This results in a comparatively large signal being generated by the product. The process used to eliminate the product signal reduces the sensitivity of the system to detect metal. The reduction will depend on the application.

Temperature has a significant effect on the electrical properties of food products, e.g. hot bread has a far greater product effect than cold bread. On the contrary, when a product is completely frozen it will generally be found electrically non-conductive and to have a much lesser effect than in the raw state. It should be noted that where a frozen product has a wet surface resulting from very slight thawing, then the benefit of the frozen state may be lost because of the electrical conductivity of the surface.

In order to be able to use a metal detector on wet (conductive) products, compensation must be made for the product effect. There are several ways to achieve this which may be used in isolation but are generally used in combination:

- *Reduce the sensitivity.* A metal detector which triggers when a product passes through it can be made to ignore the product simply by reducing the sensitivity to a point where no detection signal occurs. In practice this will result in such a drastic reduction in sensitivity. When used in isolation it is not a practical method on its own.
- *Reduce the frequency.* As shown in Figure 9.6, the *E* signal from non-ferrous metal can be reduced by reducing the frequency. Similarly the frequency can be reduced to minimize the product effect signal. This is normal practice and it will be found that detectors used on wet products will often operate at lower frequencies than a similar unit on a dry product. The latest developments include the manufacture of metal detectors having more than one operating frequency. The preferred frequency is selected by manual or automatic switching between the available frequencies to suit the product. This technique is applied particularly to applications where product is wrapped in metallized films. Some non-ferrous and stainless steel sensitivity will be lost by selecting a reduced frequency.
- *Adjust the phase (analogue systems).* This is a term applied to the adjustments which have traditionally been made manually to tune out the product signal. Referring to Figure 9.7(a), it can be seen that for a specific frequency the *P* and *E* components of the signal have values on both axis of the graph. These are shown on Figure 9.7(a) as the non-Fe, ferrous, stainless steel and product vectors. Reflecting the real life situation it will be noted that the vectors for product and non-magnetic stainless steel have similar, but not exactly the same, angular displacement, which are quite distinct from the angular displacement of the ferrous and non-ferrous metal vectors. It is this angular difference which is exploited to prevent the signal from the product completely masking the other signals. How this is achieved can be imagined as rotating the vectors around the axis until the product signal is coincident with the *P* axis.

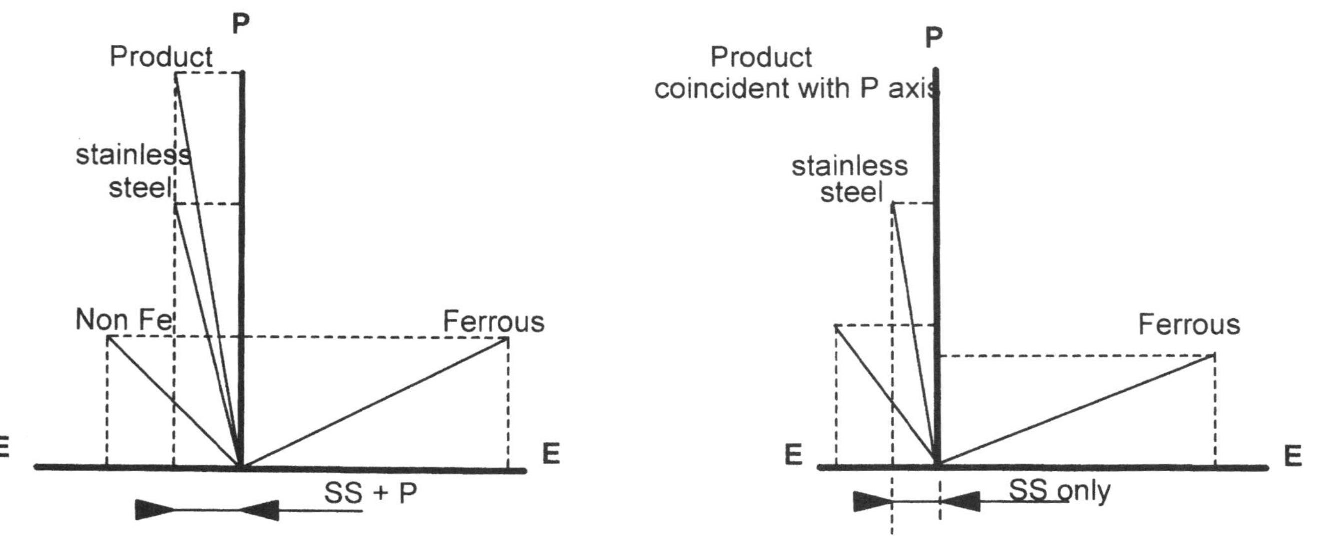

Figure 9.7 Phase adjustment.

Revolving the vectors until the product signal is aligned along the *P* axis effectively gives it zero value on the *E* axis, while leaving a reduced value for the stainless steel, non-ferrous metal and ferrous metal on the *E* axis. This value on the *E* axis represents the electrical signal available after the 'phasing' operation to register detection of a metal contaminant. It can be seen from this simplified explanation why the detection of non-magnetic stainless steel and non-ferrous metals is complicated when the product has a product effect. In practice this phase adjustment is achieved manually by turning a control. Increasingly, modern detectors achieve the same result using digital techniques (section 9.6).

(f) Metallized film

Metallized plastic film can be inspected by using specially built metal detectors using the balanced coil system. This is the type of film used extensively for packaging snack foods and has the appearance of being a shiny metal foil, which it is not. The reason being that the amount of metal deposited on the film is so small. Its thickness is measured in Angstroms and it exists as a pattern of dots rather than as a continuous film. Its effect can be phased out using conventional balanced coil metal detector technology. A simple test to decide if the film is a metallized film or a laminated foil is to measure its electrical resistance (Ω) – if the film is a conductor it will probably be a laminated foil which can only be tested in a ferrous-in-foil metal detector. An alternative is to carefully burn a small sample under safe conditions. If the ashes contain a visible aluminium film it is the type for a ferrous-in-foil unit.

The main difference between the detectors used for metallized film and normal applications is in the frequency used, which is much lower than normal. For a typical aperture of 350 mm × 125 mm, a normal frequency is in the order of 300 kHz. For metallized film the frequency used is in the order of 30–50 kHz. The result is that some non-ferrous sensitivity is lost and the stainless steel sensitivity is lower still. The difference may be as great as shown in Table 9.1.

It is quite common for metal detectors designed for use on metallized film to be constructed so that they can be switched from the conductive mode setting required to phase out the product effect of the foil to the normal non-conductive mode for normal products to obtain better sensitivity.

The same technology can be used for the inspection of some products packed in microwaveable containers, i.e. those with containers with a metallized area to increase the effects of the microwave radiation in the cooking or reheating process.

Table 9.1 Comparison of sensitivity of standard to metallized film detectors

Material	50 Khz	300 Khz
Ferrous (mm)	1.5	1.0
Non-ferrous (mm)	2.5	1.0
Stainless steel (mm)	4.0	1.6

(g) Contaminant size and shape

Industry uses the diameter of a sphere, of specified metals, as the standard to define the sensitivity of a metal detector. A sphere being round will always have the same effect on the metal detector as it passes through the aperture. On the other hand, wires and other irregular shaped objects, which are more usually the shape of real life contaminants, have a different effect on the metal detector depending on their orientation as they pass through the aperture of the metal detector.

A result of this 'orientation' effect is that a small change in rated spherical sensitivity will have a significant effect on wire detectability. For example, a particular metal detector having a maximum sensitivity of 0.7 mm ferrous sphere and able to detect 0.5 mm diameter stainless steel wires of 20 mm length under the worst conditions, but a similar detector rated at a maximum sensitivity of 1.0 mm ferrous sphere will not be able to detect lengths of the 0.5 mm diameter stainless steel wire at all in the worst conditions and nothing less than 30 mm long in the best conditions.

There are four rules for the detection of wire (Figures 9.8 and 9.9):

- Ferrous metal wires are easiest to detect when they pass through the detector with their axis at 90° to the axis of the coil windings
- Non-ferrous metals are easiest to detect when their axis as they pass through the aperture is parallel to the axis of the coil windings
- The rate of change in detectability between best and worst orientation increases at a faster rate, the closer it gets to the best orientation
- In the worst direction, the detectability of wire reaches a threshold beyond which it hardly changes, meaning that under the worst conditions a piece of wire longer than the product may pass undetected

Up until the advent of the modern fully automatic compensation circuit designs, when metal detectors sensitivity settings were frequently reduced to minimize the occurrence of false reject signals generated by electrical and mechanical drift and vibration, it was quite common to use two detectors set at an angle of 45° to each other to maximize wire detection capability. The principle being that

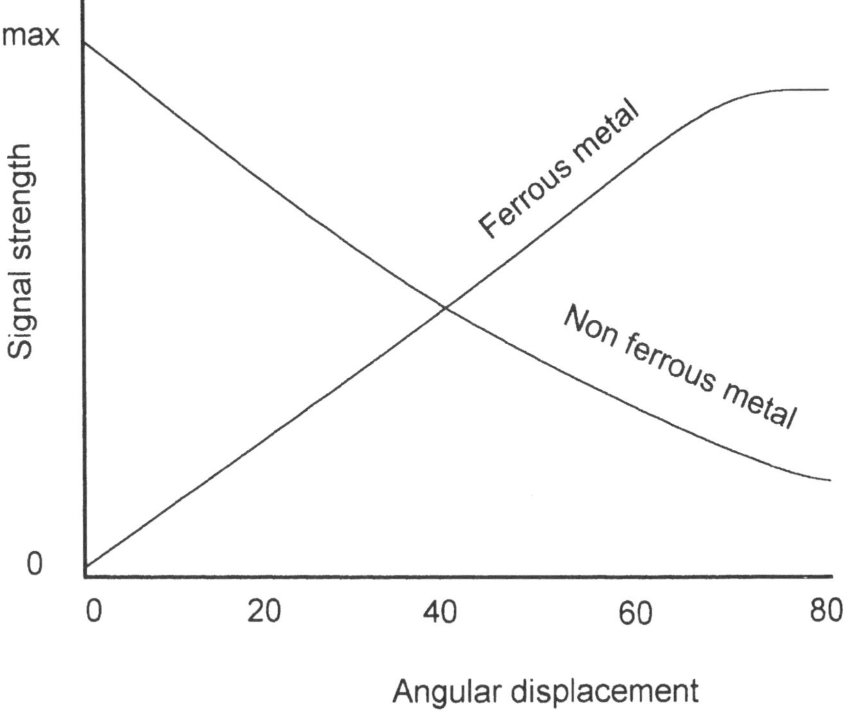

Figure 9.8 Comparative signal strength to orientation.

whatever the orientation of the contaminant, one of the two would be more likely to provide the optimum sensitivity. Improvements in technology mean this is no longer as advantageous. To locate a detector at 45° across the belt requires a significantly larger search head. In the case of a 300 mm wide belt the aperture required is not 350 mm wide but about 500 mm wide (depending on the manufacturer). The gains in sensitivity resulting from the angular settings are then offset to a great extent by the lower sensitivity of the larger search head negating in many cases any benefits gained from minimizing the effects of orientation.

(h) The environment

Manufacturers have developed closed coil metal detectors to the point where environmental factors have been either excluded completely from interfering with performance or minimized to the point where they no longer have a significant effect on performance. The electronic design almost completely eliminates mains-borne interfer-

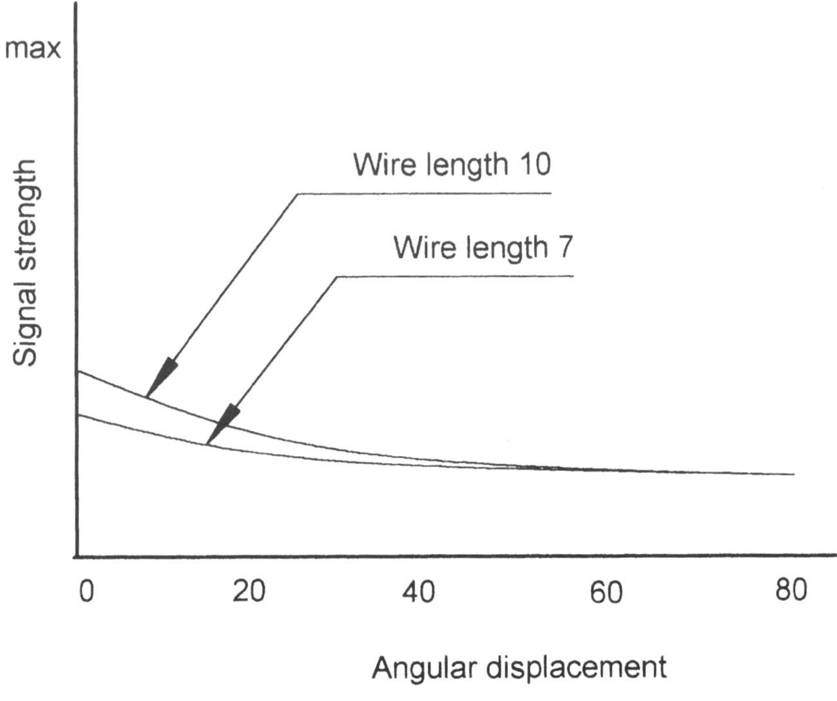

Figure 9.9 Relative signal strength in comparison to length.

ence, and external airborne interference has been minimized by improvements in mechanical design and in the development of compensating circuitry. Advances in the construction of the search heads and in the construction of control units has resulted in metal detectors being available to withstand the harshest environmental conditions and cleaning regimes. There are some environmental factors to consider when installing a metal detector, which if ignored could result in an inefficient installation.

- *Metal-free area.* The field generated in a metal detector is not restricted to the aperture or passage through the search head. The field surrounds the search head and is, therefore, susceptible to interference from the environment. The self-compensating designs of modern metal detectors makes them very tolerant of fixed and moving metal outside the aperture; however, there is a limit to the proximity that can be tolerated, generally about twice the aperture height (individual manufacturers will supply a specification for their equipment) as shown in Figure 9.10. One of the most troublesome effects is that of intermittent interference. This will often originate from the conveyor the metal detector is mounted upon, or it may be generated by another machine in close proximity. When it occurs there is no quick way to find the cause, it has to be a process of careful elimination of potential causes. The extent of the field is shown in Figure 9.10, including the area where metal detectors may interfere with each other. Manufacturers are able to minimize the difficulties presented by interference in the metal-free area to suit the some specific applications. Various means are used, e.g. detectors are now available where the metal-free area requirement has been significantly reduced by fitting a metal chute in front of the aperture to permit the installation of search heads in very restricted space.

- *Product speed*. The closed coil metal detector systems are very tolerant to product speed. It is unlikely that the normal production line speeds will affect performance of the metal detectors and it is only when speeds drop to less than 2 m/minute or exceed 300 m/minute that any problem will occur. Providing the manufacturer is aware of the details of the application, speeds as low as 0.5 m/minute and as high as 50 m/second can be accommodated.
- *Frequency offset*. Where it is necessary to mount detectors close together, then the radiated fields can cause interference with each other. This problem can be overcome by offsetting the frequency of the detectors. This is an operation for the manufacturer and normally needs to be specified when the units are ordered.

9.3.3 *Metal detector features*

Manufacturers have developed a range of techniques to remove or minimize the limitations discussed. The features available with 'analogue' designs are discussed here; other features which rely on digital electronics are discussed in section 9.6.

(a) Automatic balance

This is a technique where the balance condition of the search head and the electronics is continuously monitored and adjusted to optimize performance. This process is performed by the electronics of the metal detector. It is desirable for the rate of response of the system to be adjustable so that the rate of reaction to change is such that contamination will not be automatically 'balanced out' by the system.

(b) Automatic phase

This describes the ability of the electronics to monitor the product effect compensation setting and adjust this if it drifts from the required setting. This process has been developed to the point where

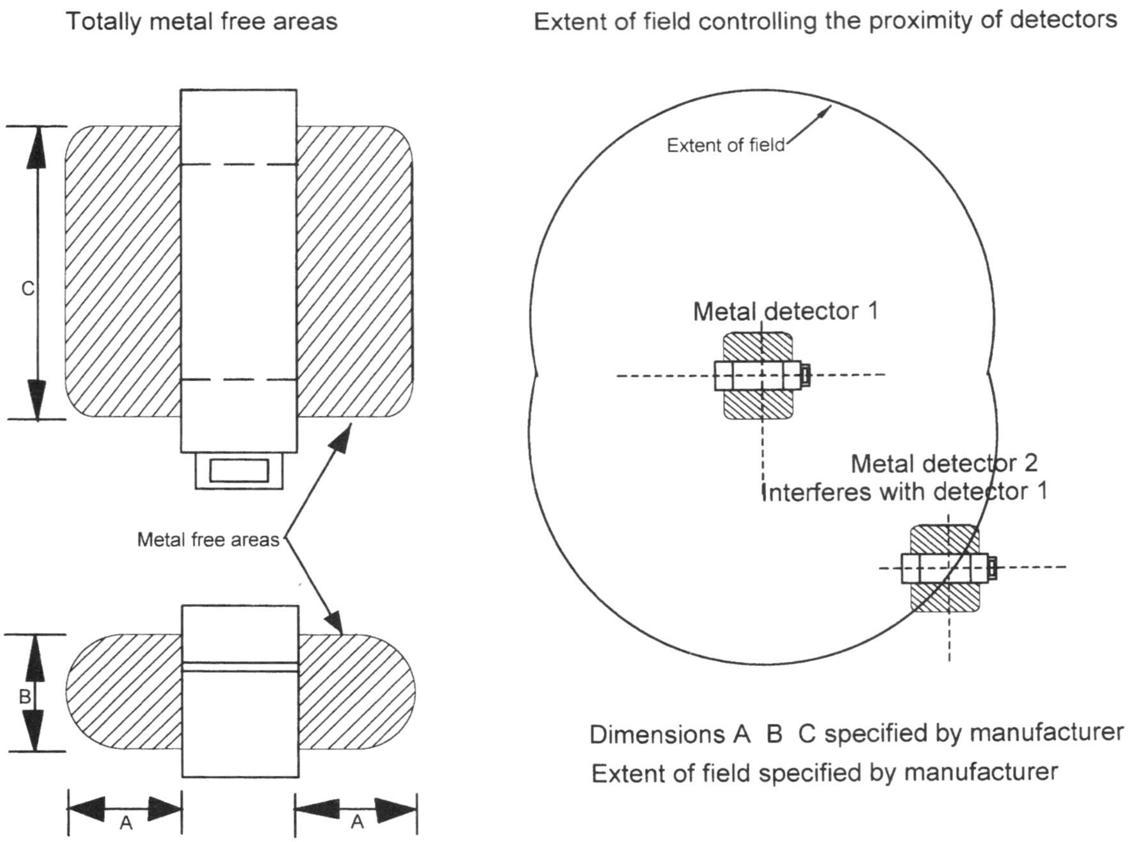

Figure 9.10 Metal-free areas.

metal detectors are able to monitor the product and automatically adjust the product setting to compensate for changes in the product consistency as well as electronic drift in the circuits.

(c) Frequency selection

This describes systems where the frequency of the metal detector can be selected to optimize performance on line. This is of particular importance on lines where metallized films are used as well as standard films.

(d) Detection mode

The original method of identifying the presence of a metal contaminant was when the signal generated by the contaminant crossed a threshold, pre-set to ignore spurious signals. The signal generated was amplified and used to operate the detection output from the metal detector. An alternative to this method was developed some time ago. This has been referred to as 'cross-over' or 'narrow zone' detection. It is important to realize that the contaminant, depending upon its size, can have an effect on the system before it enters the search head aperture. The signal generated by a contaminant as it enters the detector field has a polarity which is opposite to the polarity generated as it leaves the aperture. By using the change of polarity of a signal to instigate the detection process some false signals can be eliminated, particularly those due to vibration which generates a monopolar signal. Further, because the cross-over of polarity will always occur at a constant plane within the detector, the timing of the reject system function can be much more precisely controlled.

There are advantages and disadvantages with using the cross-over system as opposed to the amplitude system (Figure 9.11). In practice, metal contamination is normally quite unusual and may often occur as the result of equipment failure. Where a metal detector is applied to a continuous product flow which is contaminated by successive metal pieces of the same size or of increasing size, then the polarity of the signal seen at the first coil will not change. That is providing the pieces are separated by less than the width of the search head. In theory, therefore, a series of contaminants could result in only one rejection signal. Where the function is selectable on the detector, then due consideration to the potential for failure in the light of the overall quality plan should be made.

(e) Reject timing and interlocks

One of the first uses of 'digital' electronic devices was the use of shift register, counting devices, to control the timing of the reject system.

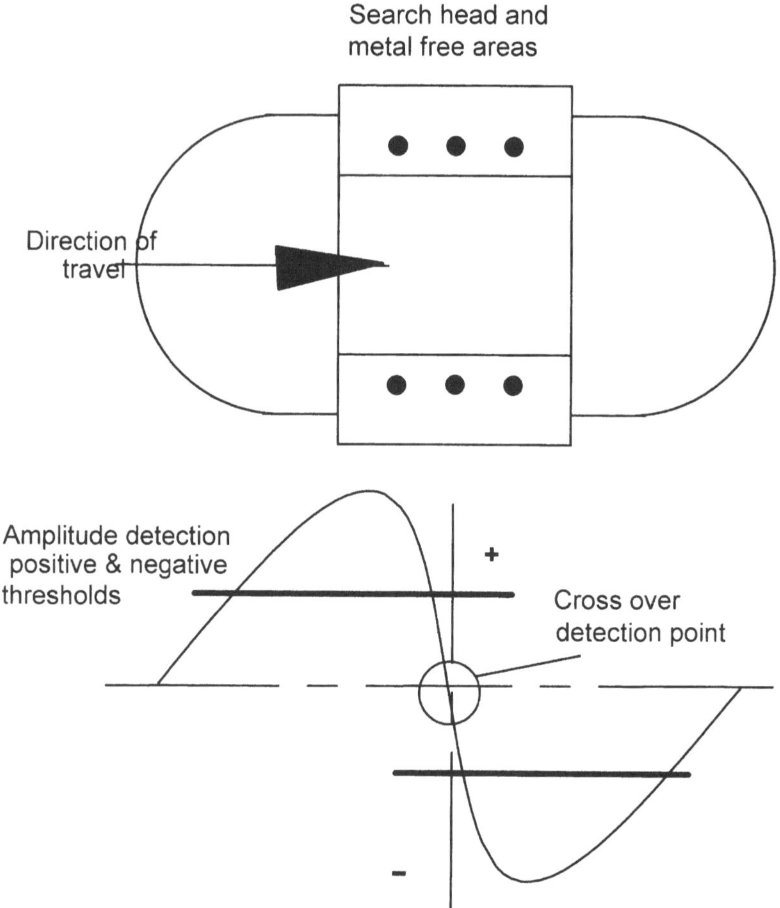

Figure 9.11 Cross-over versus amplitude detection.

This replaced analogue systems several years ago. The time controls within the detector system that govern the time delays on rejection or the time factors and constants to recognize other failures in the system are both accurate and flexible. The design of the circuits is such that the addition of external signals, from photoelectric gates or position measuring systems are easy to incorporate into the self-check and time delay systems.

Variable speed conveyor drives are fairly common as are intermittent pump operations on 'feed by demand' filling machines. A standard feature is the ability of the timing system to accept a signal from the machinery drive system in order for variable speed rates and stop/start conditions to be automatically compensated for in the reject time settings. Previously, this was accommodated by the introduction of separate variable time control devices.

(f) Overload and recovery time

The analogue circuits used in the detection process can be 'overloaded' or 'saturated' by very large signals. This has the effect of preventing them operating normally until they had recovered from the overload. Without the provision of a system to prevent this overload occurring, the recovery time could be several seconds.

(g) Self-check systems

Early self-check systems were limited in the amount of self-testing they could do. For a self-check system to be effective, it has to have the capability of testing itself in addition to the rest of the circuit for failure if absolute reliability is to be effected. As technology has progressed, more and more of the variables associated with the settings can be checked for drift outside specified levels. To meet the most rigorous quality control requirements, the systems now extend to monitoring external devices as well. This means the function and performance of the reject device (including the compressed air supply where this is a pneumatic system); the photoelectric switches used to ensure the reject bin is not overfilled (and that identified product has dropped in to it); devices used to measure conveyor movement (linked into the reject time control system); product movement or blockage sensors; to name only the most common features which can be included in a comprehensive test of the system.

When a fault is detected, ideally the system should move into a fail-to-safe mode. Where this is impractical, the system must produce an alarm for operator intervention. Whichever method is used, the metal detector test record should record the event and other records identify the repair undertaken and the decision on disposal of any product that could potentially be contaminated.

9.4 Ferrous-in-foil metal detectors

9.4.1 Applications

The ferrous-in-foil metal detectors mentioned previously operate on an entirely different principle to the balanced coil metal detector. They are used solely for the inspection of products packaged in aluminium and are only able to detect magnetic metal contaminants. They are not suitable for use with any other type of metal container.

Aluminium foil packaging is used in a semi-rigid form for 'dishes' or 'trays' for prepared dishes and similar applications. It is also used as a foil often laminated with a plastic material. Examples of the latter forms are:

- Pure foil wrappers on chocolate bars
- Pure foil lids on pots of dairy products (laminate)
- Dehydrated soup sachets made from a 'sandwich' of plastic and aluminium foil

In applications where the impossibility of using a conventional balanced coil system is not always obvious, the type of laminate can be defined in several ways:

- By passing the pack through a balanced coil metal detector where the 'product' signal will be seen to be very large and impossible to remove by adjusting the phase.
- By measuring the resistance of the material using a meter, ensuring the probes make contact with the foil.
- By carefully removing a small sample and burning it under safe and controlled conditions. This will burn away the plastic leaving the aluminium foil which is normally easy to see.

The use of ferrous-in-foil detectors has to considered against their limitation of detecting magnetic materials only. The choice between a magnet on the line before packing and the use of a ferrous-in-foil metal detector after packing need to be carefully evaluated. A magnet is unlikely to be an effective method of removing metal contamination from a solid product, e.g. a pasta recipe, but it is likely to be effective when used in a pipeline delivering the sauce (section 8.5.3).

In all cases where the final product is packaged in pure aluminium materials, the application of other equipment earlier in the process to obviate contamination is essential.

9.4.2 Construction

Ferrous-in-foil metal detectors consist of a tunnel containing a magnetic field generated by permanent magnets placed above and below it (Figure 9.12). The use of electromagnets has been superseded by the ceramic magnets.

The top and bottom walls of the tunnel of the detector are made from a steel plate behind which the magnets are mounted. This is similar to the construction of a plate magnet. The field generated by the multiplicity of magnets becomes a single magnetic face generating the field in the tunnel. The side walls are of steel construction to

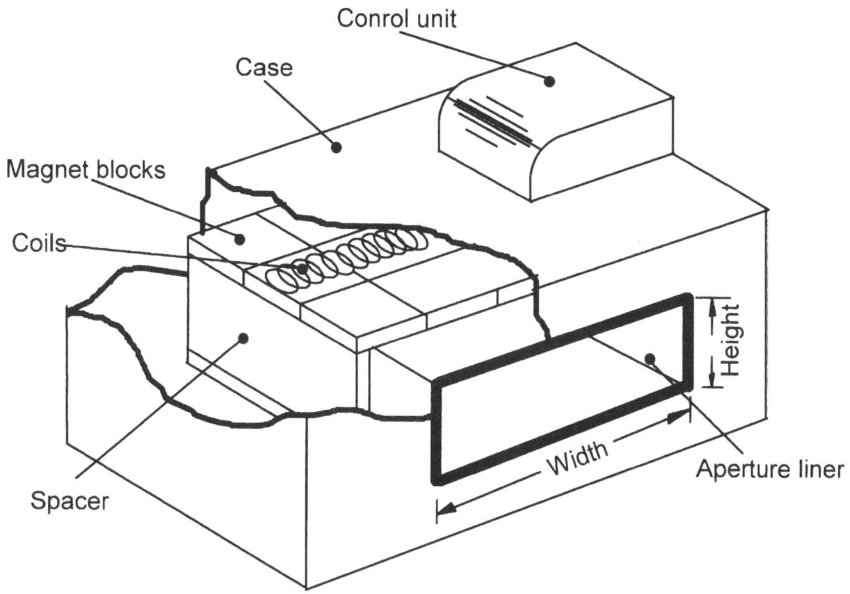

Figure 9.12 Ferrous-in-foil metal detector construction.

provide the mechanical strength needed to support the weight of the components and the magnetic forces. (Complete ferrous-in-foil metal detectors weigh considerably more than the equivalent balanced coil system.) The finished unit normally has a plastic liner fitted for appearance and hygiene. Placed along the centre line of the tunnel, as shown in Figure 9.12, are the coils which are the sensors detecting the desired signal. The complete assembly is housed in a steel box to contain the magnetic field and to prevent interference from external influences. The case is normally made from steel – aluminium is not an effective screening material for this application. Stainless steel is also used where hygiene requirements demand it. The electronic control unit is normally integral with the construction.

The magnets used are the ceramic type. These are produced in a standard block size. This is the reason there is a limited flexibility in the aperture sizes available. Magnetic forces weaken rapidly away from the surface of the magnet, limiting the maximum practical aperture height. The magnetic strength of the ceramic magnets is such that the greatest practical aperture height for ferrous-in-foil metal detectors is commonly approximately 125–150 mm.

Cost and availability have so far prevented rare earth magnets being used for this application.

9.4.3 *Principles of operation*

When a piece of metal, of a type that can be magnetized, enters a magnetic field it is magnetized and becomes a magnet, albeit a weak one. If a magnetic particle is moved over the surface of a coil then a voltage will be generated in the coil. This is the principle used for ferrous-in-foil detection.

Two things happen when a product carried in an aluminium container, enclosing a ferrous metal particle (contaminant), enters the strong magnetic field in the tunnel of the ferrous-in-foil metal detector. Electrical charges occur in the aluminium foil and the contaminant picks up a magnetic charge.

As the product proceeds through the tunnel the magnetic charge in the contaminant generates a voltage as it passes the coils.

The voltage generated in the coils is amplified to produce the detect signal.

9.4.4 *Search head dimensions*

In the same way as for balanced coil detectors, the dimensions of the frame of the detector are designed to maximize the efficiency of the assembly. The width of the system is calculated in the same way except that the tunnel width will only be available in sizes that can be made from standard block ceramic magnets used by the manufacturer. The height of the tunnel will be selected to suit the product in steps of 20–25 mm up to the limit already mentioned, although there are occasions when 200 mm high apertures may be available. The depth of the detector will depend on the manufacturer's design specifications, which will normally be related to the product length.

9.4.5 *Controls and limiting factors*

Ferrous-in-foil metal detectors do not need balancing or phasing – the only control of performance that can be adjusted is sensitivity. Sensitivity may need to be adjusted to allow for the interference effects of the packaging. The latest designs include circuits which will make this compensation automatically. The application of the units to the line will include similar timing controls for the reject system as with conventional balanced coil units. Ferrous-in-foil metal detectors are now available with some of the features of digital balanced coil metal detectors (section 9.6), including self-check systems, memorizing product settings, internal performance memory and facilities to be connected to a central data logging system.

The electrical charges in the aluminium can interfere with the effect generated by the contaminant. These changes reflect changes in the size and shape of the packages, differences in sealing, and changes in the thickness of the aluminium material. The effect may reduce sensitivity in some cases.

9.4.6 *Sensitivity*

As previously stated, the units are only able to detect magnetic materials, in the main steel particles. Some stainless steel items can be detected, although this will be found to be mainly fasteners (nuts and bolts) and detectability can only be established by test. Ambient temperature is unlikely to effect performance providing it is in the range –5 to 40°C. Although in some circumstances higher sensitivities can be achieved, 1 mm Fe or greater is generally the norm for sensitivity.

9.5 Eddy current loss detectors

9.5.1 *Applications*

There is a range of metal detectors available which work on a different principle designed specifically for the plastics industry. These are generally manufactured by companies specializing in this area or the manufacture of metal detectors for non-food applications. These are referred to as eddy current loss detectors. They are included in this chapter because plastic packaging is used in various forms by the food industry and thus it is equally important that the same precautions for freedom from contamination are applied by the plastic industry.

There are three basic applications:

- The inspection of material in drop-through mode
- The inspection of material being transferred under vacuum or pressure in pipes
- Conveyor belt applications

Many of the applications are for machinery protection.

9.5.2 *Principles of operation*

The principle of operation is that a coil is wound round a tube or chute, surrounding the passage the material flows through. The coil is connected to an oscillator which supplies an oscillating current, in the range 200–400 kHz. This generates an electrical field within the coil (and the chute). See Figure 9.13.

A metallic object lying within an oscillating electrical field will draw energy from the field, generating eddy currents on the surface of the metal particle. This has the effect of reducing the frequency, which the electronics of the system is able to sense to generate a detection signal.

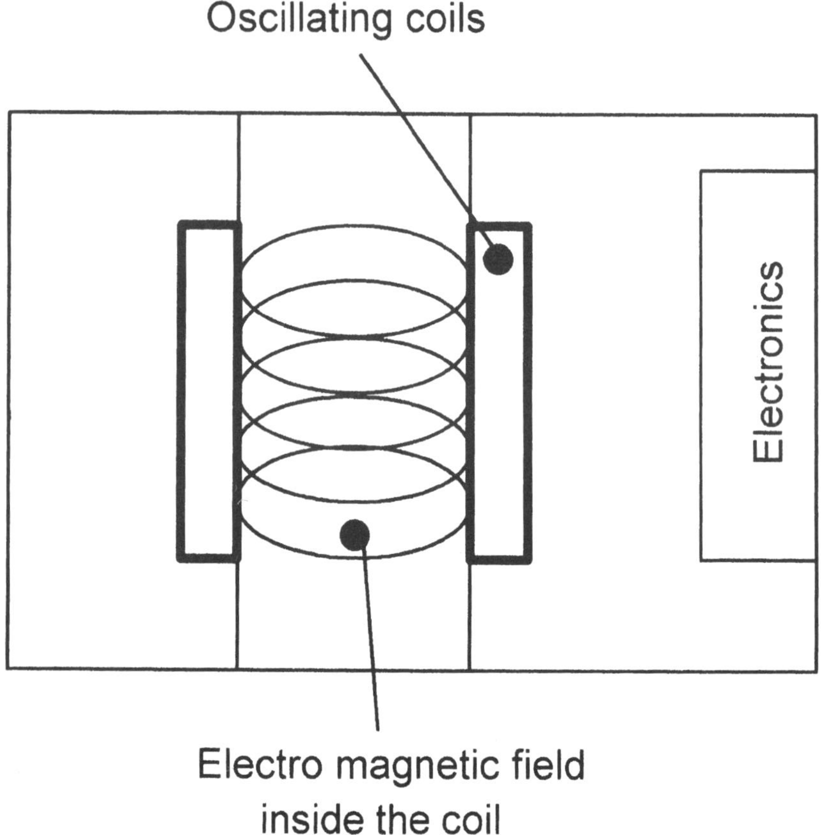

Figure 9.13 Eddy current loss metal detector.

The loss of energy is proportional to the surface area of the particle – a flat, thin particle will have the greatest surface area in proportion to weight of material and is the easiest shape to detect. Ferrous metals have higher eddy current losses than non-ferrous materials such as copper and aluminium. This means these systems are better at detecting steels.

9.5.3 Controls and limitations

The complete system is a single unit housing the control electronics, the reject system and chute. Some of the systems separate the search coils from the control electronics and the reject mechanism, and there are versions available designed for use on conveyor belts.

The units are equipped with a single control to regulate sensitivity. The units are available with self-check systems able to monitor electrical/electronic faults, mechanical failure of the reject system, loss of air pressure and power failures via a relay contact which can be used to instigate an alarm.

9.5.4 *Limitations and sensitivity*

Maximum sensitivities and capacity of the drop-through systems illustrated in Figure 10.15 are given in Table 9.2.

Because of their method of operation they are unsuitable for use on any 'wet' products.

Table 9.2 Capacity and sensitivity of eddy current loss detectors

Nominal pipe diameter (mm)	Maximum capacity (kg/hour)	Maximum sensitivity (Fe)
25	350	0.3
50	1900	0.5
70	5000	0.7
100	8000	1.0
200	23000	2.0

9.6 Digital metal detection technology

9.6.1 *Introduction*

The basic principles of operation of balanced coil metal detectors apply to the latest digital detectors, although some of the limitations have been reduced or overcome by the use of digital electronic techniques. Digital technology has also enhanced the capabilities of metal detectors to monitor their performance, including that of reject systems attached to them. The introduction of digital electronics has also made it possible for metal detectors to store product settings in memory for instant recall, to provide printed reports on performance and to talk to central computers. These additional features and the application of digital technology to reporting systems are discussed separately.

The additional features now built into the latest metal detectors fall into two distinct types:

- Those associated with improvements in sensitivity
- Those affecting the reliability and performance of the system

9.6.2 *Improvements in reliability by digital technology*

(a) Metal detector set-up

The setting up of metal detectors could be difficult, requiring time and experience to achieve the optimum settings. The great advantage of digital systems is not only that they are able to carry out the setting up adjustments themselves, but that once settings are established they can be stored in memory. The changeover requirements are, therefore, much easier, requiring in the main no more than calling up the particular product. Coupled with automatic testing, the operation and supervision of metal detectors becomes much easier.

(b) Signal discrimination

Technology has been developed that allows the metal detectors to recognize some signals and to ignore them. This technology is particularly applicable when the product under test contains a component the metal detector will 'see'. An example being the chemical agent used to absorb any oxygen left in a pack after gas flushing. This material will be seen by the detector; however, using digital technology the signal can be excluded from the detection process.

(c) Self-check systems

Self-check systems can be set to monitor the frequency of detection in a period of time or as a ratio of the number of products. An alarm signal can be provided when preset levels are exceeded.

9.6.3 *Improvements in performance*

(a) Sensitivity, mode and phase setting

Digital technology has made the automatic control of phase, the selection of conductive or non-conductive mode and the setting of sensitivity practical features of normal metal detectors. It also allows these three features to be interlinked so that the metal detector is able to select and achieve optimum settings. Drift away from these settings by the electronics is monitored and compensated for automatically, as is drift in product effect during the course of a production run. This automatic setting process normally results from a specific 'teaching' process after which the data is stored in memory for instant recall. Compensation for drift is an automatic process. The result is that the detector will keep itself operating properly for extended periods minimizing the need for frequent testing and monitoring.

(b) Noise reduction

An important feature of digital systems is their ability to analyse signals and to eliminate unwanted signals. The situation is analogous to hearing: when the environment is quiet we can hear easily, when there is a lot of background 'noise', traffic or machinery, etc., it becomes difficult or impossible to hear and we miss information. A common feature of electrical and electronic circuits and systems is that they generate 'electrical noise'. They also pick up electrical noise from interference from the environment, associated machinery and the mains power supplies. Digital technology allows a significant proportion of the noise in a circuit to be eliminated, particularly that which is constantly present. Techniques also exist to eliminate signals with parameters outside prescribed limits. This provides protection from some transient problems. The overall result is that the digital metal detector can be set to run at higher levels of sensitivity without noise from the environment causing instability and false signals. This makes the metal detector far more reliable as well as more sensitive.

(c) Removal of product effect

The signal generated as a piece of metal passes through a three-coil system increases as the product approaches the first balance coil and then reduces until it passes the centre or drive coil. It then crosses the zero line, changing polarity and increasing until it reaches the second balance coil and then reducing back to zero as it moves away. Digital technology makes it possible for the metal detector to recognize when the signal is generated by a product as opposed to a metal contaminant and to eliminate this from the detection signal output processing.

(d) Removal of bulk effect

It is possible, using similar programming techniques, to eliminate a secondary effect, sometimes described as bulk effect. The cause of this effect or signal is not fully understood, but the signal is generally associated with larger and denser products. The signal generated is a monopolar signal, of greater or lesser degree depending on the product, which, unless it is removed, limits the operating sensitivity of the system.

9.6.4 *Automatic quality testing*

Traditionally metal detectors have been tested at specified time intervals by the line or quality personnel. These times have generally been set on arbitrary instructions of every 20 minutes or every hour or some other specified period, most of which has been based on the requirements of old analogue metal detectors which were very susceptible to drift and failure. Modern systems with all the automatic features now available do not need such frequent testing, although as with any quality control tool they must be tested at established intervals and the results recorded. Since the introduction of digital electronic systems it is possible for the systems to be programmed to sound a warning at predetermined intervals when a performance test is required. Failure to carry out the test within a specified time will lead to the system going into 'fail-to-safe' mode and a record being made that the test was not carried out. The facility also exists for the metal detector to recognize when the test is carried out with the correct test sample. The system can also demand sequential tests with different test samples. Utilizing the facilities of the system can include identification of the operator performing the test and recording of the results. Where the test is not carried out at all or not to the required specification, then the metal detectors can be arranged to trigger alarms or 'fail-to-safe' with the data being recorded.

9.6.5 *Data storage, display and hard copy reports*

The introduction of digital technology has allowed the operation and performance of metal detectors to be recorded automatically, and for this information to be available at the detector or at a central control point. It is also becoming possible to change product settings remotely. The major limitation with all these facilities is that they are all manufacturer restricted. As yet there is no industry standard for data interchange or data recording; therefore, it is not yet easy to have metal detectors from more than one manufacturer working within the same control system. There are specialist software houses who may be able to write programmes to link the information from more than one brand of metal detector together as well as incorporating data from other devices. The complexities of such a solution will be considerable and the installation and maintenance complex.

There are two main types of system available.

(a) Single detector data storage, display and hard copy

The operator is able to read a variety of information in the display on the control panel of the metal detector. A typical control panel for a modern digital metal detector is illustrated in Figure 9.14.

The metal detector has the facility to store product parameters for up to 20 products. This can include details of mode, phase sensitivity, reject timings, product name, etc. The details of the product test function are also stored in memory. The stored information can be viewed in the display panel on the control of the metal detector. Details of current product settings, detect signals and the quality test function may also be viewed in the control panel display. The metal detectors can operate in isolation in the same manner as the traditional analogue units.

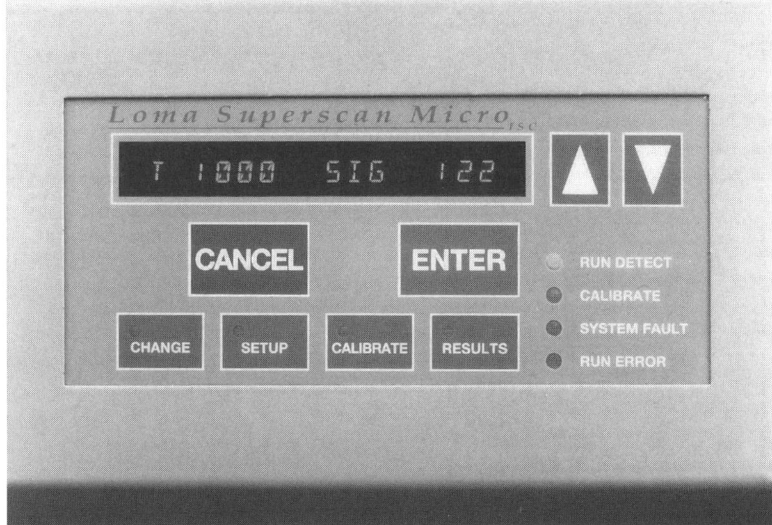

Figure 9.14 Typical digital metal detector control panel. (Courtesy Loma Engineering Ltd.)

Where there is only one metal detector in operation, for instance in a small business, the costs and complexity of a full system may be beyond the resources of the business. There is still a need for hard copy of the information to help in the record keeping requirements of quality control systems such as ISO 9000 or to meet the needs of demonstrating 'due diligence'. This can be simply achieved by linking a printer to the metal detector and recording the information available. The operator can take all information from the metal detector and produce hard copy reports on a printer linked by an RS 232, RS 432 or 20 mA current loop serial link system. This means even the smallest manufacturer can capture the performance records of his/her metal detectors in hard copy form very economically. A typical report produced from the Loma Superscan Micro$_{ISC}$ is shown in Figure 9.15.

(b) Multiple metal detector data storage and hard copy

The introduction of digital metal detectors is a comparatively recent innovation which will continue to develop. There are various levels of collecting, storing and manipulating the data available from metal detectors, and other equipment, of which two options are described in the following:

- Collecting the raw data from numerous devices and displaying it on a central computer in its original format using the metal detector manufacturer's protocol and interface. In this case the data is

LOMA SUPERSCAN MICRO METAL DETECTOR	
PV TEST REPORT	
Time 10.22.00	Date Mon 09 JUL 1995
Machine Identification	M 27599
Product Number:1	Name: Frozen Peas
Prompt: 10.15.00	On: Mon 09 JUL 1995
Operator Identification	ABC
Test sample Ferrous	5 x 1.00
Test sample Non Ferrous	5 x 1.00
Test sample Stainless St	5 x 1.00
Threshold detection: 1500	False:3000
PV Test prompt:	Off/Time or batch

PV Test successful
or
No samples
or
PV Test not actioned

Figure 9.15 Example of single detector printed record. (Courtesy Loma Engineering Ltd.)

taken from the metal detector, or detectors, and stored in the memory of the computer for recall as required. This is a single step up from the use of a printer linked to the metal detector. The information can be taken from the computer and printed out.

- Collecting the data from the same devices but manipulating it in the central computer to provide structured reports in formats to support the recording requirements of quality assurance programmes and legal requirements. In addition where the manufacturer supplies other equipment, for example checkweighers, this data can be incorporated into the system. The data is stored in the central computer system.

It is also getting easier to incorporate additional external information into the systems; however, this so far mainly applies to simple go/no-go voltage-free contacts which indicate if a machine is operating or a link is in a specific position – it does not include variable data. Adding information from other sensors provides further information and analysis of a production process.

Details of product settings, performance information, quality information, etc., can all be stored and observed from a central point. The results can be manipulated to suit the individual enterprise and tabular or graphical reports produced.

This is all automatic and continuous, and provides much more detail and information than manual systems, which helps continuous improvement programmes as well as ensuring detailed records are always available should they be required.

10

Mechanical handling and rejection systems

10.1 Introduction

None of the detector systems discussed will be effective unless it is incorporated into a mechanical handling system which has the dual purpose of delivering the product to the sensor and removing any part which the sensor identifies as 'contaminated'. These systems are often referred to as 'conveyors', a term which does not fully describe the function of the system. The mechanical handling system is required to deliver the material in a form which the sensor can accommodate, arrange the material to minimize losses in the rejection process and provide a means of diverting contaminated material from the system, all in a manner which matches the process and provides interlocks and controls to ensure fool proof operation. The greater part of the technology used for this purpose has been developed for metal detector systems and while much of this chapter refers to applications with metal detectors, the technology can be applied to other types of sensors. Vision systems which use specific patented diverter devices are dealt with in Chapter 12.

A metal detector on its own is non-functional, it requires the product under examination to move through it in order for the detection process to work and then it needs a system to remove the product from the line.

Metal detectors are available in almost any size to suit an application, which when multiplied by the variations of types and styles means almost any application can readily be fitted with a metal detector to suit. There is a similar breadth of mechanical handling systems produced, many of which are designed and built to suit a specific application, to ensure the user can obtain exactly the specification he/she needs to obtain an optimum result.

The design and construction of the mechanical handling systems is of equal importance to the sensor. Mechanical handling systems have two main components in addition to the metal sensor, the transport system and the rejection system. It should be noted that a rejection system is essential if the sensor is to provide the optimum protection.

Mechanical handling systems fall into three categories:

- Conveyor systems
- Free-fall product
- Liquids

A conveyor system will consist of a belt driven by a motor, mounted on a support which carries the metal detector (Figure 10.1). Normally there will be a rejection system and some form of container to hold rejected items. There may or may not be additional sensors, product control devices, automatic cleaning equipment and various electrical controls and interlocks. All of these items are available in various forms to suit individual applications.

10.2 Construction

All conveyor systems have to conform to the 1995 Machinery Safety Act in the UK and carry the CE mark for sale within Europe. This

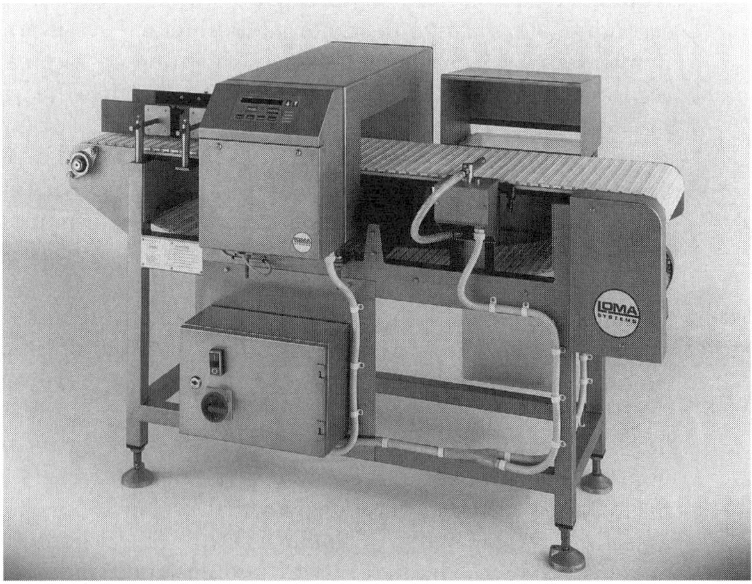

Figure 10.1 Typical metal detector and conveyor system. (Courtesy Loma Engineering Ltd.)

standard lays down minimum safety, electrical noise and hygiene requirements.

A metal detector on a conveyor system presents a potential cleaning problem. The belt passes through the detector supported on a deck which has to be clear of the inner surface of the aperture. The result is a void which is very difficult to clean. There are conveyors available which allow the best tension to be released to allow acess to this point. Cleaning this space must be considered.

A conveyor framework can be stainless steel or painted steel material depending on the demands of the application. When considering the suitability of designs care should be taken to ensure the mechanical construction minimizes dirt traps and that all hollow sections are sealed by welded caps, not push in plastic fittings. Electrical safety, which will be to the approved standard, must include the use of conduit and enclosures for connectors and sensors, etc., that do not compromise the hygienic requirements of the installation.

As previously mentioned metal detectors are susceptible to radiated electrical interference and a potential source of this is the conveyor system (Figure 10.2). These are sometimes referred to as 'earth loops'. Electric motors and switches radiate electrical signals which the metal construction of the conveyor 'picks up' just like a radio aerial. These signals do not affect the metal detector as long as the signal is constant. As soon as it changes it will momentarily affect the metal detector and cause a false signal. The main cause of this is metal components of the conveyor making intermittent electrical contact. This causes an interruption to the continuity of the field radiating around the frame. The radiated field is normally ignored by metal detector but when it becomes intermittent it can cause a false signal by the metal detector. Wherever possible all metal to metal joints on conveyors should be welded, where this cannot be then they must be positively insulated.

To minimize the effects of radiated electrical fields and metal interfering with the metal detector field, both fixed and moving must be kept a specified distance away from the metal detector. The metal detector manufacturer will provide specifications of the metal free area and mounting requirements of his/her metal detectors (section 9.3). These must be adhered to for maximum performance. This is of particular importance when fitting metal detectors to process machines.

Even with the advanced automatic control systems built into metal detectors it is important to ensure that vibration is kept to a minimum. Not only can vibration generate false signals it can also affect the construction of the metal detector, in the worst case loosening fasteners and damaging electronic components.

In selecting the size of the search head to use in a particular situation the first priority is to ensure it will accept the product. It is also

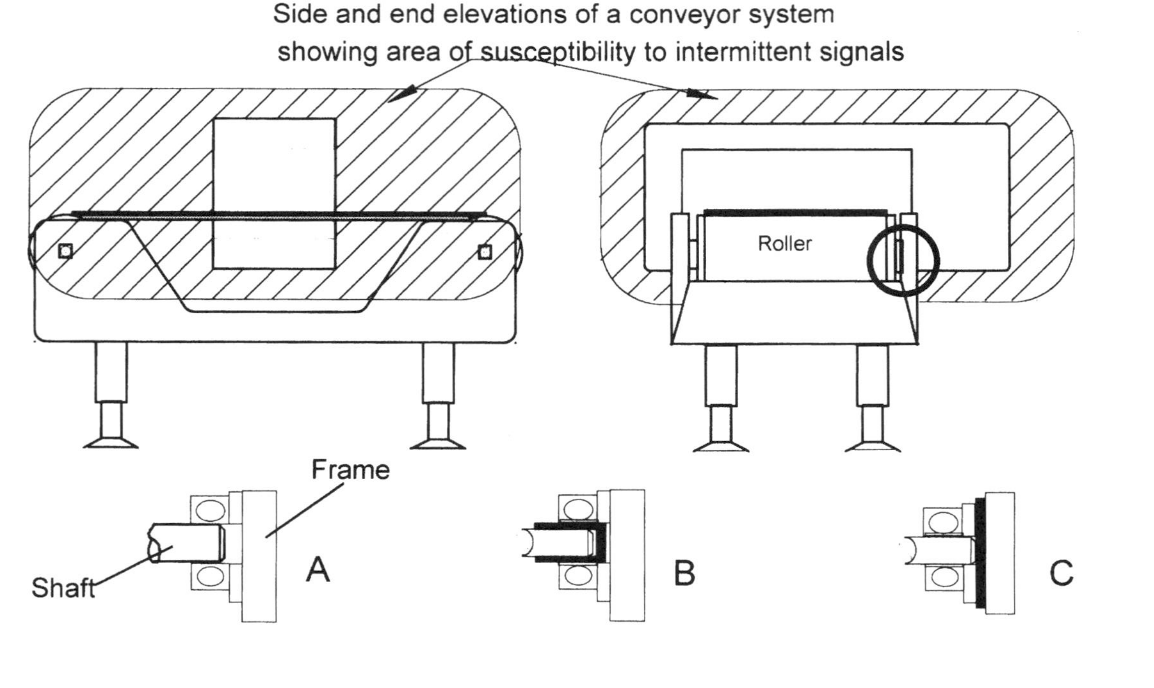

Figure 10.2 Intermittent joints.

necessary to ensure that it is wide enough to be clear of the belt passing through it, with some additional clearance. In case the belt wanders off track, about 25 mm clearance is needed on each side, as this can very quickly cause severe damage to the metal detector. Where there is any danger of products striking the search head if they are 'off centre' on the belt, strong crash barriers or diverters should be mounted in front of the metal detector for protection.

The rollers over which the belts travel ideally should be non-metallic or plastic coated to prevent metal or rust pick up on the belt which will cause false signals. Stainless steel is often a suitable substitute.

By definition the aperture and a space either side of it have to be kept free from metal. This means that the only material available to support a belt is plastic. Plastic running on plastic is a source of static electricity which cannot be prevented by using anti-static belting. A belt support material needs to be used that minimizes this effect.

Electric motors are the normal method used to drive conveyors. Drive can be provided by hydraulic motors and air motors although these will only be used in very special circumstances. To provide additional flexibility in the systems electronic variable speed drives are being used more and more. When selecting these care must be taken to ensure they do not interfere electrically with the performance of the metal detector. When selecting the type consideration should be given to the facility available to use a signal from the metal detector to select the speed setting of the variable speed controller.

10.3 Transport belts

Not all belts are suitable for use with metal detectors:

- *Belts with anti-static material* incorporated in them will normally be unsuitable as the joint will be found to cause false detection signals and variations in the consistency of the anti-static system may also interfere with detector performance.
- *Slat belts or belts made from moulded plastic* sections when they are connected by metal pins for obvious reasons. While there are many applications where moulded section belts are very useful care must be taken to ensure the material is neutral to the metal detector, some pigments will affect metal detectors, and that the plastic used in the mouldings is free from metal contamination.
- *Wire belts* are never suitable.
- *Belts joined with metal clips* are never suitable.

Metal contamination of a belt is a condition that can be extremely difficult to cure once it has occurred. Before fitting a new belt to a metal detector conveyor it should always be checked by a metal detector to ensure it is not contaminated. Manufacturers of belts should be able to supply belts for metal detectors and where these are to be stored they should be carefully packed to prevent contamination in storage. Whenever welding is carried out near a metal detector, the belt should be covered for the duration of the job then carefully cleaned before being run again.

This leaves a wide variety of belts that can be used. In addition there are options available to assist with product handling that are useful when installing metal detector systems. It is recommended that any belts purchased for metal detectors be ordered to be free from metallic contamination and suitable for the purpose. Once delivered, belts should be stored in sealed wrappers to prevent contamination. Before installing the belt it should be carefully passed through the metal detector, stretched out to its full length and lying as close to the base of the aperture as possible, to test that it is free from metal contamination

Wherever possible the belt path needs to be designed to make changing as simple as possible. Where flat belts are used it is beneficial to have these run twice through the aperture as this makes replacement easy, a pre-joined belt can be used rather than the complexities of trying to weld a belt on site in production if it forms a closed loop round the detector aperture.

Flat plastic belts are the most common type used. The type will be selected to meet the duty requirements of the application and can vary from thin single ply cloth belts to heavy duty plastic laminated three-ply materials. Colour is often a matter of personal preference and white has traditionally been the norm; however, blue belting is now available that is very suitable for loose product transfer, where, should any damage occur, the colour makes it much easier to find visually.

Modified flat plastic belts are also used in several modified forms. They may be 'trough' by causing the edges to rise as they pass over the working surface of the conveyor to provide a guide and prevent spillage of loose products. They may have 'flights' welded to them to provide a positive lift to product where the belt is elevated, an essential feature to control time for rejection. They may have sides welded to them – either convoluted or overlapping sections to prevent spillage on loose products:

Flat plastic belt joins are important to the performance of the metal detector. The join must be made under clean conditions – there is nothing worse than finding a sliver of metal has been welded into a join. The join must be made by welding or adhesive not by metal clips or stitching. Where adhesives are used, they must be of a type which does not interfere with the metal detector. The best joint form is a finger joint where this can be achieved, but otherwise it is advisable to make the join at an angle across the belt rather than at 90° as this can sometimes generate a false signal, particularly with thicker belts.

The drive to flat plastic belts depends on the amount of radial contact between the belt and the drive roller, rather than simply tension to the belt. To prevent metal contamination from the rollers affecting the belt they are normally covered in plastic. To achieve correct tracking one or more of the rollers will be crowned, i.e. its outer surface will be barrel shaped rather than cylindrical, the amount of crowning being about 3°. Provision will be made in the construction to adjust the roller axis in relation to the centre line of the conveyor to ensure the belt runs on track.

Intralox belting is a relatively new system to be adopted by the metal detector industry. The material is made up of injection moulded plastic sections, linked together with plastic pins. Drive is provided by a sprocket system giving positive drive and preventing side slip or 'off track' problems. Intralox belting is extremely durable, positive in its drive action, less prone to moving off track and because of its modular construction easy to repair on the machine. It is also available in a variety of colours. There are various styles of moulding designed for various applications to make transfer positive and/or to maximize hygiene, as such it is ideal for use on raw meat in particular. All the additional features such as side walls and flights are available with the system.

Slat band belting is the type which has been traditionally used in the handling of metal cans and glass jars. The all metal type is totally unsuitable but it is possible to obtain the belting in plastic with plastic connector pins. It comes in a restricted range of widths, basically designed for the can and glass industries, and providing care is taken in its selection, it is useful on bottle and jar applications. Drive is similar to the Intralox system.

Rope belting, usually made from a polyurethane material, has applications on some products. It consists of a round plastic rope that is wrapped around a grooved drive and return roller, with support as required, which is welded in situ. The ropes are spaced at intervals across the width of the conveyor.

Belt support is important as it must not be allowed to rub on the aperture liner. While modern detectors will probably tolerate this without generating false detection signals, the wear will damage the detector. Therefore, the belt needs to be supported while it passes through the metal detector, for the specified metal free area. This is usually achieved by using a length of non-metallic material supported on plastic legs if required. Care needs to be taken in the selection of the plastic material as the plastic belt rubbing on it will generate static electricity. Wood is an ideal material, but is not recommended for food applications; an alternative is the brown cloth resin laminate commonly used as an electrical insulator which is available in sheet form. There are situations where even this will leave some static electricity which can usually be discharged by fitting stainless steel strips on the surface connected to earth to conduct the charge away from the belt.

10.4 Roller conveyors

These are sometimes used for handling large or heavy packs. These will have the section passing through the search head and metal-free area constructed from plastic roller section. This section is normally for idler rollers only so that reject timing relies upon gravity or pushing from following items. To establish positive timing, a system of sensors is required to follow the product from the metal detector to the reject point to ensure rejection is synchronized to movement. It should be noted that this method is often used for manual feed, using a simple alarm system to identify metal contamination for subsequent manual removal.

Roller conveyors are also used for human and vision system inspection processes. In these applications the rollers are driven and spaced apart, causing the rotation of the rollers to impart a rotary motion to the product under inspection. This ensures that all the surfaces of the product are exposed to the line of vision. Travel along the length of the conveyor is achieved by moving the rollers along a horizontal path as they rotate.

10.5 Vibratory conveyors

These are unsuitable for use with metal detectors, partly because they normally need to be made from metal in order to achieve the mechanical properties to make the product flow and partly because the effects of the vibration transmitted to the metal detector will tend to cause damage.

10.6 Product transfer

Having decided on the type of belt to be used the question of transfer from the existing system to the metal detector conveyor and off again has to be considered. How this is to be achieved will depend upon the construction of the feed system and the metal detector conveyor and the type of product.

Figure 10.3 illustrates the gap that exists when end rollers of different sizes are brought together. They cannot touch, as this will cause damage. The gap D in the drawing represents the unsupported distance separating the working surfaces of the conveyors. This dimension needs to be less than one-third (30%) of the product length if smooth transfer is to occur. Figure 10.3 shows how this can be achieved by the introduction of extra rollers or the use of a 'knife edge' which can be made down to 10 mm if necessary. Where the gap is long then a series of rollers can be used which only need to be powered when separation of product is necessary and the gap top to be bridged is greater than the product length.

For certain applications it is necessary to stand the metal detector conveyor at the side of the existing conveyor, for example on glass jar lines. The method of transfer is illustrated in Figure 10.4.

Finally, a dead plate can be used to bridge the gap between conveyors instead of a roller section (Figure 10.5).

Both a dead plate and a roller section can be used to accommodate changes in conveyor heights providing the transfer will work under gravity.

10.7 Product spacing

Transfer from the production conveyor onto the metal detector conveyor provides an opportunity to adjust the spacing or the depth of the product as well as providing an opportunity to align the product. This facility can be used to reduce the volume of product necessary to reject in order to achieve rejection of a contaminated item, and it can also be used to separate and align products for subsequent operations, e.g. check weighing or packing.

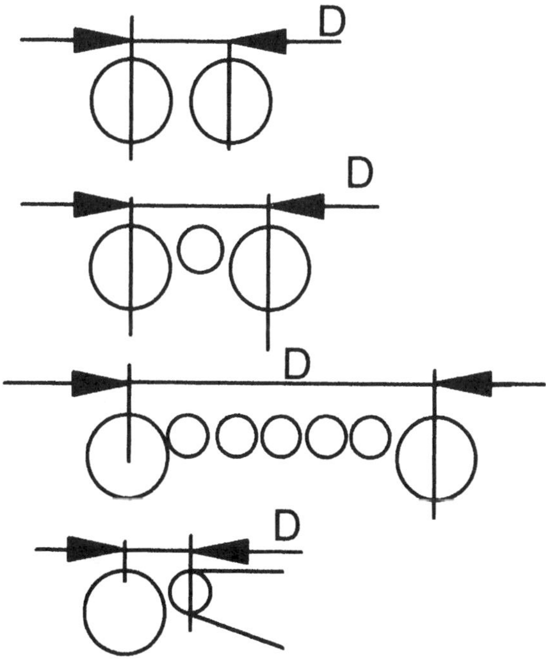

Figure 10.3 Roller transfer.

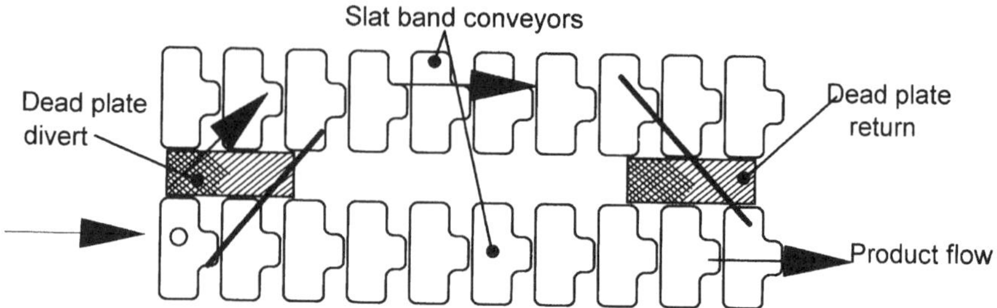

Figure 10.4 Slat band cross-transfer over a dead plate.

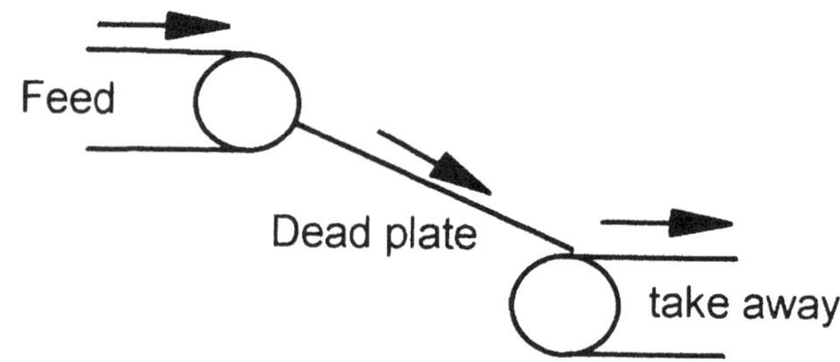

Figure 10.5 Dead plate transfer.

By adjusting the relative speeds of the conveyors, products can be 'opened up' or the burden depth be reduced, or the opposite (Figure 10.6). By the addition of guides and levelling bars the product can be made to move on the conveyor in a preferential manner.

10.8 Rejection systems

10.8.1 Introduction

This section deals exclusively with the types of rejection systems used with conveyors. While the main thrust is their application to

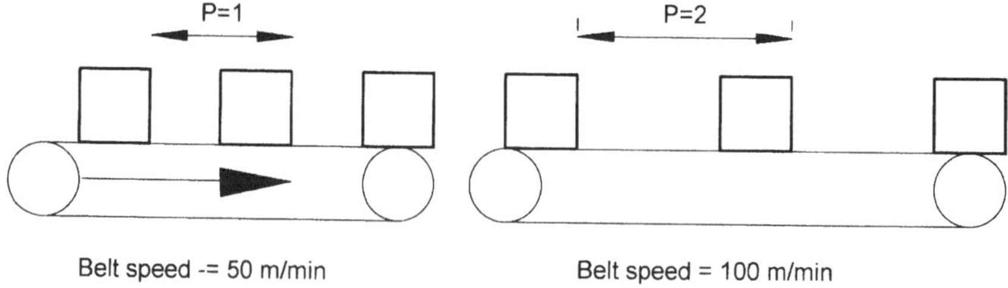

Figure 10.6 Separation by conveyor speeds.

metal detectors, the same data and information will apply regardless of the type of sensor generating the reject signal. Other systems are described in section 10.10.

10.8.2 *Manual rejection*

There are numerous automatic methods of rejection available, and the choice will depend on the product and line speed. It is recommended that an automatic positive rejection action always be used, although there are circumstances where the use of manual methods may be considered.

10.8.3 *Automatic rejection methods.*

The various methods are summarized in Table 10.1.

Reverse belt rejection is mainly used for loose dry product. There are two ways of achieving the result. One is to simply reverse the belt back through the sensor for a fixed time period, allowing the contaminated section to drop into a collection bin. The second is to take the rejected material from the conveyor and feed this onto a second smaller conveyor fitted with a similar detector, repeating the reverse rejection operation when the contamination is detected. This has the advantage of reducing the waste and isolating the contamination for identification. Provision can usually be made to return the good product to the production stream automatically.

Alarm and belt stop (Figure 10.7a). For manual rejection it is possible to use the relay output of the metal detector to trigger an audible and/or a visual alarm to warn that a contaminant has been detected by the system. This can be supported by a signal to automatically stop the belt. A reset switch is then used to stop the alarm and restart the conveyor. This type of system should only be used where production volumes are low and there is no practical alternative method economically available. Operator training and motivation are critical to the efficiency of the system.

Air blast rejection (Figure 10.7b). This is the most common type of rejection system used for small packed items and it can even be used on heavier products such as loaves of bread. Depending upon the product, registration may or may not be required.

Air collector and arm diverter systems (Figure 10.7c and d). These can be adjusted to operate gently, diverting product with a minimum of shock, making them suitable for glass bottles and jars, providing the action is to divert the container smoothly onto a storage area. Alternatively, they can be used to divert product off the conveyor into a side mounted rejection bin. They are limited in operating

Table 10.1 Summary of rejection systems and their applications

Figure	Type of system	Metal detection	X-ray systems	Glass container inspection	Suitable for	Not suitable for	Max belt width	Belt speeds	Cost
10.7(a)	alarm and belt stop	✓	✗	✗	all		any	slow	low
10.7(b)	air blast	✓	✓	✗	light packed items	loose material	350	fast	medium
10.7(c)	air collector arm	✓	✓	✗	light packed items	loose material	400	fast	medium
10.7(d)	air diverter arm	✓	✓	✓	light packed items	loose material	400	medium	medium
10.7(e)	air kicker	✓	✓	✗	light packed items	loose material	250	medium	medium
10.7(f)	belt sweep arm	✓	✓	✗	heavy packed items	loose material	500	low	high
10.8(a)	heavy duty kicker	✓	✓	✗	heavy items	loose material	500	slow	high
10.8(b)	progressive diverter	✓	✓	✓	medium size items	loose material	500	slow	high
10.8(c)	three lane diverter belt	✓	✓	✓	delicate products	loose material	250	medium	high
10.9(a)	simple flap	✓	✓	✗	all light material		1000	medium	medium
10.9(b)	diverting chute	✓	✓	✗	light dry materials	wet or sticky or heavy materials	500	medium	medium
10.9(c)	driven flap rejection system	✓	✓	✗	packed items	medium size packs	400	slow	high
10.10	drop end	✓	✓	✗	packed items loose		2000	medium	high
10.11	retract band	✓	✓	✗	all		2000	medium	high
Not shown	reverse belt	✓	✓	✗	all	any	Slow	low	

speed but because of the way they work product registration is not normally required

Air kicker systems (Figure 10.7e). These are only suitable for a limited range of applications. The effectiveness of this type of system is limited by the need for the separation between products being sufficient for the kicker plate to be able to travel out and back across the belt without fouling on products either side of the item identified for removal. Product registration is normally required.

Belt sweep systems (Figure 10.7f). These are advanced forms of kicker systems which use a rod-less cylinder mounted over the belt. The advantage of these is that the width of the system is not excessive as the cylinder travels along an internal guide within the cylinder rather than being mounted on the end of a rod. These systems can normally be set to make a single motion across the belt on rejection with the subsequent detection signal instigating a rejection stroke in the return direction. They are very useful for large products but do require product registration.

Heavy duty kicker (Figure 10.8a). Heavy products are often carried on roller conveyor systems. Plastic roller conveyors, which can be passed through a metal detector search head, are available for a limited range of product weights. Where the load capacity of the plastic roller sections is insufficient then the product has to be transported on a belt. Driving a heavy weight product off a belt will often lead to belt damage through it being forced out of line by the action of the reject device. In these cases a separate metal roller section can be installed after the detector. This provides a practical solution to the removal of heavy products without damaging the conveyor. A kicker-type reject can then be fitted, locating the pneumatics under the roller section and bringing an arm through between the rollers to drive a pusher. These systems can be used for heavy sacks of material and are equally useful for handling large boxes of products.

Delicate products require careful handling to minimize waste and in the case of glass to prevent contamination of the product. There are a range of systems suitable for these requirements of which the simplest is a belt diverter. This is simply an arm angled across the conveyor surface which diverts product onto a parallel conveyor. Similar to the system shown in Figure 10.4 for slat band conveyor systems.

Progressive diverters (Figure 10.8b) are usually pneumatically operated. They consist of a special purpose conveyors with a transport surface constructed from 'rods or bars' along which plastic diverter plates slide from side to side. The bars move along the machine while the plastic sections are pneumatically directed to a point across the width of the system designed to deliver the prod-

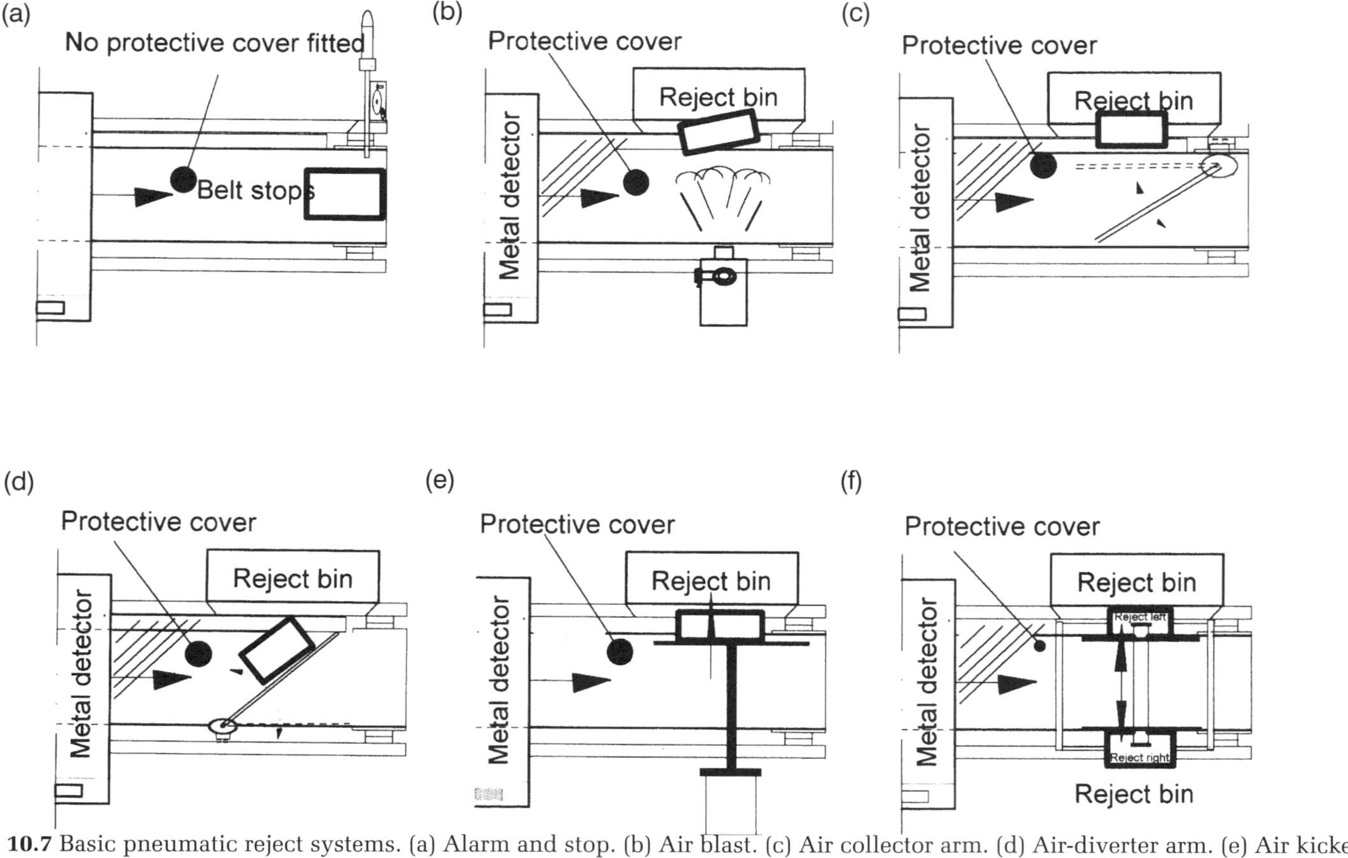

Figure 10.7 Basic pneumatic reject systems. (a) Alarm and stop. (b) Air blast. (c) Air collector arm. (d) Air-diverter arm. (e) Air kicker. (f) Pneumatic sweep arm (double action reject operation).

uct in channels for subsequent disposal. The smooth action of these systems is very useful for product that can spill if subjected to sudden movements.

Twin/triple lane diverters (Figure 10.8c) operate by using a diverter arm to deflect product onto one of two or three belts following the metal detector belt, effectively diverting the product into lanes for subsequent disposal. These systems are very useful for glass containers or product that can spill as the reject motion is smooth.

Flap rejection systems are used where the product is 'loose' or small. Examples are pharmaceutical tablets, sweets or loose vegetables such as peas. There are several ways the principle can be applied and the following are three examples.

The most simple (Figure 10.9a) is to have a two-part inclined flap mounted slightly below centre of the output roller of the conveyor. Product slides across the two flaps until rejection is required when the moveable section of the flap is raised, diverting some product out of the main stream. This is the least costly method which with the addition of side guides can be used for a variety of products.

Where the material is very 'powdery', e.g. dried diced vegetables, then an enclosed type of system is required to minimize dust. The system illustrated in Figure 10.9(b) shows how a chute can be arranged to swing to provide a smooth control of rejection while containing the product.

When the product is a packed item or a fairly large individual item which will not slide, then a driven system is used as illustrated in Figure 10.9(c). In normal flow conditions the product is transferred from the detector conveyor to the take-off conveyor by the powered intermediate conveyor section. On rejection this lifts, allowing the identified item to be dropped out of the line.

Drop-end systems (Figure 10.10) are very useful for handling loose products such as biscuits or chocolates on wide belts. They are also an alternative method for rejecting large products such as sacks. The system is arranged so that the end of the conveyor section drops through a distance up to approximately 200 mm, guiding the product to a receiving area below the normal take off conveyor. This process is carried out smoothly without damaging the product.

Retracting band rejection systems (Figure 10.11) are very positive in action. The principle is simply that when required the end roller is pulled back, opening a gap in the belt allowing an identified product to drop out of the production line after which the gap is closed. The construction of the system is quite complex and costly. For small items the technique is almost the perfect solution but for large items there is always a problem of space under the mechanism which may be insufficient to hold a reasonable number of products. They can be used on belt speeds up to 45 m/minute and made to fit on very wide

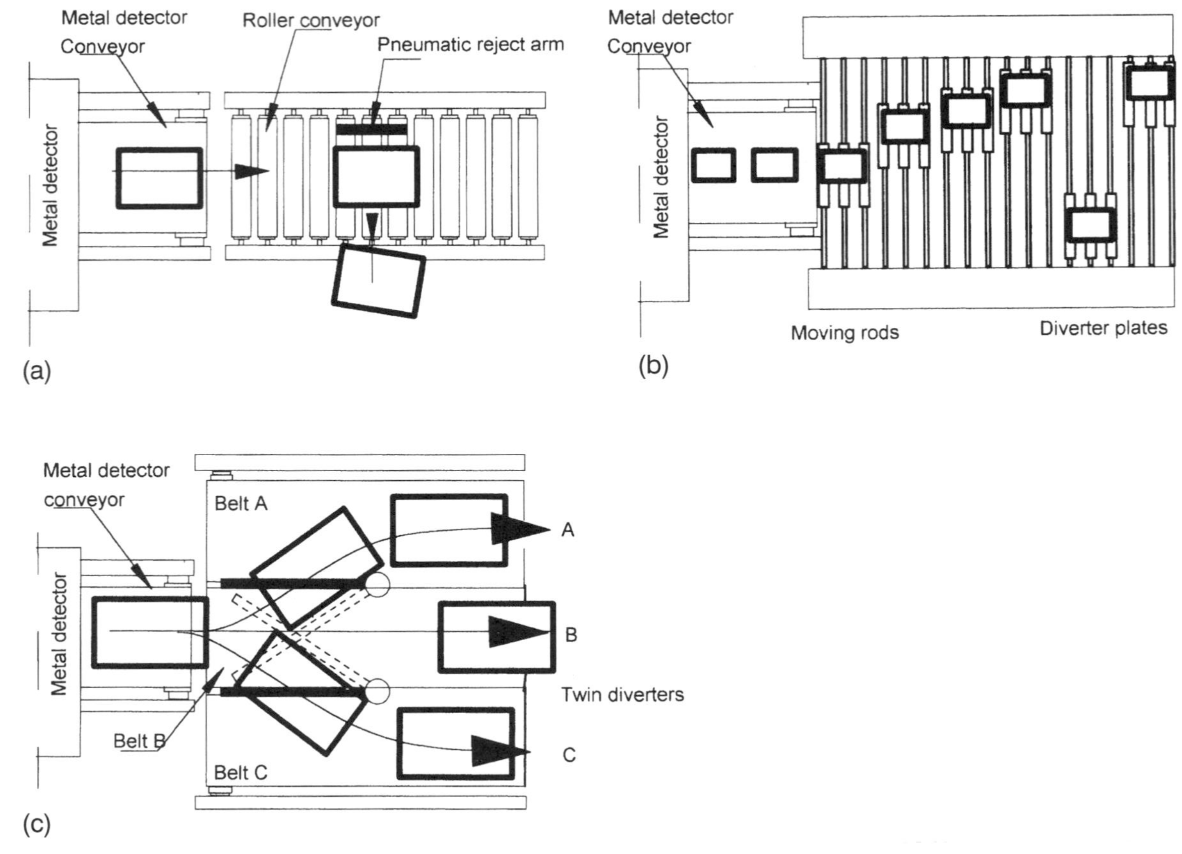

Figure 10.8 Heavy duty rejects. (a) Heavy duty kicker. (b) Progressive diverter system. (c) Three-lane diverter.

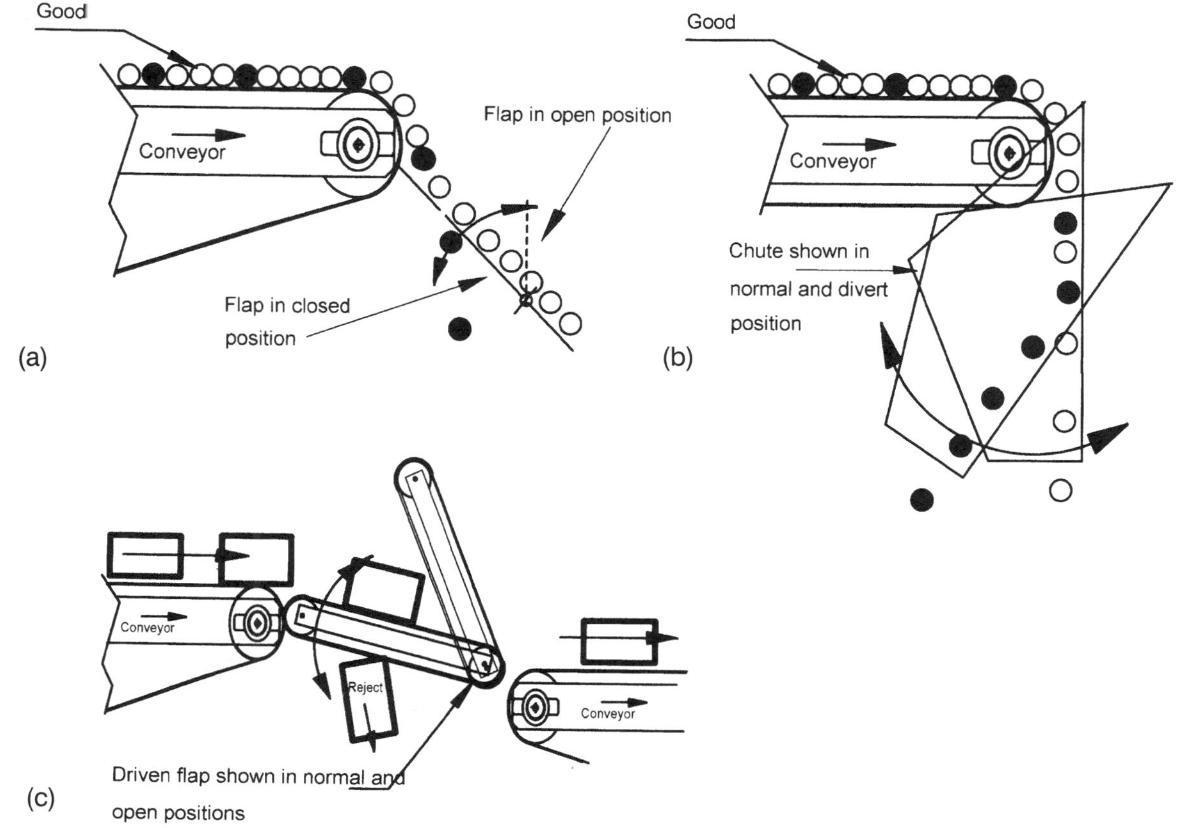

Figure 10.9 (a) Simple flap system. (b) Diverting chute system. (c) Driven flap system.

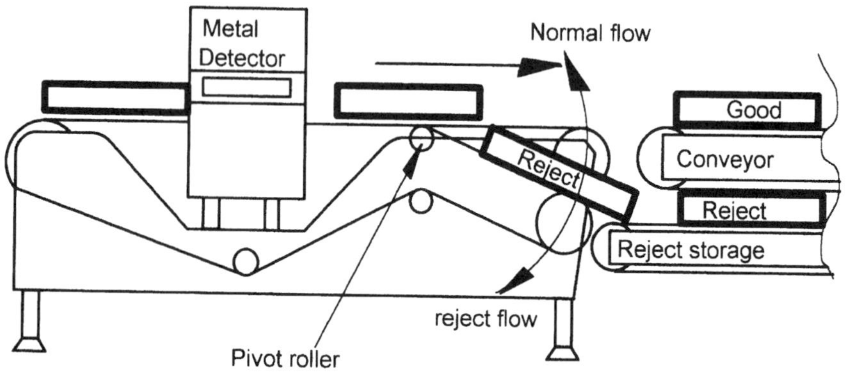

Figure 10.10 Drop-end rejection system.

belts, although on any application where the belt exceeds 500 mm width the fitting of an automatic belt tracking system is normal.

10.9 Reject timing – introduction

The operation of a reject system is normally controlled by time. First, the time from detection to the opening of the reject, shown in Figure 10.12 as 't', then the time the reject gate is held open shown on the drawing as 't2'. For any of the reject systems described to operate properly these times must be synchronized to the product speed. In many cases this is quite simple, but in some applications, e.g. where belts stop and start or machine speed varies, it is more complex and a method of measurement of position is needed. The size of the product will also influence the accuracy of timing of the reject. There are different solutions available to overcome these problems.

10.9.1 Belt speed

The speed of the metal detector conveyor belt may be linked to a machine drive causing it to vary or to move intermittently. In these circumstances a sensor is required to monitor the movement of the belt and to control the delay timings to synchronize with the product movement. This is achieved by fitting a device to the drive system, shown in Figure 10.12 as the 'digital counter', which is normally a pulse generator of some type. The reject delay time is then controlled by a system of counting pulses to control the reject action as opposed to time. This relates belt travel directly to the operation of the rejection device to ensure correct operation of the system. Most modern metal detectors will have the circuitry necessary to automatically adjust reject timing built in and only require the addition of a pulse generator.

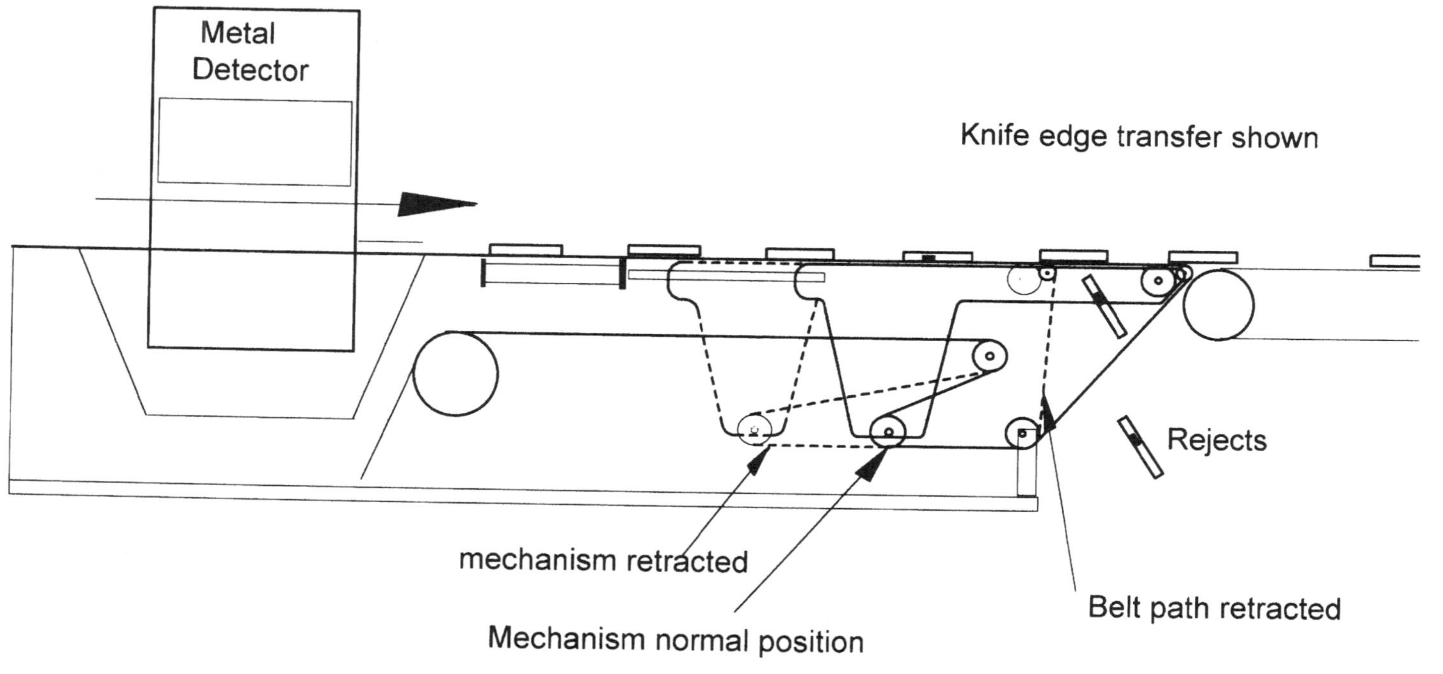

Figure 10.11 Retracting band mechanism.

10.9.2 *Product size*

Figure 10.12 shows a product 500 mm long with a contaminant 'A' located on the leading edge and a contaminant 'B' on the trailing edge. The position of the contaminant within the length of the product affects the time between detection and rejection which may be sufficient to allow contaminated product to pass without being rejected.

For example, if the system in Figure 10.12 had the following specification:

Belt speed	30 m/minute or 500 mm/second
Dimension 't'	1000 mm
Pack length	500 mm

If the contaminant is located on the leading edge of the pack 'A' then by setting the time delay 't' to 2 seconds (the time taken for the leading edge of the pack to travel to the rejection point) and holding the rejection open for 1 second 't2', any pack having a contaminant on the leading edge will be rejected. In practice allowances are applied for absolute security.

However, if the contaminant is located on the trailing edge of the pack 'B' the pack would be completely past the rejection point in 2 seconds and not be rejected.

For many applications where pack length is not so large in comparison to the length of the system, this problem can be overcome by reducing the time delay between detection and start of rejection, and extending the time the reject is held open to cover the worst situation. However, the alternative is to use an additional sensor to detect the position of the product, and to use the signal from this to control the detect and reject times. This is illustrated as the photoelectric register on Figure 10.12. In this case, the detection signal is used in a simple logic circuit to utilize the signal from the register to initiate the operation of the rejection system.

10.9.3 *Contaminant separation*

In setting the time delays for rejection, consideration must be given to the effect of a continuous stream of contaminated product. This is not likely to occur with packed products but may occur with loose products. To ensure that the reject system is able to reject all the contamination the reject open time must be set to take off a length of at least the width of the search head and it must be designed so that sequential signals add to the reject open time, thus ensuring adequate safety in the reject operation.

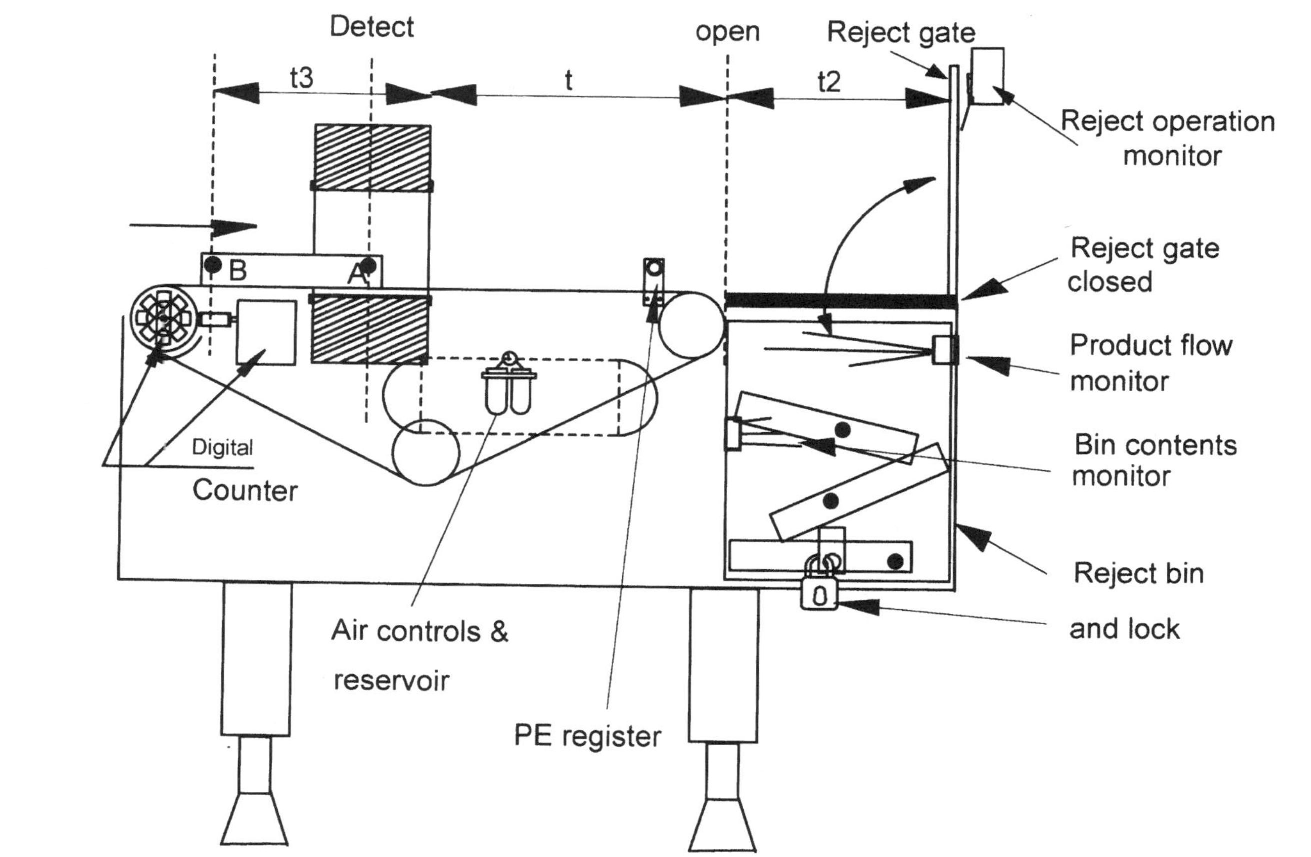

Figure 10.12 Reject timing.

(a) Reject function – basic operation

The continuous operation of the reject system is essential to the performance of the system. Most reject systems are pneumatically operated. Because the reject operation, unlike a belt tracking device for example, only operates very occasionally, they are prone to suffer from the effects of corrosion and dirt unless they are regularly operated to keep them clean; normally the routine quality assurance test process will be sufficient for this purpose. They also rely on there being a sufficient volume of air present at the correct pressure to function.

In normal factory environments this may be difficult to achieve all the time. Therefore, it is recommended that wherever a reject system is pneumatically operated there should be an airline filter and lubricator fitted to the incoming air supply, and an air pressure switch to monitor and 'fail-to-safe' if air pressure drops.

The quality assurance process needs to include monitoring of the level of lubricating oil in the air lubricator and emptying the filter of the system fitted to the machine.

Where the reject system is liable to be required to make a series of reject operations, which is in most cases, then tests must be made and the results recorded to establish that the air supply volume is sufficient for the purpose. Air blast systems, which use a large volume of air, will frequently be found to have an insufficient air supply for more than a limited number of sequential operations. Where this is the case it is essential to fit an air reservoir on the machine to provide the volume required.

Having established the system is fully operational under normal conditions, then the use of a sensor or sensors to monitor the operation of the reject system is required. This facility will normally be available as an extension of the self-check system built into the foreign body detector.

(b) Reject function – complete operation

The operation or motion of the reject device can normally be checked by incorporating a switch into the system activated by the mechanical operation of the reject device. This can be linked back to the foreign body detector self-check system, which may be able to not only detect and record the motion of the reject but also to check that the motion occurred at the specified time. Failure to operate will normally be used to signal an alarm and put the system into a 'fail-to-safe' position if possible, either through the self-check system or by direct connection. This will ensure the reject operation has taken place but there are occasions where this may be insufficient for absolute control of the reject operation.

The inherent dangers of reject system failure not covered by monitoring the operation of the reject are associated with failure of the contaminated product to be collected in the reject enclosure. This can occur because the enclosure is full, in which case the reject will operate but the product will fail to enter the rejection bin and remain in the product stream. Alternatively, failure of the reject system to drive the contaminated product off the belt properly will result in it failing to be gathered into the reject enclosure. These situations can be monitored by incorporating a sensor to monitor the level of product in the enclosure, typically a photoelectric switch device, or by using a sensor to note the contaminated item passes a particular point. Where these systems are used they should be linked back to the foreign body detector or used to signal alarms directly.

10.9.5 Reject enclosures

As previously stated, the use of an automatic reject system is essential and the rejected material must be held in a sealed enclosure. Removal from the enclosure should be by duly authorized personnel. The reject enclosure must satisfy the potential requirements of the application. First, of all it needs to be of a suitable shape, i.e. with dimensions large enough to allow product to move or fall freely within it. Secondly, it needs to be large enough to accommodate sufficient product for the normal day-to-day operation and a routine emptying procedure should be implemented and recorded. Thirdly, the entry needs to be clear and smooth, and engineered so that contaminated items cannot normally balance on the edge and then subsequently be taken away. In the case of conveyors with side mounted reject bins the edge of the conveyor should be chamfered to encourage the material to drop clear. Access needs to be provided to remove contaminated product, usually by an exit drawer or by sliding out a drawer, either of which should be locked. Some foreign body detectors may have provision for the opening and closing of the reject bin to be monitored and recorded by the self-check monitoring circuits, providing both records and the potential for 'fail-to-safe' in the event of unauthorized opening.

10.10 Specialist metal detector applications

10.10.1 Introduction

There are applications for metal detectors that require the use of specific solutions. These include the handling of materials falling under gravity, such as grain, or liquids being pumped through a process. There are also applications where metal detectors have been designed to suit the specific needs of the application, e.g. in the snack food industry. Metal detectors also have applications in the industries supplying packing materials to the food industry, some of which utilize special types of metal detectors. These are the subject of this section. Metal detectors are also widely used in the pharmaceutical and tobacco industries, using the same techniques as those discussed in this book.

10.10.2 *Granular and powder materials*

Granular and powder materials includes cereal grains, salt, sugar, cocoa powder, dry soup ingredients and similar free flowing materials found in the food industry and plastic granulates in the packaging industry.

Where granular or powdered materials have to be inspected for metallic foreign body contamination there is generally no difficulty in using a metal detector, even at very high speeds. There are applications where metal detectors operate on product speeds up to 50 m/second. The complexity lies in the mechanical handling and rejection system design required to prevent spillage and dust – both factors precluding the use of conveyor systems. Raw material can be presented in two ways, either falling on an inclined plane or falling vertically under gravity. The solution is to pass an enclosed chute through the aperture of a metal detector and arrange for a flap to divert the flow when metal is detected.

Inclined-chute systems are the simplest to deal with mechanically and will generally be based on the systems described in section 10.8.3 and shown in Figure 10.9(a). The product falls through the metal detector search head, which is mounted at an angle to the horizontal to coincide with the angle of an inclined chute which may be rectangular or circular. When metal is detected the flap located after the detector is raised and causes product to flow out into a second chute or reject bin. Rejection time is set up using the conventional timing system. Operation of the flap reject and divert action can be checked using modified versions of the systems used for conveyors (section 10.9).

Where product is falling under the force of gravity then rejection becomes difficult due to the speed needed to operate the reject system. The overall height of these systems is dependent upon four factors:

- Product speed at which the material enters the system
- The response time of the metal detector
- The response time of the system actuating the reject
- The distance the reject has to move

Table 10.2 demonstrates the effects of changes in the free-fall height into the system and the reject system response time on the overall system height. The effects of the response time of the metal detector can be largely ignored for modern equipment. The response time of the system actuating the reject, shown as the system response time in Table 10.2, is based upon arbitrary figures. The distance the reject has to travel will affect the situation in practice but has been ignored in the example.

The solution to this problem that has been adopted is to manufacture systems that require the initial velocity to be controlled so that an acceptable overall system height is achieved. Some manufacturers keep the pipe round as it passes through the detector and some offer the larger sizes with rectangular chutes, the objective being to limit the amount of travel the reject system is required to make and to achieve better sensitivity as a result of having a smaller dimension.

Where the system utilizes a rectangular passage or chute through the metal detector then generally better sensitivity will be achieved as the metal detector has a smaller dimension equating to aperture height in a conventional application. Table 10.3 gives the theoretical equivalent capacities of rectangular systems in terms of pipe sizes.

However, in deciding to select a rectangular-chute system for the advantages it gives it must be remembered that the dimension inside the chute will be significantly smaller than that of the aperture of the metal detector. In most cases the manufacturer will design the chute so that it does not contact the metal detector aperture. Adding this clearance to the thickness of the material used for the chute results in the clear passage being reduced. As can be seen in Table 10.3 the capacity of the rectangular systems is generally less than that of a round system of the same nominal size. Final specification of capacity will depend on the flow characteristics of the material.

Table 10.2 Drop-through metal detector reject system heights

Reject system response time (seconds)	Free fall infeed height (m)	Overall system height (m)
0.30	0.00	0.44
	0.25	0.77
	0.50	0.91
	1.00	1.11
0.50	0.00	1.23
	0.25	1.78
	0.50	2.01
	1.00	2.33
1.00	0.00	4.91
	0.25	6.01
	0.50	6.47
	1.00	7.12

Table 10.3 Drop-through system capacity

Nominal pipe size (mm)	Rectangular equivalent[a]	Approximate capacity[b] (kg/hour)
25	Na[c]	350
40	Na[c]	400
50	Na[c]	1400
75	Na[c]	2000
100	Na[c]	6000
150	Na[c]	13000
200	Na[c]	24000
100	200 × 50	3900
125	150 × 100	6000
150	200 × 100	10000
175	300 × 100	14000
200	350 × 100	20000

[a] The rectangular equivalents are given as a guide only.
[b] The capacity quoted is based on free flowing plastic granulate with an even flow rate.
[c] Not applicable.

When considering the introduction of a drop-through system (Figure 10.13), the specification of the pipe size is essential if the system capacity is to be sufficient. Where the product already flows in pipes the solution is simply to introduce a system which has the same capacity; however, where this experience is not available, the simplest way to specify the pipe diameter is to find the answer by test using samples of pipe of varying sizes.

Where the product is a powder as opposed to granular it may have a tendency to form a bridge, this may result in a blockage in the system. When working with this type of material it will be found that there is a critical minimum dimension of pipe that can be used without bridging and blockage occurring.

The rejection system of most drop-through systems is operated pneumatically. It is of critical importance when installing these systems that the air supply is not only of sufficient pressure but also volume. Experience has shown that when detection does occur it is regularly found that there will be a sequence of detections. These require rapid continuous operation of the reject and will put an exceptional demand on the air supply. It will be found that where these systems are installed an air reservoir should be located immediately prior to the connection to the system that is large enough to ensure the reject system will operate correctly.

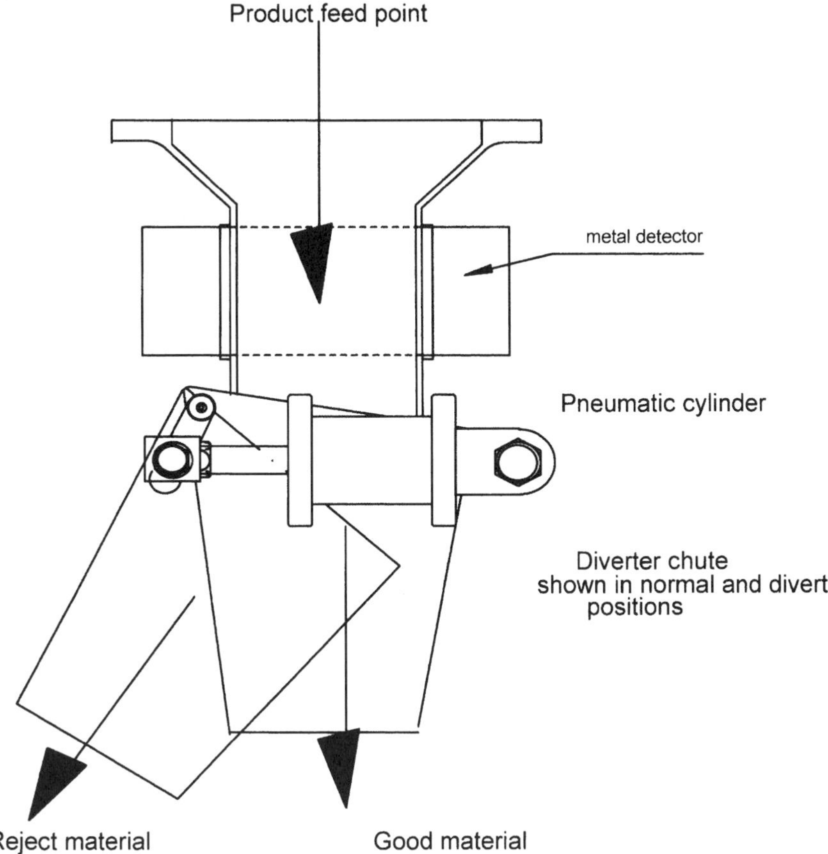

Figure 10.13 Drop-through metal detector system.

The systems can be set up using sensors attached to the reject mechanism to be able to utilize the same automatic test functions as ordinary metal detectors described in section 9.6

Quality testing is more difficult than for conventional conveyor systems as it is necessary to introduce a contaminant into the flow and observe its rejection. The system should be arranged to allow this check to be carried out with adequate precautions to prevent the test sample contaminating the product by accident. If it is not rejected as a result of the test procedure then there is a fault in the system and steps need to be implemented to withdraw product after the metal detector has been found to be inadequate.

Where the system is to be introduced into an inclined position then the design of the reject system is easier as the flow rate will be less. There are several methods adopted for these applications using rectangular or circular chutes, which in some cases may not be totally enclosed, and reject valves of varying levels of complexity selected to suit the needs of the system, a simple design is shown diagrammatically in Figure 10.14. This uses a standard diverter valve automated for the purpose.

Most manufacturers make a dedicated version of the inclined-chute systems aimed principally at pharmaceutical applications but which finds applications in the food industry on similar products, e.g. in the confectionery industry.

The units utilize a small rectangular search head operating at a very high frequency (section 9.3) and incorporating a built-in electrically operated reject system. Construction is normally totally in stainless steel with plastic chutes that are easily removable for cleaning. Very high sensitivities are achieved, particularly to stainless steels often quoted of the order of 0.2 mm or less. These can be connected to central computer systems.

The capacity of the systems is limited by the size of the clear passage through the aperture – of the order of 10 000 tablets/minute depending on the tablet and the model chosen.

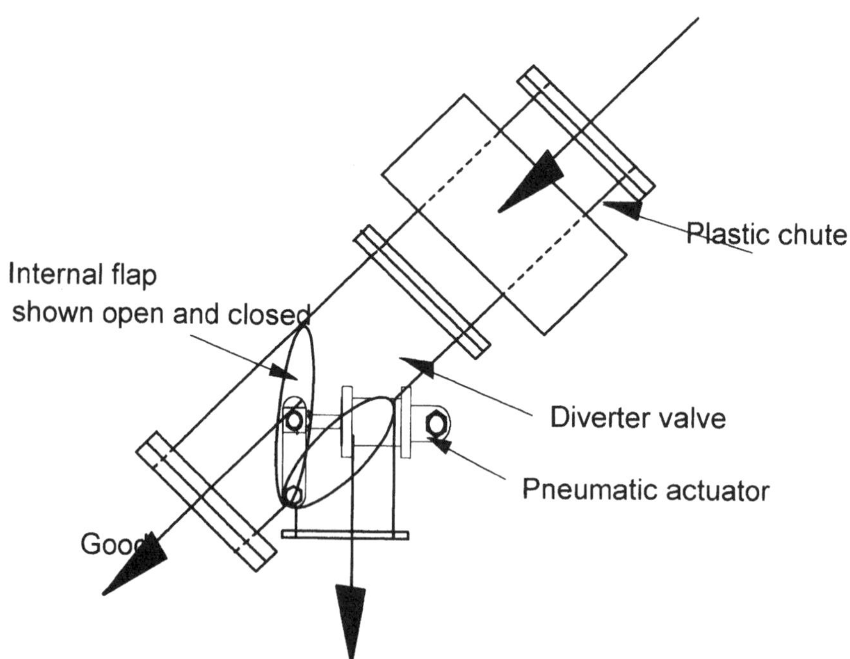

Figure 10.14 Inclined drop-through system.

10.10.3 *Plastic industry applications*

Plastics are used extensively for packaging and need to be free from metallic contamination either as loose scraps of metal inside the pack or as embedded contamination in the material. Failure to control packing materials may result in product contamination or 'false' rejections – the latter arising from the detectors reacting to contamination trapped in the packing material.

The principle of operation of metal detectors designed primarily for the plastic industry is described in section 9.5.

In most plastic manufacturing operations some of the material is recycled. Waste is produced by the process, as 'sprue' from injection moulding, or products that have failed to meet the specification and are to be reworked. Before the material can be reused it has to be reduced to a granular form.

To protect the granulators from damage by tools, etc., metal detectors are fitted to the delivery conveyors supplying the waste or scrap material. Damage to the machines is both costly and has the potential to be a source of contamination.

The granulated material is either stored in bins or transferred under vacuum to a separate storage point. Metal detection systems are available to fit to the delivery pipes to detect and reject metallic contamination preventing it passing further on into the process.

Finally, the regranulated material will be fed into the extrusion or moulding machine where a combined metal detector and reject system shown in Figure 10.15 are located. The main advantage of the eddy current loss machines is that they are capable of detecting metal even when the product passes through them extremely slowly or with intermittent motion.

10.10.4 *Paper and board industry*

Cardboard and reclaimed paper products are often contaminated by small pieces of metal, particularly aluminium foil. When packages manufactured from these materials pass through a metal detector this contamination will be picked up and generate rejection signals. The position is exacerbated by the packing material being closest to the coil, by definition, and experience has shown that with corrugated board it is often necessary to set a rejection threshold at 2.5 mm Fe in order to prevent false signals. This is clearly unsuitable for most food applications.

Some board manufacturers, mainly in the USA, use a special type of metal detector on the board production lines to monitor contamination in order to minimize this problem for the user. The type of

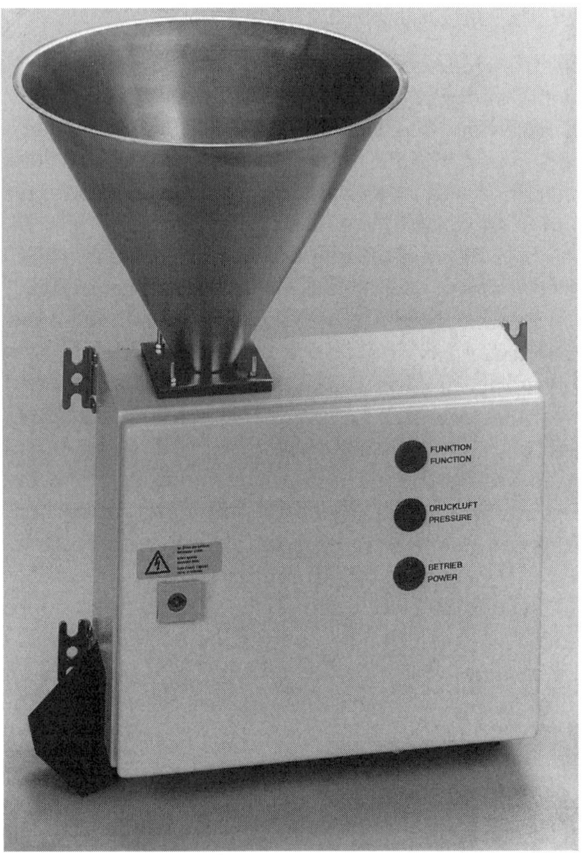

Figure 10.15 Special purpose gravity separator. (Courtesy Pulse Technology Ltd.)

metal detector used is an open-faced, balanced coil unit, often referred to as a single-face or single-sided detector. These units were originally designed to protect machinery in the carpet industry. Sensitivity is limited to an area close to the face to prevent interference by the machinery around it. Sensitivity is of the order of 1 mm Fe or equivalent. These signals are counted and used to establish acceptability or otherwise of the material.

10.10.5 *Liquids in pipes*

The inspection of liquids, slurries and pastes carried in pipes requires systems designed for the purpose. The technique is only practical up to 100 mm (4 inch) pipe sizes, and requires a length of plastic pipe, necessary to carry the product through the search head, connected to the existing pipeline and the installation of a metal detector and a diverter valve (Figure 10.16). Similar systems are used with X-ray machines.

The systems are suitable for use with products such as sauces, jams, meat pastes and ice cream. They can be used with liquid chocolate, but because of the need for a water heating jacket around the pipe passing through the metal detector may cause false signals, it is preferable that the pipe and the valve to be heated by a water jacket are kept clear of the metal detector aperture.

(a) System construction

Pipeline systems comprise a plastic tube to carry the material through the metal detector. The selection of the plastic is critical as it not only has to have the physical strength to withstand temperatures up to a maximum of 100°C and pressures up to 7 bar which occur in pipelines, but must also be suitable for contact with foods.

The plastic material is connected to the existing system at one end and to the reject valve at the other. This may involve the fitting of stainless steel adaptor pieces to the plastic to provide the strength for

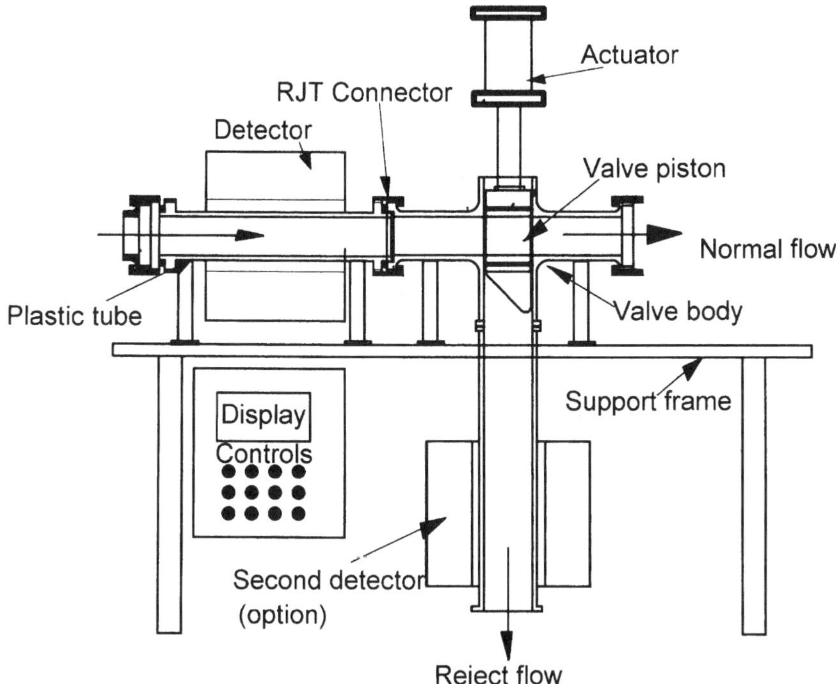

Figure 10.16 Pipeline system.

a conventional 'Tri Clover' or 'RJT' connector to BS 1864 or for connection to the specific fittings of a machine.

The metal detector is a conventional unit usually utilizing a separate search head and control unit. The aperture size being selected to suit the particular pipe size.

The reject valve connected to the plastic tube is normally either a piston type as shown in Figure 10.16 or a rotary plug valve type which is not illustrated. They both have the same function of closing the normal flow passage and diverting the flow into a reject passage in such a manner that the material flow continues and does not leave a 'plug' of material that is not rejected, which is a danger with twin butterfly valve systems. The bodies of the valves are manufactured from stainless steel with food grade plastic components and pneumatically operated. The piston valves have some capability to 'chop' some meat products for clean separation of the flow. It is most important when selecting a valve that access for cleaning is easy and that the internal form is as free from grooves, etc.

For some applications, particularly on the larger pipe sizes over 100 mm (4 inch), twin butterfly valves are used, one to stop the normal flow passage and one to open (and close) a reject passage. The application has to be carefully considered to ensure all material is rejected.

The complete assembly will be mounted on a framework suitable for the application, and including the control unit electronics for the metal detector, air line cleaner, filters and lubricators, etc. As most applications will be wet and arduous, the construction will generally be in stainless steel and to IP 66 standards.

(b) Specific detection problems

Most liquid products will be found to be electrically conductive and, therefore, will have a product effect which has to be cancelled out by the metal detector phase control system. Unfortunately, this is complicated by the nature of the application where the product will in theory keep the pipe full all the time, which tends to result in the out of balance signal of the product being cancelled out as both detection coils continuously 'see' product. If this was the case then setting up would be relatively easy and high levels of sensitivity would be achievable. Unfortunately, in practice starting and stopping the process results in the coils being subject to different amounts of product (and signal). Products are rarely truly homogenous, and air bubbles and voids appear in the product, all of which will result in the detector sensing the change in product as it passes each coil and if set incorrectly will give rise to false signals.

In practice the detector has to be set up to eliminate the product signal in the same way as a normal metal detector. This is best achieved when the system is 'off-line', using a sample that can be passed through the detector mimicking the passage of a discrete product carried on a belt. Automatic product compensation systems can be used during this operation; however, but once the system is operational they become ineffective. Using this process eliminates the problems of start/stop, homogeneity, bubbles and voids from the detection process but not the rejection process.

(c) Reject timing

While modern detectors can be connected to the pump drive system to automatically adjust reject timing to accommodate start/stop situations, because product flow in pipes is laminar setting the time delays for the operation of the reject system is not as straightforward as for conveyor systems.

Materials flow in pipes is laminar, i.e. the velocity profile is parabolic. The material at the geometric centre of the pipe flows at a faster rate than that at the pipe wall where in theory the flow rate is zero. Theory would, therefore, seem to dictate that to ensure rejection of a contaminant, because the flow at the wall is zero, the only way to ensure rejection is to stop the flow and dismantle the system for washing out. The theory could also be interpreted to mean any contaminant located at the wall of the pipe would never move along the pipe run to the detector in the first place. Because the laminar flow pattern is complicated by variations in the product, air bubbles trapped in the product and turbulence generated as the material passes over interruptions to the smooth walls of the pipes, all the product eventually flows through the system albeit at varying flow rates.

To minimize the effect of the complex laminar flow pattern it is preferable to locate the reject valve as close to the metal detector search head as possible. A calculation can then be made of the shortest time a contaminant will take to travel from the metal detector to the valve using the approximation that the speed at the centre of the pipe is twice the average flow rate. In these applications the use of 'cross-over detection' systems, discussed in section 9.3, is advantageous. This figure is then used to set the time delay between detection and the valve opening taking into account the valve operation time.

Example

Flow rate F	= 10 l/minute
Pipe diameter D	= 50 mm
Reject valve operation time T_1	= 0.75 seconds
Distance from detection point to valve L	= 150 mm
Product speed (average) S	= $F/\pi D^2/4$ per minute

	= 84 mm/second
Time to travel distance T_2	= L/S
	= 1.79 seconds
Adjust by a factor of 2	= 0.9 seconds (rounded up)
Reject valve open time delay	= $T_2 - T_1$
	= 0.15 seconds

It is recommended that a safety factor of 10% be taken from the calculated figure, making the time delay setting before the valve opens, which in this case means in practical terms the delay time should be zero.

The calculation for the time the valve should stay open cannot be calculated with such certainty as the time taken for the material closest to the surface of the pipe to reach the reject valve becomes infinite. In practice a factor of 0.25 times the average speed can be used for initial tests. In the example this is:

Valve open time	= $T_2 \times 4$
	= 7.2 seconds

In this time period a volume of 0.11 litres would be rejected. *Whether this is a suitable time delay can only be ascertained by experience and test.*

(d) Twin inspection systems

Where the time delay setting of a single metal detector system proves to be so unpredictable that the reliability of the system fails to meet the requirements of the quality control programme then the alternative is to use a second metal detector mounted on the reject flow line, as shown in Figure 10.16. The time delay to open the reject valve is calculated as shown, but the signal to close the valve is derived from the detection signal generated in the second search head when the contaminant passes. Because the contaminant may have an orientation effect that precludes its detection in the second search head, a time delay and alarm should be used to prevent excessive amounts of product flowing out of the line. In this event a decision has to be made on dispersal of the material rejected after the system has been stripped and cleaned to ensure any contaminant is not lodged in it.

X-ray machines commonly take the contaminated material and pass it back through the system in a smaller pipe for re-examination and recycling.

10.11 Twin-head conveyor systems

There has been a tradition of using two metal detectors for applications where wire sensitivity is important. The principle used has been to place the detectors across the belt at an angle of 45° forming an angle of 90° between them. The objective has been to increase wire sensitivity by having two chances to see a wire in the most favourable orientation. While this is true, the loss of sensitivity due to the extra length of the apertures works against the objective and with modern stable sensitive metal detectors is not significantly more sensitive than a single detector placed at 90° across the belt.

10.12 Vertical form fill and seal machines

With the introduction of metallized film, the application of metal detectors on products packed in the material, particularly snack foods, presents problems of achieving a level of sensitivity to meet the demands of the process. The metal detector manufacturers have developed a range of metal detectors having a very slim depth dimension (Figure 9.1) with separate control units designed specifically to overcome this problem. The units are mounted below the

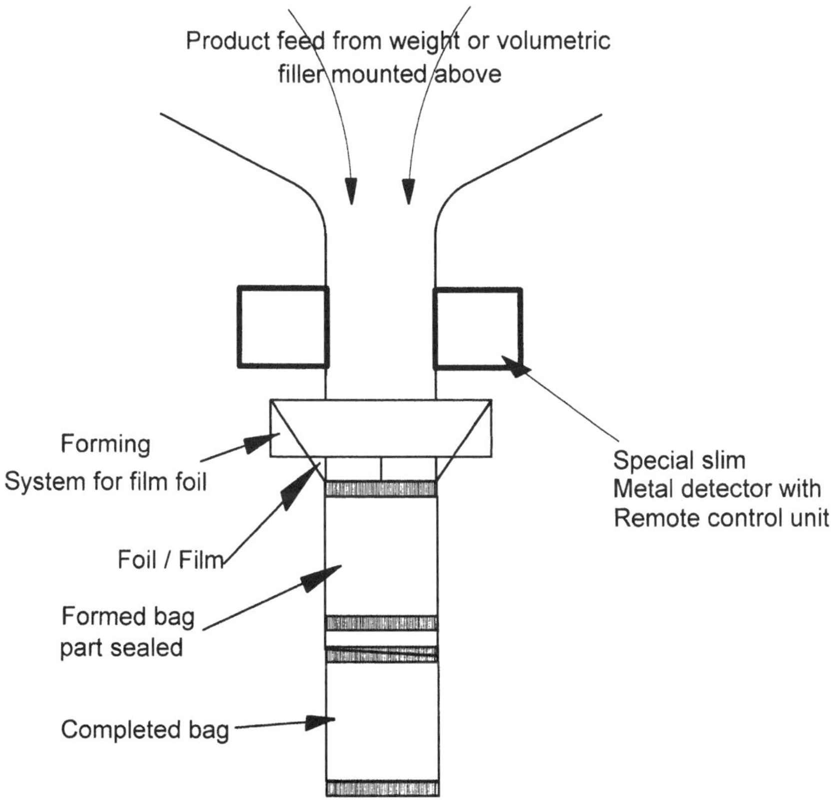

Figure 10.17 Form fill and seal detector.

weight or volumetric filling heads and above the bag maker. Any metal passing through them is detected and the reject signal is either used to operate a synchronized rejection device or to stop the machine 'fail-to-safe' arrangement. The set up is shown diagrammatically in Figure 10.17.

11

X-ray detection systems

11.1 Introduction

In the food industry there has been a requirement to find all foreign objects or undesirable material in foodstuffs. X-ray systems provide one step forward in that quest, but do not provide the complete solution. This chapter outlines the principles of X-rays and how they work. It then reviews the machine technologies available to the food industry followed by more recent developments. X-ray detection systems were initially installed to combat two specific applications, i.e. that of looking for broken glass in glass jars and the other finding bones in meat products, in particular chicken. Both applications can have significant consumer reaction – the problem of glass in baby food caused major repercussions.

X-rays were initially used in the medical field, and some of the earliest systems were very crude and were open systems with no protection for the operator. In the 1950s there was even a program to routinely X-ray pregnant woman and mobile units were set up. This was abandoned once there was an increased understanding of the risks of too much exposure to high levels of X-rays. The main symptom from over exposure is that of X-ray burns. X-rays have been used for non-destructive testing work for many years. Their use has been significant in the inspection of welds or material joints for critical mechanisms which may undergo high stress levels or be crucial to the safety of a process. One of the earliest reported food applications was that for inspecting for bones in fish by Frascatore and Holston in 1955.

It is this key property that allows one to use the technology to selectively detect foreign bodies in food. The range of foreign bodies that can be detected includes:

- Glass fragments
- A wide range of metals both ferrous and non-ferrous

- Stones
- Bones
- Hard dense plastics
- Certain rubbers

An advantage of X-rays is that they can be used to detect foreign bodies or defective products in the pack but also within many different types of pack which include cartons, cans, glass jars and foil trays. One of the most important applications is that of detecting glass. Glass is commonplace in many factories in the form of packaging such as bottles and jars, and therefore there is a high risk of possible contamination.

11.2 The technology

X-ray technology is a relatively old technology being first discovered by Röntgen in 1895. They were called 'X-rays' because at the time it was not known what they were. He had some photographic plates that he had wrapped and stored carefully to avoid exposure in the laboratory where he worked. However, when he came to use them he found they were fogged. Rather than just discard them he set out to find out why they had fogged. After a while he found a gas-discharge tube which he had been using for low pressure/high voltage work to be the only likely cause. He then discovered that this tube emitted a form of radiation that penetrated materials such as paper, wood, rubber and glass. He experimented further and found that the radiation even penetrated aluminium up to 1.5 cm thick. He then had a problem determining whether X-rays were a stream of particles being emitted or whether they were in a wave form. It was not until 1912 that it was discovered that they were electromagnetic waves with a very short wavelength.

Since the discovery of X-ray radiography many applications have been proposed, notably in medical, dentistry, chemical analysis and non-destructive testing applications. Within the food area, in 1896 it was suggested that ionizing radiation might be used to kill micro-organisms. It was not until 1921 that Schwartz in the USA filed a patent for the use of X-rays to kill the parasite *Trichininella spiralis* found in meat. Since then there has been considerable research into the irradiation of foods and many systems are now used. There are strict guidelines and regulations on the use of and operation of such processes which are specified in section 11.12. Other forms of radiation tend to be used today for irradiation of foods, such as gamma-rays that are a lower cost than X-rays.

The research on food irradiation and medical radiology has served as a good base for the safety of X-rays used in inspection systems. The levels of radiation used in food processing range from 0.05 kGy for inhibiting sprouting, up to 50 kGy for the bacteriological sterilization of certain foods. In 1970, the International Food Irradiation Project was established to investigate the wholesomeness of irradiated foods. A number of Joint Expert Committees on Food Irradiation (JECFI) were also set up to investigate the same area. Results and discussions led to the JECFI concluding in 1980 that an overall average dose of 10 kGy presented no toxicological hazard or any special nutritional or microbiological problems.

The major uses for irradiation within the food industry are for:

- Extended shelf life – killing of spoilage organisms
- Disinfestation of crops – spices, herbs, cereals, etc.
- Killing of pathogens that produce foodborne diseases
- Inhibiting ripening, germination or sprouting

The major specific applications of ionizing irradiation to foodstuffs have been the following:

- Sterilization of herbs and spices
- Inhibition of sprouting in potatoes, garlic and onions
- Disinfestation of dried fruit and cereal grains
- Control of spoilage, parasites and pathogens in meat, seafood and poultry

The source of radiation for some of the above has been from radionuclides such as cobalt-59 and cesium-137 rather then X-rays.

11.2.1 *Background*

The first and most fundamental question most people would think of asking is – what is an X-ray? Most people have experienced going to the doctor or dentist and having to sit or stand still for a while whilst an X-ray is taken. X-rays are waves, similar to that of light, but are of a much shorter wavelength than light. Figure 11.1 shows the electromagnetic spectrum, from this it can be seen that the wavelength of X-rays falls between that of UV light and γ waves.

The next question which is often asked is – how does one produce an X-ray? X-rays are produced by colliding accelerated electrons or cathode rays, with a target or walls such as electrodes of a discharge tube. The generation of a standard X-ray system is not much different today. They can be produced by the rapid deceleration of electrons and this is achieved, as in the earliest system, by firing electrons at a tungsten target.

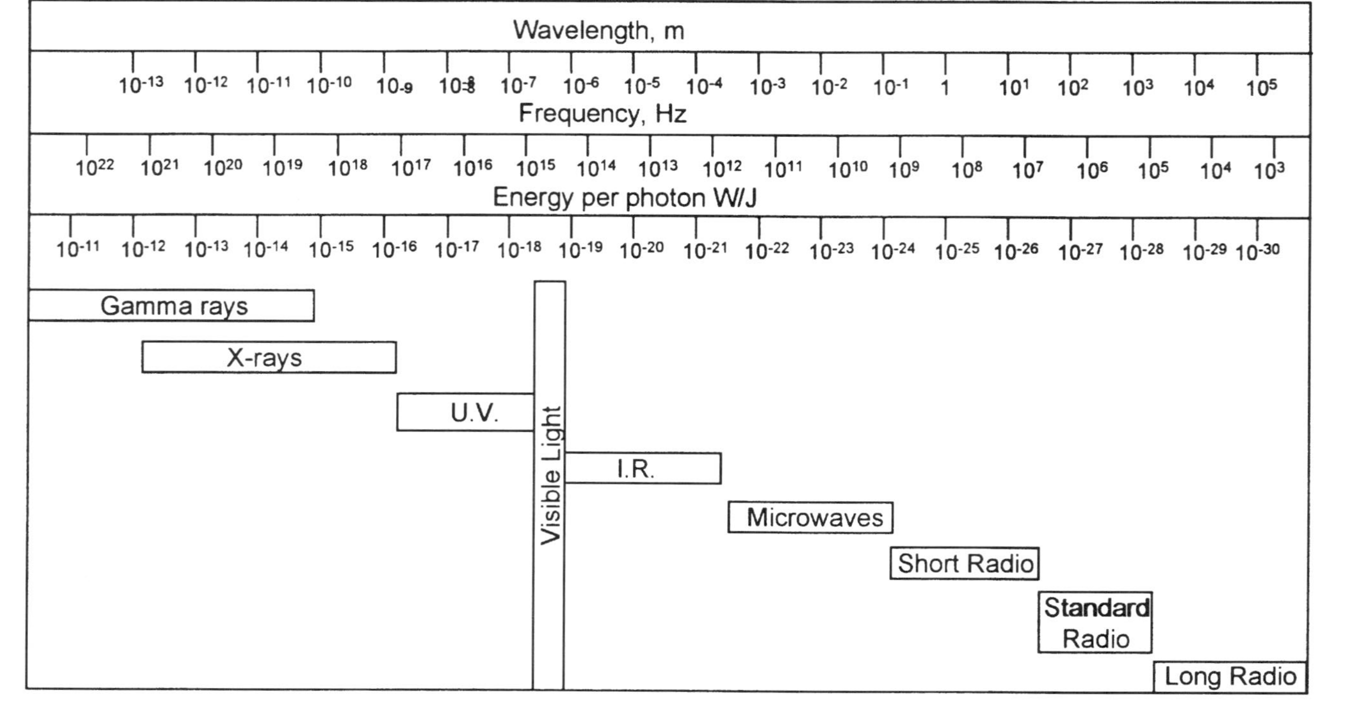

Figure 11.1 The electromagnetic spectrum.

11.2.2 *Generation of X-rays*

Initially electrons have to be produced and this is achieved by heating a tungsten filament. The filament is heated to a high temperature by passing a small voltage (about 10 V) through it. Metals are good conductors as they have free electrons. Having free or loosely held electrons, it is possible on heating to increase their energy. Increasing their energy creates a greater force than the attraction of the positive ions in the structural lattice of the tungsten. Therefore, when a metal such as tungsten is heated to a high temperature the electrons are 'boiled off' and escape. This is termed thermionic emission. This effect is similar to that of a cathode ray tube as used in a television system.

However, just allowing electrons to be 'boiled off' does not create X-rays – the electrons have to be accelerated and impacted on a tungsten target. The acceleration is achieved by creating a very high voltage between the filament and the target. The filament and target are housed in a glass vacuum tube, often called a Coolidge tube, which is subjected to as higher vacuum as possible, so that there is no gas to interfere with the flow and collide with the electrons. The pressure will normally be of the order of 10^{-5} mmHg. The high voltage (40–100 kV) accelerates the electrons sufficiently so that when they impact on the target X-rays are emitted. The use of an a.c. supply means that on the half-cycle that is positive the electrons will be colliding with the target and creating X-rays, but on the negative half-cycle nothing will happen. This system is quite convenient as it means the tube acts as its own rectifier. Figure 11.2 shows an illustration of a typical X-ray tube.

As a result of the electrons bombarding the target it becomes extremely hot and, therefore, has to be cooled. Cooling is achieved

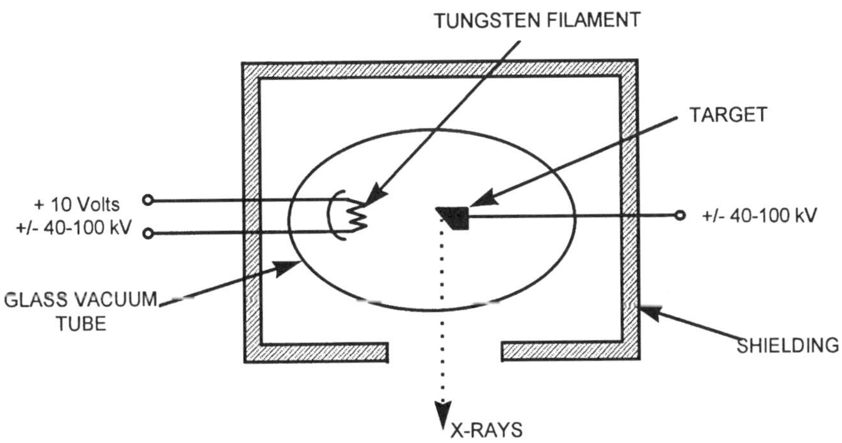

Figure 11.2 A typical X-ray generator tube.

by manufacturing a hollow target through which oil or water can be circulated as a coolant. It is important that the tube design is correct as it will determine the maximum peak kV regardless of what current is applied. The kV must not be too great so as to exceed the dielectric strength of the insulation. The maximum mA will depend on the tube filament design and the maximum electron emission from the filament.

The amount of power is usually measured for a system by multiplying voltage by current, for X-rays this is expressed in slightly different terms. The power/energy is expressed in heat units (HU) rather than joules. The radiographic exposure is taken as:

$$HU = kVp \times mA \times seconds$$

11.2.3 *Properties of X-rays*

Materials react differently when they are exposed to X-rays and it is these differences in response that one can exploit. As electromagnetic waves, there are some specific features that the X-rays themselves possess and these are the following:

- Ionize gases
- Fluoresce materials
- Change photographic films or emulsions
- Can be reflected and diffracted by crystals
- Penetrate materials
- Travel in straight lines
- Cause photoelectric emissions from metals

Chemical changes can take place and one specific reaction that does occur is that of the oxidation of ferrous sulphate in solution to ferric sulphate. This reaction can be used as a means of measuring the quantity of X-rays absorbed. Organisms can be affected by X-rays. This can cause living cells to be damaged or to die, genes can be affected and mutations can occur. Many of these effects, managed well and controlled, can be put to use to kill bacteria or irradiate malignant tumour cells.

The shorter wavelength and higher frequency of X-rays allows them to penetrate materials. If materials are placed in the line of the X-rays they will absorb the X-rays, and the amount of absorption will be dependent on the structure of the material, atomic number, density and the energy of the X-rays. Materials of a high atomic number will absorb more than a lower atomic number. This means that dense materials absorb more X-rays than less dense materials. Therefore those softer less dense materials such as packaging materials, pastry, milk and meat are penetrated more readily, whilst dense materials such as metals, glass and bones are not penetrated but reflect and scatter the X-rays. As X-rays travel in straight lines and are not deflected by electric or magnetic fields they are very suitable to be used as an inspection field.

X-rays can be used to detect metals such as iron, tin and copper in an inspection field with relative ease as these metals are dense. A major advantage with X-rays is that they can be used to detect stainless steel – this is a major benefit as the majority of food processing equipment and systems are constructed from stainless steel. It is possible with certain X-ray inspection machines to detect metal wires down to just a few millimetres in thickness. Materials such as glass and stones can be detectable down to sizes as little as 1 mm using high resolution machines. Bones are more difficult to detect as this depends on the properties of the material or product they are located in and the nature of the bone such as its size, shape or density. Bone is variable in density and chemical nature; it can also be attached to less dense ligaments or tendon which are often less visible as their density can be very similar to that of the product they are located in.

Other materials such as certain insects, paper and cardboard, stalks, stems, certain fruit stones, soft plastics, etc., can be detectable by an X-ray system; however, when they are embedded in a product they are less detectable by standard, on-line X-ray inspection systems. This is often because the machine's power has to be increased to 'see through' the product and this reduces the resolution at the lower end and makes the system less sensitive to lower density materials.

Inspecting products in their packaging is possible for a number of food pack materials such as foil containers, cardboard, certain plastic trays, polystyrene trays, etc. Some of the more advanced and higher power systems can inspect through plastic containers, glass jars and some cans, albeit with reduced effectiveness. One has to check the capabilities of specific machines to evaluate their limitations, and also what resolution will result and what contaminants one is likely to identify.

The X-ray machine's capabilities, accuracy and level of detection vary according to the machine manufacturer, type, model, product to be examined, speed of detection, contaminant(s) to be detected and the technology used by machine. Therefore, one cannot generalize about the performance of X-ray systems.

In addition to inspection systems, other properties of X-rays have been used in analysis including emission, absorption, low angle scatter, diffraction, fluorescence, k-capture, electron probes and soft X-ray systems. Some of these analytical systems were first used as early as 1912, in particular the discovery of the diffraction properties of zinc compounds and copper sulphate.

11.2.4 Dosage levels

The effect of X-rays on food has been well researched because of the use of ionizing radiation in the processing of some foods. The dosage level of X-rays is important from the food safety angle but also the effect on the quality of the foodstuff. The level of dose is measured in the unit of the gray (Gy). It is defined as the dose of radiation corresponding to the absorption of 1 joule of energy per kilogram of the matter through which the radiation passes [1 kGy (kilogray) = 1000 Gy; 1 Gy = 110 rad].

One can define the overall average dose by integrating the effect over the volume of the sample as given below:

$$D = \frac{1}{M} \int p(x, y, z) \mathrm{d}(x, y, z) \mathrm{d}V$$

where D is the overall average dose, M is the total mass of sample treated, p is the local density at the point (x,y,z), d is the total absorbed dose at the point (x,y,z) and dV is the (dx,dy,dz) derivative volume fraction.

The dosage received by the food is very low from an X-ray inspection machine and considerably less than that which food is exposed to during irradiation. Food is only exposed to X-rays for a very short time during inspection (normally about 1 second). Food may be inspected several times but the dosage will still be small as the total exposure time will only be a few seconds.

11.3 Fluoroscopy

The early X-ray inspection systems used fluoroscopy as a means of displaying a real-time image and enhancing photographic images. The system was developed to move away from the expensive and slow method of photographic plates. It was found initially that if phosphor were exposed to X-rays it would fluoresce. The effect of fluoroscopy 'screening' was that a visible image could be seen on a simple coated screen. This then enabled screens made of phosphor to be utilized. It was later found that other materials such as calcium tungstate, zinc cadmium sulphide and caesium iodide also exhibited this fluoresce effect.

The early machines were designed such that there was a lead glass window in the door which could be used to view the back of the phosphor screen through a lens and mirror arrangement (Figure 11.3)

The technology of fluoroscopy has been developed further as an off-line system. The system utilizes X-rays produced from a standard X-ray tube as described above. The X-rays are used to bombard the

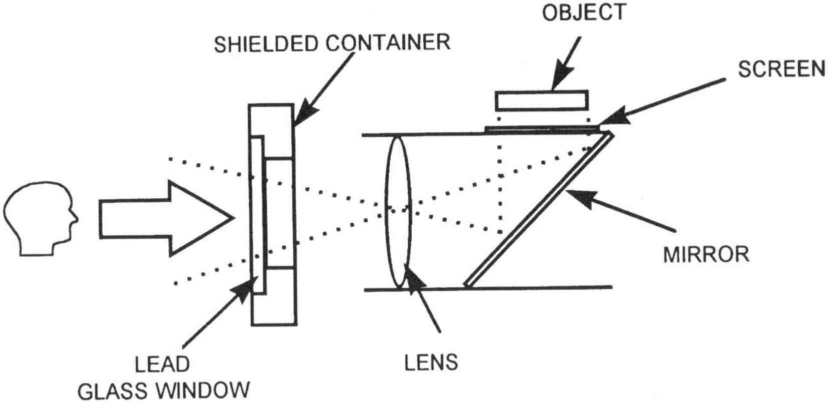

Figure 11.3 Early lead window inspection machine.

product sample which is located in a holder usually made of plastic or aluminium. The effect of using a high energy source of X-rays is to produce secondary X-rays from the sample being analysed. These secondary X-rays are characteristic of the elements that make up that substance. The secondary X-rays are collimated by directing them through a set of capillary tubes which are usually made of nickel. The collimated X-rays are targeted onto a crystal which has a known spacing. From Braggs equation we know that:

$$n\lambda = 2d \sin\theta$$

where θ is the angle between the incident and refracted beams and the planes, d is the interplanar spacing, and n is an integer.

The collimator may be made for parallel plates or from capillary tubes – their dimensions are usually 3–10 cm and they are positioned 0.1–0.5 mm apart.

11.4 Line scan X-ray systems

The most common form of X-ray foreign body inspection system is the line scan system. One of the earliest reported uses of X-ray inspection in the food industry was in 1965 by 'Cloetta', a Swedish confectionery company. They used the system to inspect each carton. The system was a 140 kV fluoroscopic system and the operator was able to see the image on a fluorescent screen. They inspected 3000 cartons a day and had an average of six rejects per day. Other early uses of the technology were for inspecting bread, sweets, baby foods and sausage meat.

In 1970 an on-line scan system was developed by Rank Precision Industries who were contracted by a British food industry consortium (NRDC) to construct a prototype machine based on this technology. The group was prompted into doing something following the increase in reported cases of consumer complaints which rose from 7000 in 1967 to 9000 in 1970. There was general concern over the increase – it had also been seen that contaminants such as stones, bone and glass were being reported, and these were obviously not detected by metal detectors. The technology then was adopted by the food industry in the 1970s. The reason for the development of the line scan type system were several fold. The most important was to be able to provide a real-time system which could operate at high speed. Another was to reduce the cost of an on-line X-ray system to an affordable level. In the USA at about the same time Borden Inc. developed a continuous X-ray inspection system.

This early system consisted of an X-ray generator (Figure 11.4) which operated at 40 kV. This was a standard X-ray generator using a high voltage vacuum tube system.

Rather than use the full beam of the ray produced from the target, the X-rays were channelled through a narrow diverging beam. The aperture was 17.78 cm (7 inches) high and 15.24 cm (6 inches) wide. A linear array of 96 photo-detectors were located along the 6 inch length. The conveyor speed used was 36.6 m/minute. This system was then used to test the feasibility, suitability and sensitivity for foreign body detection of small metallic balls, solder, lead, stones and

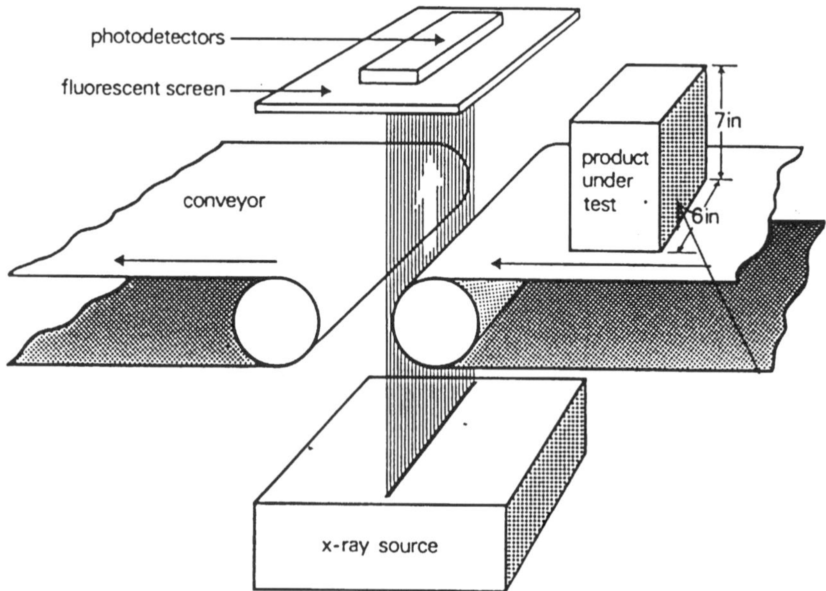

Figure 11.4 Typical linear array X-ray system.

glass. They found that the technology was not as widely applicable as they had hoped and decided to proceed further.

A number of inspection equipment companies have now taken on this technology and sell machines for on-line inspection. The system has not changed significantly in principle from the early design but has become more advanced as technology has progressed. A typical line or linear array system will now have:

- An X-ray generator (50–100 kV)
- A linear array of 1536 (or more) photodiodes each of a size of 0.5 × 0.5 mm
- A scanning time of array between 6 and 800 times per second
- A speed of conveyor of approximately 20–40 m/minutes (some machines are significantly faster where scan time is faster or resolution less critical)

The system operates by placing the product on a conveyor belt. The conveyor then passes through the machine and within the machine a beam of X-rays is directed onto the belt. The X-ray column is projected vertically and perpendicular to the product; the product on the belt then passes through this column. The X-ray detectors (photodiodes) are usually located above the product being inspected and opposite the source of the X-ray column on the other side of the belt. It is important that the belt is constructed of a material which is transparent to the X-rays. The photodiodes are capable of detecting the level of X-rays that fall on them and, therefore, the absorption can be measured.

The elements within the linear array have a typical surface and are of about 0.5 × 0.5 mm dependent on the particular system. There are usually 512, 768, 1024 or 1536 elements within the array. The size of the elements could be smaller and this could potentially improve the performance of the machine by increasing the resolution. The photodiodes, which are coated with a scintillator layer, are exposed to X-rays for a set period of time so as to accumulate the X-ray dose. The information is then recorded, and the detectors reset and available for the next dose. This accumulation and recording can occur very rapidly, approximately 1 millisecond and the data processed within the same cycle time. The output from the individual detectors is converted from X-ray generated photons to an electrical signal which can then be used to determine what level of grey will be displayed for individual pixels on the screen which represent the output from individual photodiodes. The electrical signals from the array are transferred to a multiplexing circuit thus converting the array into a serial signal. This operation in many systems is carried out using a charge-coupled device (CCD) analogue shift register. The CCD multiplexer has a broad dynamic range and a very low noise readout.

The analogue output data can be converted to a digital format and can then be stored. Outputs from the array of detectors can be added to form a matrix and the matrix can then be displayed as a two-dimensional image on a visual display unit (VDU). The quality of conversion from the photonic to electronic output can have a significant effect on the quality of the image. The key factors are the signal-to-noise ratio, the dynamic range and the level of sensitivity. The number of different levels of grey scale will be determined by the number of data bits used in the digital signal processing. An 8-bit can give as many as 256. It is widely acknowledged that humans can only detect 12 levels of grey scale.

When a food material passes through the column of X-rays it is scanned and an image is built up within less than 1 second. The image will normally show an outline of the food and if there are dense materials they will show up by being darker then the rest of the image. Many linear array systems use a threshold to detect whether there is a contaminant in the product.

Figure 11.5 shows an picture of a typical linear array machine. Figure 11.6 shows a graph of the output from an array – where there is some dense material this is indicated by the sudden drop.

A drop below a certain threshold will trigger a reject mechanism which will remove that item from the line. With a threshold system it is important to decide at what level to place the threshold. A high threshold which is close to the natural product absorbency level could trigger many false rejects; however, one set too low could allow contaminated product to pass through undetected. Figure 11.6 shows an example of an output of the threshold and a peak illustrating a contaminant is present.

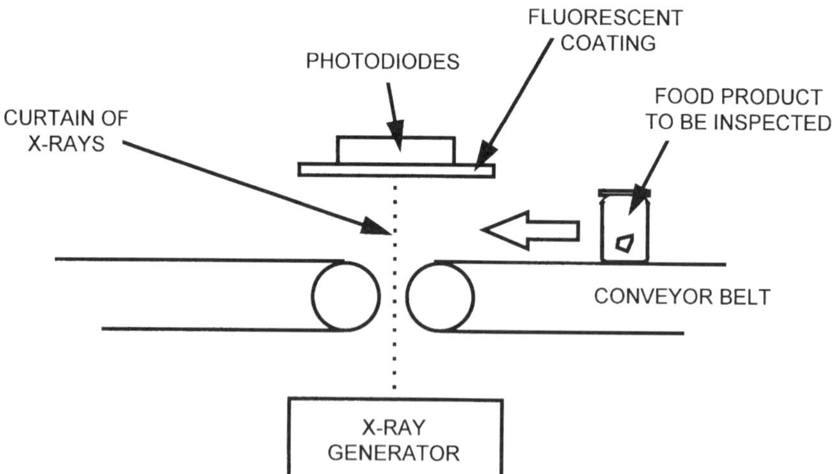

Figure 11.5 Diagram of a typical linear array X-ray system.

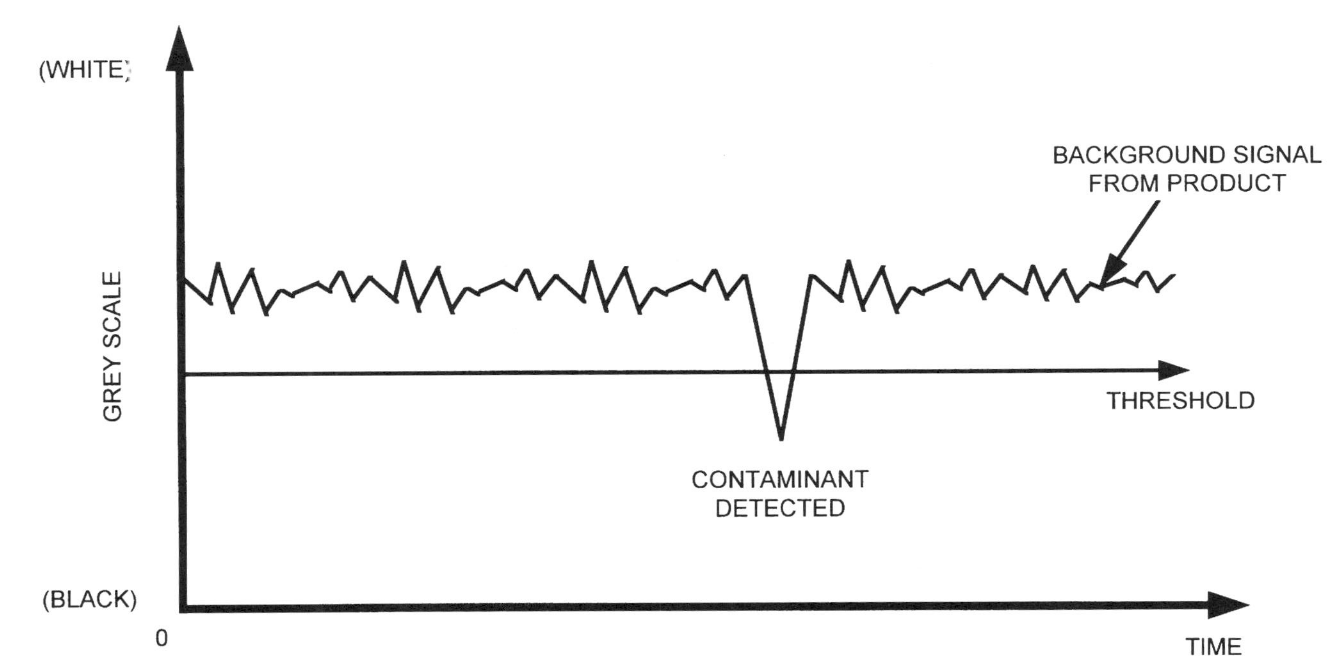

Figure 11.6 Graph of typical output from a linear array system.

This balance is critical for some products with very low densities, but is not an issue if the contrast is great between the food product and any contaminant such as stone or bones. However, often the product will have a natural variance, maybe in thickness, and this could have a significant effect on the performance of the system.

Detecting bones in chicken meat poses this kind of problem as the thickness of the meat could create the same level of X-ray absorption as that of a thin bone – a threshold system would, therefore, not be able to differentiate between the thick meat and the bone. In order to help resolve this particular issue some equipment companies have developed higher resolution systems and others use more sophisticated image analysis techniques such as morphology.

The machine that houses the X-ray source and detection system has to be well sealed to prevent any leakage of X-rays. The outside construction is usually of stainless steal so as to be sanitary. The inside has to comprise of shielding, this is usually lead as it is an effective shield and easy to work with.

11.5 Image intensifier X-ray systems

Originally, medical X-rays were produced by exposing a fine grain X-ray film to the X-rays and then developing it. Like photography, the best quality images were produced by setting the focal length to obtain the correct focal spot size. Images were often blurred due to incorrect settings. The images also had to be developed and this often took several hours. For many situations it was impractical to wait several hours and, therefore, real-time X-ray systems were developed. These allow the operator to view images as they occur and give the ability to view the object or subject from different angles.

Figure 11.7 shows a typical schematic of an image intensifier system. The system comprises of the following main components:

- A cubicle
- X-ray source/gun
- A turntable and rack for adjustment
- An image intensifier
- A CCD camera
- An image processing system

The image intensifier type of system is often used for diagnostic or inspection purposes for specialist equipment or components which are used in the medical or electronics industries. This type of X-ray system provides a good clear image, but there is a finite time required to allow the image to be illuminated on the intensifier screen. The system is, therefore, normally used in a static mode where objects are placed in the X-ray cabinet and then observed

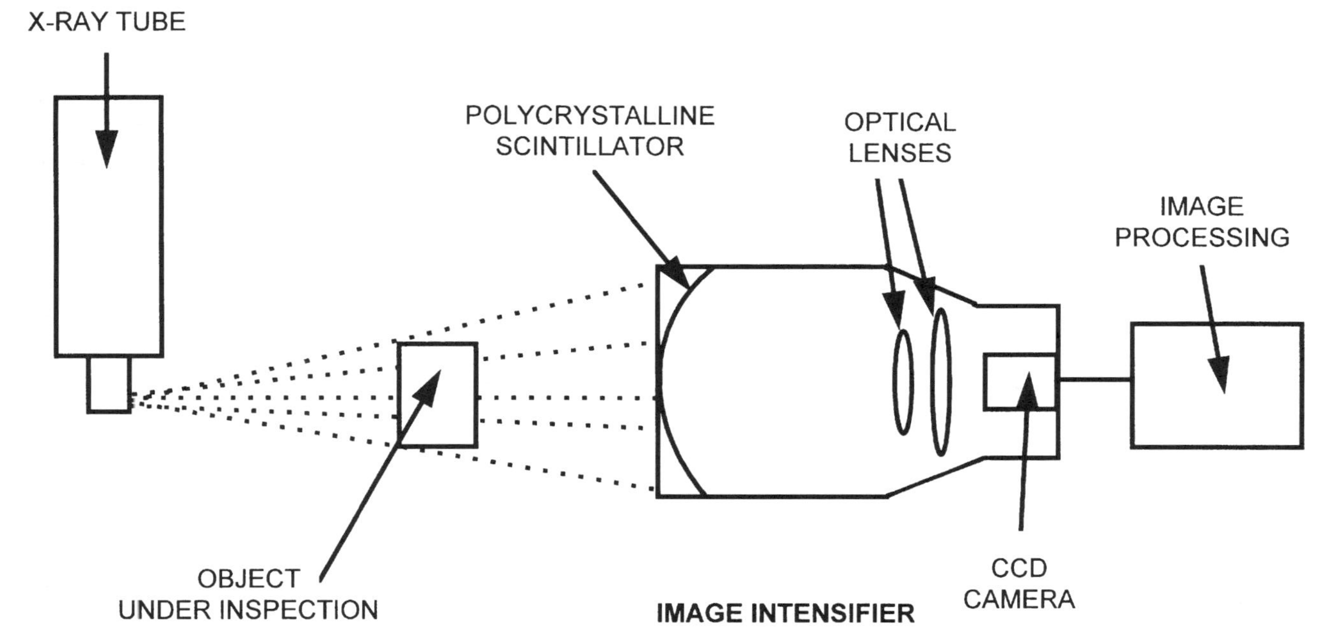

Figure 11.7 A typical image intensifier system.

after a short time has elapsed – objects are manipulated as necessary on a remotely controlled platform. The system, although operating in real-time, does not, therefore, lend itself particularly well to high speed continuous operation in a factory situation.

The image performance will be governed primarily by the focal spot size. The focal spot is the main contributing factor to the *unsharpness* or clarity of the image. The *unsharpness* can be quantified by the following equation:

$$U_g = \phi c/(F - c)$$

where U_g is the unsharpness, F is the distance from scintillator to focus, c is the defect to scintillator distance and ϕ is the diameter of the focus.

In order to obtain the best performance, having selected the appropriate X-ray source, scintillator and screen, one has to select the correct power (mA and kV), frequency (wavelength), and the value of c and F. Filters can then be used to optimize the image processing techniques. There are many standard algorithms available for these processing techniques.

There continues to be developments in the area of scintillators and the use of alternative materials to improve the sensitivity, and, therefore, the quality of image achieved.

11.6 Pulsed X-ray system

An alternative method which has not been fully exploited is the use of a pulsed X-ray system – this has the potential of allowing an image intensifier type system to be used for on-line inspection. An image intensifier normally requires the X-ray source to be on for a relatively long period of time (several seconds) which then renders it too slow for on-line inspection.

A pulsed system, as it suggests, uses an X-ray source which is pulsed for a very short duration, normally less than 1 second. The power level of the system is often higher than a linear array. The pulse period is sufficient to allow the scintillated screen to illuminate and the image to be captured. The image can then be processed whilst the next pulse is taking place. This system then allows images to be produced and analysed very rapidly giving cycle times of less than 1 second allowing line speeds of at least 60 objects per minute.

11.7 Morphology and processing of X-ray images

Lower cost X-ray systems tend to use the line scan system and just detect that there is a peak and set a threshold to determine whether the peak is inside or outside the noise level. This system can be effective for some contaminants but not all as there are situations where products may vary in thickness, shape, density or size, thus requiring the threshold to be continuously changed along with the power to enable the same level of detection of foreign objects.

Image processing techniques have been significantly developed over the past decade. Once an image is produced it is possible to carry out many mathematical functions (some of these are explained more fully in the section on vision inspection).

A morphological system (morphology being the study of the form of animal or plant materials) is a more sophisticated method of inspection. Rather than just using a threshold, the system can be used to look for particular features of an image. Filtering techniques can be used to assist with this. Electronic templates can be made which can be overlaid on the product to filter particular product features. This can be used for jars and cans where the end sections could prevent objects from being visible by X-rays. In subtracting a template from the image obtained one can then clearly observe the differences in a much clearer field. Having a clearer field of view allows one an improved field of vision and, therefore, better resolution. The example in Figure 11.8(a) shows an image of a bag of peas – if the regular shape of the peas is subtracted as shown in Figure 11.8(b), a contaminant is easily visible.

If specific contaminants are being inspected and they have a specific or even unique shape, size or density it is possible to utilize this knowledge within the inspection system. The process that could be used is to wait until the threshold system detects an abnormal reading, and then use a secondary image processing technique to analyse

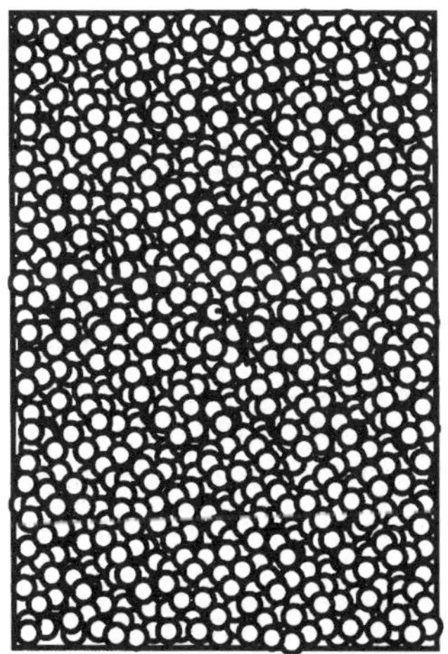

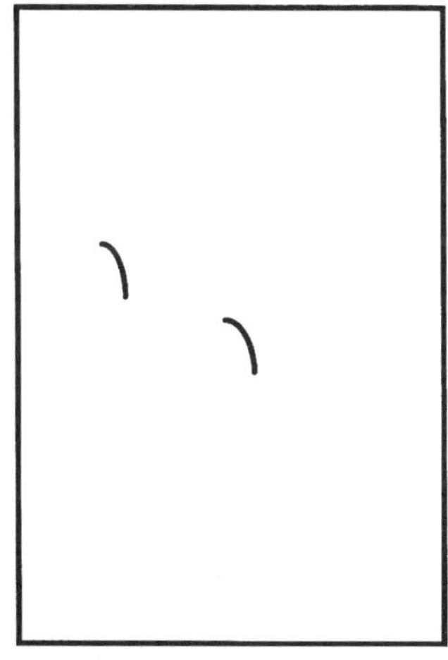

Figure 11.8 Example of an image processing filter.

the area around the suspected item and compare the image with a stored shape or size. A simple algorithm will allow one to count the number of pixels in a particular region which are of the same intensity (density). One can then use this as a measure of area or one could then calculate the area from the outermost pixels with the same grey scale. For specific products or contaminants this technique can work extremely well.

As an alternative to using a stored image of the contaminant for certain regular food items it is possible to form a stored profile which can then be used as a filter. This could be used for items such as grains, sweetcorn kernels, peas, etc. Once the regular items or items of the same geometry have been subtracted from the image it will then be possible to detect any contaminants 'hiding' within the regular product.

Product textures as well as shapes could be used to enable the inspection system to intelligently differentiate between what is a product shape or texture and what is not, and therefore deduce it must be a contaminant. Such use of image processing can be expensive as the processing has to be carried out rapidly if it is to operate on-line at acceptable line speeds. The costs are associated with the computing power required. A drawback to such technology is that food products change and for each product it would be necessary to create a new suite of software profiles. Although, if this could be automatically carried out the problem could be overcome.

The use of a morphological type approach can allow one to utilize X-rays for more than just foreign body inspection but also to check fill levels, damage to product or packaging and missing items or accessories.

11.8 X-ray scatter systems

X-ray scatter is an alternative form of X-ray analysis to that of absorption.

More recently, alternative types of X-ray systems have been developed in order to improve the performance and detection level, and reduce false detection rates, all at a lower cost level. The X-ray scatter system is a different approach to the use of X-rays in detecting foreign objects. There are a number of researchers working on this type of technology, but as yet no industrial production machine has been developed.

11.9 X-ray computer tomography (CT Scan)

The use of computer tomography has increased rapidly as computers have become more advanced and data processing times significantly reduced. Computer tomography allows the mapping of parameters in a two- or three-dimensional space.

One use of this technique is to use X-ray absorption. Beer's Law can be used to represent the X-ray absorption process:

$$\mu_a = \mu_s f_s + \mu_w f_w$$

where μ_s is the X-ray absorption coefficient, μ_w is the X-ray absorption coefficient of water, f_s is the volume fraction of pure solids and f_w is the volume fraction of pure water.

With fresh fruit, water is a major component and this controls the level of absorption and the signal observed. It is possible to use X-ray tomography to map the X-ray absorption coefficient μ over regions of the fruit or vegetables. This then allows one to observe small differences in structure. These techniques could potentially be developed to provide on-line analysis. The techniques have been developed by many workers for off-line quality inspection of apples, peaches, citrus fruits, etc.

11.10 Choice of X-ray system

There are now a reasonable number of X-ray systems available from different manufacturers. Most use similar technologies but some have specialized for detecting particular contaminants. In procuring a system it is important to understand the limitations and constraints of the system. Table 11.1 shows some of the typical key features which could be used to indicate the 'state of the art' machines which are available at the time of print.

The line speed indicated is that of the belt speed and the resolution is the smallest object detectable which is normally in terms of a spherical stainless steel ball.

One of the difficulties the food manufacturer faces is that in order to achieve the best results from the system one has to know the nature of the materials passing through it and to set the X-ray machine to the optimum settings in order to achieve the best inspection results. Some of the typical applications for X-ray inspection systems are shown in Table 11.2.

Table 11.1 Some typical key features of an X-ray machine

Type of System	Line speed (m/second)	Resolution (mm)	Cost (£)
Basic linear array	10 m/second	1.0 s/s ball	35000
Advanced linear array	30 m/minute	0.8 s/s ball	80000
Scintillator array	up to 75 m/minute	0.1 wire 0.5 s/s ball	+100000

Table 11.2 Some typical X-ray inspection applications

Contaminant	Products
Bones	boned chicken portions, meat cubes, pies, ready meals and mince
Glass	baby food, milk bottles, soft drinks, beers, wines and spirits,
Stones	vegetables, fruit and cereals
Wood and EVM	vegetables, fruit, cereals
Plastics	meats, confectionery,

Table 11.3 Machine design factors affecting X-ray system performance

Controlling factor	Key issues
Machine	speed of line operating conditions – power, resolution of machine – threshold setting reject mechanisms
Contaminant	type of contaminant – chemical composition size and shape of object density
Product	type and variation of product, size, thickness and shape density packaging material – layers of packaging

In order to select whether X-ray technology is suitable and what performance could be expected, one has to consider some key factors as shown in Table 11.3. These factors will be critical as to whether the systems will be effective but also to determine the level of performance which is likely to be attained from the system.

11.11 Operational and machine design aspects

Generally, those machines that have been developed are all very similar in design. Many have been applied to belt systems to be used to inspect bones in de-boned poultry meat.

The machines are designed as a complete unit with a conveyor mechanism as an integral part of the machine. The product is placed on one end of the conveyor, either manually or by an automatic transfer from another belt. The product passes through the machine and the machine then indicates if the product is contaminated or not. It is possible to link the reject signal directly to trigger a reject mechanism (Chapter 10). For meats the contaminated piece is usually removed manually. For glass containers an automatically triggered reject system is used in most cases. This is due to the higher speeds for glass containers, usually several 100s per minute, whereas a poultry or meat system would operate at 60–100 pieces per minute. The jars are rejected into an accumulation area. Some systems allow the jars to pass through the X-ray inspection machine a second time in order to reduce the number of false rejects.

Figure 11.9 shows a typical meat inspection X-ray detection machine and Figure 11.10 illustrates an X-ray machine used for the inspection of a product contained in a glass jar.

11.12 Safety of X-rays

Generally, X-ray inspection systems are very safe as they are designed with safety in mind. The main concern that operators have is the level of leakage they may be exposed to. Most machines will leak a small amount of radiation, a typical level is 1 μSv. At this level the operator will be safe. Some companies prefer to tag operators with radiation badges as this allows a measure of the level of exposure. Machines are built to a very high standard and have many safety features so it is most unlikely there will be any leakage, but precautionary measures are always wise. Due to the low levels of radiation used there is no residual radiation.

The X-ray systems are housed in lead-lined boxes which prevent any leakage. As the X-rays travel in straight lines the systems can be

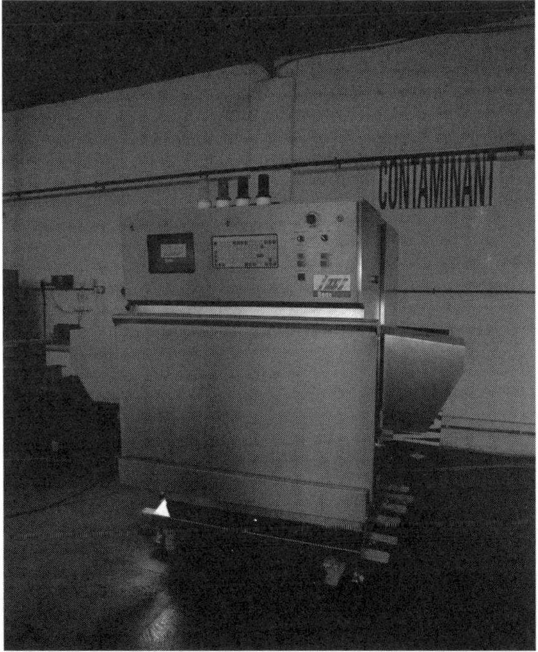

Figure 11.9 A typical meat inspection X-ray machine (IMS).

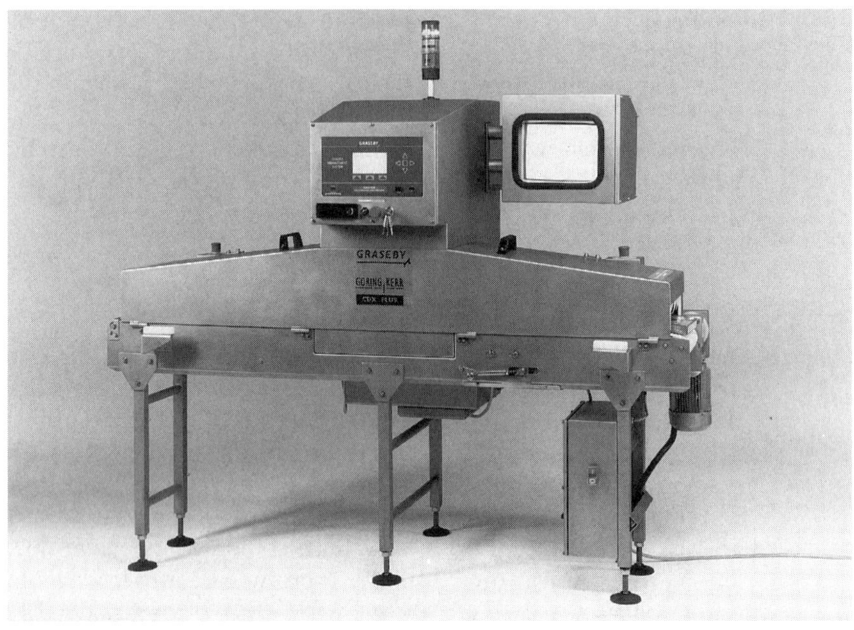

(a)

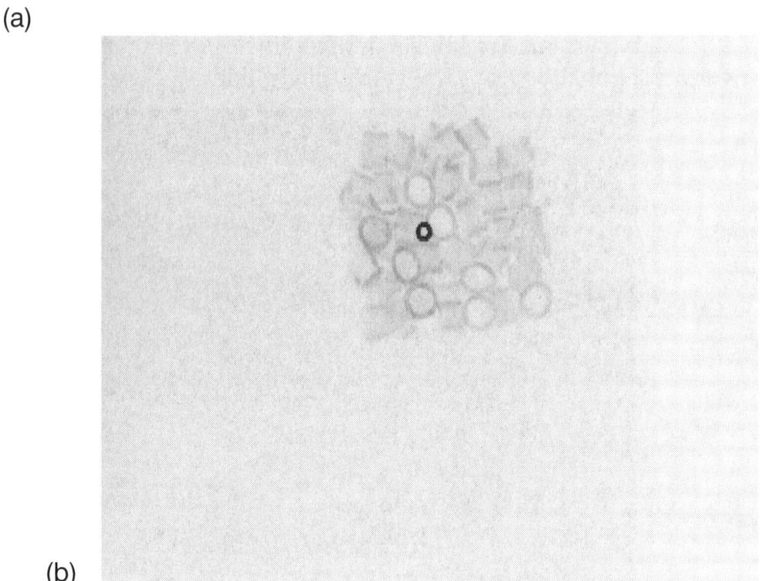

(b)

Figure 11.10 (a) X-ray machine for inspecting product in a glass jar (GKI). (b) Typical X-ray image (Elbicon).

designed using conduits to allow for cables in and out of the protected area without any leakage. Where a conveyor is used it either has to be raised or lowered after it enters the machine or an X-ray

Table 11.4 UK Ionizing Radiations Regulations 1985 specific doseage levels

Person	Age	Type of exposure	Level (mSv)
Employee	18 years plus	whole body	50
trainees	under 18 years	whole body	15
other persons	any age	whole body	5
Employee	18 years plus	individual organs and tissues	500
trainees	under 18 years	individual organs and tissues	150
other persons	any age	individual organs and tissues	50
Employee	18 years plus	lens of the eye	150
trainees	under 18 years	lens of the eye	45
other persons	any age	lens of the eye	15

protective curtain or double curtain has to be used. The machine has to be designed such that its safety mechanisms have built-in interlocks which prevent the machine being opened whilst the X-rays are on or started whilst the machine is open. Machine manufacturers also build in a number of other safety features to ensure that the machine does not overheat or fail in an unsafe mode.

11.12.1 Regulations

There are very specific regulations for the irradiation of foods. For example, the UK Food Regulations (Control of Irradiation) 1967 (amended 1972) states

> *No person shall in the preparation of any food subject it to ionizing radiation ...*

and

> *This regulation shall not prohibit the subjection of food to more than 50 rad (0.5 Sv) where the energy delivered does not exceed 5 000 000 electron volts.*

More recent legislation under the UK Ionizing Radiations Regulations 1985 state specific dosage levels (Table 11.4). These levels relate to doses over a calendar year.

There are also a number of general requirements which state that every employer should take all necessary steps to restrict so far as reasonably practicable the extent to which his/her employees and other persons are exposed to ionizing radiation. Employees also have a duty to ensure they do not knowingly expose themselves to ionizing radiation and should make use of any personal protective equipment provided.

Under the UK Health and Safety at Work Act 1975 employers have a duty to ensure the health, safety and welfare of all their employees. In Germany, the regulations do not allow foodstuffs to be irradiated using ionizing radiation. However, Article 47a of the Foodstuffs and Commodities Act allows products processed in one Member state to be sold in another Member state if they are a member of the European Economic Area (EEA).

The maximum level of 50 rad was also stipulated in a WHO Memorandum in 1990. The regulations state that escape from the system can be up to 1 mSv/hour, which is less than that which is emitted by some television sets.

X-ray systems are very safe and there is no cause for concern if safety guidelines are adhered to. The main concern for an operator is that the exposure limits are not exceeded. As the levels used are so low one would have to be directly exposed to the X-rays in order to feel any adverse effects such as radiation burns. The normal level of X-ray radiation for a foreign body detection machine would be of the order of 10–20 mrad compared with approximately 10 000 mrad for a human X-ray and 1 000 000 rad as a typical exposure for irradiating food. A typical medical X-ray system, e.g. a chest X-ray, will utilize a 150 kV/1000 mA compared with the 100 kV/1 mA typical food inspection machine.

In the USA, the Food Drug Administration (FDA) regulations under Part 179 of Title 21 of the Code of Federal Regulations (21 CFR) gives provisions for the use of irradiation of foods for production, processing and handling. The regulations are slightly different to other countries and the key figure is 1000 mrad – if the level of radiation is less than this no declaration has to be made on the food pack and the maximum dose allowable for inspection purposes is 50 rad. As mentioned above, the normal order of magnitude for inspection is several orders less that this limit.

The level of leakage permitted from an X-ray machine is 2.5 μSv/hour. Most manufacturers' machines fall well below this and are normally less than 1.0 μSv/hour. For added operator safety, operators could wear radiation badges which can be used to indicate if there is any leakage from the machines, although this is normally considered unnecessary as we are exposed to higher levels of natural radiation (which is 2.3 μSv/hour). There are a number of different badge types, but the most common is a photographic film type. This consists of a photographic film coated by two layers of emulsion and enclosed in a thin light protected housing. When the badge is exposed to radiation a latent image forms on the film – when developed, the level of darkness can be measured using a densitometer.

References and further reading

Anon (1973) X-ray unit detects minute glass particles, metal, stone (Borden Inc.). *Food Processing*, **June**, 47–48.

FAO/IAEA/WHO (1981) *Expert Committee on The Safety and Wholesomeness of Irradiated Foods*. WHO Technical Report Series No. 659, Geneva, Switzerland.

FDA (1997) *Regulations under Part 179 of Title 21 of the Code of Federal Regulations (21 CFR)*. Food Drug Administration, Washington, DC.

Frascatore, A. J. and Holston, J. A. (1955) Bone detection in fish by X-ray examination. *Commonwealth Fisheries Review*, **17**(11), 1–11.

HMSO (1967) *Food Regulations (Control of Irradiation)*, amended 1972. HMSO, London, UK.

HMSO (1975) *Health and Safety at Work Act*. HMSO, London.

HMSO (1985) *The Ionizing Radiations Regulations No. 1333*. HMSO, London.

HMSO (1986) *Report on The Safety and Wholesomeness of Irradiated Foods*. Advisory Committee on Irradiated and Novel Foods, HMSO, London.

HMSO (1989) *Irradiation of Foodstuffs*. House of Lords Select Committee, HMSO, London.

WHO (1990) *Memorandum*. World Health Organization, Geneva.

12

Vision systems

12.1 Introduction

The term 'vision systems' includes all the machine systems currently available which use light from both the visible and invisible spectrum in order to discriminate between foreign bodies and the food product.

The food manufacturer's objective is to supply products completely free from foreign bodies or as close to that objective as possible. It is what the consumer sees that decides how well this objective has been met. To achieve the same sensitivity and resolution as the eye is a technical challenge. In clear air, a candle flame is just visible, to the eye, at a distance of 10 miles: thus, 10^{-14} parts of light produced by a single candle is sufficient to stimulate vision (Fischler and Firschein, 1987, p. 214). However, for the reasons discussed in Chapter 14, human inspectors in the production process will not achieve the objective stated.

Secondly, the consumer senses foreign bodies in food through his/her sense of taste and touch as he/she eats the product. Some foreign bodies are hardly distinguishable visually from the food but are easily, often objectionably, sensed during eating, e.g. hairs and pieces of bone, particularly fish bone.

Modern machine-based vision systems achieve high levels of efficiency for the detection and removal of foreign bodies for many applications. Because they can respond to ultraviolet (UV) and infrared (IR) they are able to distinguish some contaminants by their visual properties that are indistinguishable to the human eye but which would be noticed by the consumer eating the product.

Work on the replacement of human inspectors by vision sensors could not start until the first photoelectric devices appeared at the end of the last century. The first patent for a colour sorting system was filed in 1907. The first practical colour sorters started to appear in the USA during the 1930s, in response to cost pressure, to replace human inspection of Michigan pea beans. The early machines were slow and dedicated to a specific product.

The first machines designed in Europe, by Gunson's Sortex, were introduced in the early 1950s. The first application was on peas, where rates of 100 lb/hour were attained. The introduction was justified on cost savings achieved by reducing the number of inspectors required, not on increased cleaning efficiency. It was accepted practice in those very early days to use a small human inspection team after the machine to carry out a final inspection/clean operation. At that time 'electronics' as we understand the term today did not exist. The technology available at that time was unable to achieve the reliability and sensitivity commonplace today.

Advances in machine vision systems have been the result of the development of technology in general and specifically that of photodiodes to replace earlier devices, the rapid development of charge coupled device (CCD) camera technology and the development of computers capable of processing massive amounts of data at very high speeds. In 1997 Herbert Fraenkel of Sortex Ltd estimated the cost impact of the developments in solid-state electronics has resulted in a 10-fold increase in efficiency when calculated in terms of the tonnage that can be sorted related to the capital cost of the systems.

Automatic vision systems are used in a wide variety of applications within the food industry including the detection and removal of foreign body contamination. There are several areas where they perform this purpose while at the same time looking for other faults, such as wrong colour in, for example, raw vegetables or for damage to the sealing ring on a glass container. These are not strictly foreign body contamination problems but as they are often carried out at the same time that contamination is removed they will necessarily be touched on. Specific foreign body applications include the detection of shells in nuts, residues left in containers, glass contamination in glass containers, glass and stones in rice, pods and stems in vegetables, and many more.

12.1.1 *Types of vision systems*

Within the context of foreign body control and prevention there are two types of task that can be carried out by machine based vision systems. These are the inspection and sorting of raw materials for contamination from extraneous materials, degraded material, shape and infestation as well as foreign bodies in general; the inspection of containers, particularly glass containers including recycled bottles, for production faults, damage during storage and transport, and contamination from various sources.

12.1.2 *Machine vision – special techniques*

As previously stated, machine-based vision systems are able to recognize the response of product to IR and UV light, and to work with laser light sources that are either dangerous to the human eye or outside its range of sensitivity. Machine-based vision systems detect the presence of certain faults and contaminants using these techniques. Table 12.1 lists some of the more common techniques and applications.

Laser light is able to penetrate some materials and the associated processing systems are able to measure the amount of the transmitted light absorbed by the product – thus providing discrimination based on the optical properties of the material, not reflection or colour.

When vegetable material is exposed to IR the reflected image appears at the white end of the grey (monochrome) scale. Other materials such as those of animal origin and stones will appear at the dark end of the scale, thus permitting automatic discrimination. Vegetable material which has started to rot will also appear darker than fresh material.

UV has the property of making some materials fluoresce, thus making it particularly useful for the detection of infested coffee beans. It is also useful for the detection of deer faeces which are a common contamination in the American cranberry crop and which are sometimes collected by the harvesting process used by that industry.

Instead of using the systems to measure reflected light, transmitted light can be used to measure transparency – the technique employed to find and remove the coarse undesirable parts of an onion which are opaque compared to the transparency of the good material.

Table 12.1 Special techniques used in machine vision systems

Material	Contaminant	Technique
Glass containers	washing liquids	HF
Black currants	deadly nightshade	laser light absorption
Tree nuts	shells	IR
Prepared mixed vegetables	snails and animal contamination	IR
Prepared mixed vegetables	stones	IR
Coffee beans	infested beans (stinkers)	UV
Cranberries	deer faeces	UV
Onions	root and stem	transparency

12.2 System components

The vision system process may be broken down into blocks of activity which can be identified as:

- The feed system: product presentation
- Illumination and background
- The sensor
- Processing the information and decision making
- Rejection

This is a simplification of a complex process that is in a state of continuous development. It is by no means exhaustive but provides a basis to describe the main features of vision systems.

12.2.1 *The feed system: product presentation*

In order for a product to be inspected visually, whether by human inspectors or machines, it has to be presented at the inspection point in such a manner that the whole surface is exposed to the sensor.

The method used will depend upon the application and the volume of material to be processed. Some materials, such as cereals, flow easily while others, such as diced raw vegetables, do not. Container inspection requires specific techniques. The main classifications are:

- Single stream of product in a chute
- Wide stream of product on a chute
- Product supplied by a conveyor system
- Container inspection

The various styles of machine which are described in section 12.6 tend to be associated with only one of the above methods. Details of their operation are discussed in section 12.6.

12.2.2 *Illumination and background*

Information about an object is supplied to the sensor by the light reflected or transmitted by the product. Cameras and sensors respond to a specified part of the 'light' band in the electromagnetic energy spectrum (section 11.2). This spectrum includes the band visible to the human eye, as well as the IR and the UV bands.

The principle of human sight is that light from the object being observed passes through the lens of the eye. An iris is located behind the lens which opens and closes to control the amount of light allowed to pass. The lens focuses the light onto the sensing surface (the retina) where the light is converted to signals which are transmitted to the brain via the optic nerve. The brain provides the information of size, shape, colour and movement the human inspector uses to carry out his/her task.

In vision systems the eye is replaced by a camera or sensor. The camera lens focuses the light from the object onto the detector which converts the light energy into an electrical signal proportional to the amount of light. This signal is processed, usually by a computer, to generate an output signal, which in the case of vision systems for foreign body detection is used to drive the rejection device. Both the eye and machine can only see the surfaces exposed to the direct line of sight. The use of multiple sensors to achieve all round images from the product is a technique used by machine systems to optimize results.

Both the human eye and vision systems are affected by the level of illumination. Just as with the human eye, there has to be enough light to enable the features to be distinguished. The light has to be of a colour that does not camouflage the product. The light must not be excessive or generate reflections. All factors which will hide the object to be viewed. The advantage of cameras over the human eye is that they can be constructed to 'see' using the IR part of the spectrum, which enables cameras to distinguish certain objects more clearly than the human eye.

Machine vision systems have a light source built in to provide the illumination required to optimize visibility. It may be incandescent, fluorescent or laser light sources, which can be selected to be polychromatic or monochromatic. The selection of the light source has a direct bearing on performance.

The object will normally be viewed against a background. The colour and reflectivity of this are an important factor in what the system is able to see. The background colour must be optimized to suit the specific objective. When differentiating good from bad product simply by colour, the background colour will normally be adjusted to match the colour of the good product. The setting and calibration of the colour background is relatively straightforward for monochromatic systems, but becomes increasingly complex when the system uses more than one colour. The calibration of background colour was a manual process that adjusted the contrast of the background to suit the product. This has been superseded by an automatic learning process using specified samples.

Consideration has to be given to the effects of ambient light on the sensor where the camera or sensor is not totally enclosed. Variations in ambient light intensity and colour may be sufficient to alter the accuracy of the result. Most modern systems have built-in compensation circuitry which continuously monitors the light illuminating the product and provides feedback compensation signals to the system. It must be recognized that while these systems are capable of compensating for large variations in ambient lighting conditions there is a limit to the range they will cover. When installing machine vision systems it is advisable to place them where the effects of strong sunlight are excluded or where stroboscopic lights cannot effect them.

To obtain the optimum results, the method of illumination has to be considered. The principle methods of illumination are:

- *Diffuse lighting*. In this case the light source is placed behind a diffusing screen. This method is useful where surface characteristics are important
- *Backlighting*. In this case the light source is placed behind the object so that a silhouette is seen by the camera. This is particularly useful where shape is important.
- *Structured lighting*. In this method points, stripes or grids are projected onto the surface of the object. The benefits of this technique are that (i) it is possible to obtain three-dimensional information from the way the light pattern is distorted and (ii) it establishes a known pattern on the object from which variation can be recognized.
- *Directional lighting*. In this case the light beam is controlled and directed onto the object to highlight surface defects by the scatter of the light.
- *Laser systems*. Laser light is a highly collimated beam of light immune to interference from ambient light sources.

12.3 Vision sensors

There are five basic methods of machine vision available:

- Photodiodes (single-point systems)
- Vidicon cameras
- Line scan cameras
- CCD cameras
- Laser scan systems

12.3.1 Photodiodes

Photodiodes have replaced the gas filled or vacuum tube photocells and photomultipliers that were originally used by the early colour sorters. A photodiode is a light sensitive electronic component which produces an electrical signal proportional to the amount of light falling on it. Most consist of a semiconductor *pn* junction (a type of semiconductor construction) housed in a container designed to collect and focus light onto the semiconductor material. By selecting a specific type of semiconductor material the response to light of a specific frequency range can be optimized, e.g. indium antimonide is one of the materials used for the IR spectrum.

A monochromatic system uses a single diode which will react to a single wavelength of light. Monochromatic systems work by measuring the 'brightness' of an image on the grey scale. They respond to changes in grey scale values, not the true colour of the object When sorting peas a single photodiode sensor will be unable to distinguish between a pale yellow pea which is undesirable and a green pea which has white spots that is acceptable. Neither will it be able to distinguish between dark green peas and peas with a red content in their colour.

By utilizing two photodiode sensors, making a bichromatic system, with two different specifications for the diodes, then the system will respond to two wavelengths of light. By measuring the ratio of the output from the two diodes a decision on colour can be made based on the ratios of each wavelength present.

Trichromatic systems are an extension of the same process, increasing the ability of the system to distinguish colour. Having a diode which is responsive to the IR or UV spectrum increases the capability of the system to distinguish good from bad product and foreign bodies.

12.3.2 *Vidicon cameras*

Vidicon cameras have been replaced by CCD cameras – a relatively new technology which overcomes many of the problems associated with the use of vidicon cameras. The operation of the vidicon camera is covered here as a basis for comparison with CCD systems to define why these new systems are finding increasing uses in industry. Vidicon cameras use a scanning system similar to the raster scanning system used in a consumer TV set (Figure 12.1).

The operation of a vidicon tube camera expressed in very simple terms is as follows. Light reflected from or passed through an object is focused by a lens onto a screen. The screen is coated with a transparent metallic film to which a positive voltage is applied. The metallic film in turn is coated with a photosensitive material (the target layer) which changes its resistance in proportion to the light energy striking it. The tube is surrounded by coils which are used to focus and deflect the electron beam generated by the electron gun to generate the raster scan. The raster scan is the continuous path the point of the electron beam travels as it moves across and down the

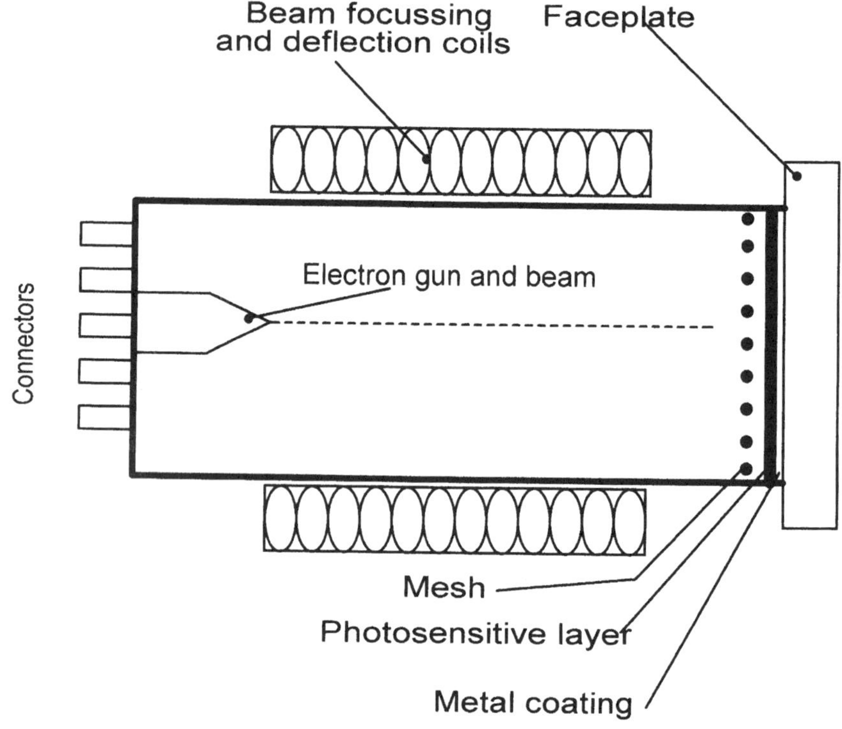

Figure 12.1 Schematic representation of a vidicon tube.

charged layer. The effect of bombarding the target layer with electrons is to generate a positive charge on the outer surface and a negative charge on the inner surface, i.e. it becomes a capacitor. Light striking the target layer reduces its resistance and allows electrons to flow to neutralize the positive charge in proportion to the light at any particular point on the target layer surface. The next time the beam scans the surface, the charge is replaced which causes a current to flow in the metal plate. The current is proportional to the light intensity – by measuring the current value and knowing the position of the scanning beam the circuitry of the camera produces a video signal proportional to the light energy of the image.

The vidicon camera has several limitations when used for industrial control applications. The use of a flat surface with a deflected beam can cause some geometric distortion in the resulting picture or data. The synchronization of the scan is critical. Errors in components or variations caused by temperature effects on the components can interfere with perfect synchronization. The whole assembly is complex and costly to manufacture. The electron gun requires high voltages to work and the heat dissipated by the gun requires the tubes to be warmed up before coming into operation. The provision of external cooling may be necessary where the application is subject to higher ambient temperatures. The system can be subject to 'burn in' when an image is viewed for a lengthy period of time. The average life of a camera tube is in the order of 1000 hours, after which it will require replacement.

12.3.3 *CCD cameras*

The lens of a CCD camera and its associated iris focus the image of the object onto a sensor, which is a matrix of minute photosensitive elements, photosites, from which a complete picture of the object in view is eventually generated in digital form. CCD is an acronym for 'charge coupled device', a term which describes the function of these cameras. Each photosite is a combination of a light-sensitive layer and a storage layer. Light strikes the photosensitive layer generating a charge which is stored in the second layer. Scanning each photosite in turn and reading the value of the stored charge provides electrical information of the image while at the same time discharging it ready to be charged again. The electrical charge collected sequentially at each photosite during the scanning cycle is amplified and passed to the processor. This process is similar to the raster scan made by vidicon cameras, but it is a solid-state electronic technique.

The value at each photosite can be identified by giving it a reference on the x- and y-axis, and this value can be related to a grey scale value. Hence a picture of the object under observation can be described digitally. Camera resolutions from 32×32 to 1024×1024 elements are available. The greater the number of elements, the finer the resolution. With modern equipment the image may be taken in monochrome or full colour. See Figure 12.2.

The advantages of CCD cameras are that they are robust, do not generate heat in their operation, do not suffer from geometric distortion and, because scanning is a continuous digital process, do not suffer from the same inherent weaknesses as vidicon systems. CCD cameras do not require changing at regular intervals as do vidicon cameras.

12.3.4 *Line scan cameras*

A line scan camera is a single line of photosites instead of the matrix found in conventional CCD cameras. This makes them particularly suitable for use where material is travelling under the camera on a belt or in free flow under gravity. The photosites are scanned at up

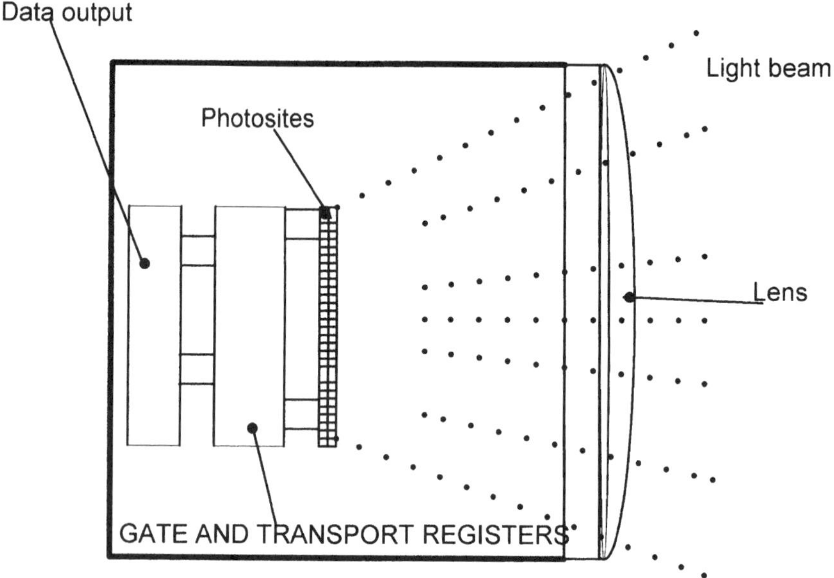

Figure 12.2 Schematic representation of a CCD camera.

to 2000 times per minute providing a very accurate image of the product.

A line scan camera which utilizes only one set of photosites is limited to a monochromatic, grey scale view of the image. By using cameras having more than one set of photosites the processor is able to measure changes in colour using a similar principle to that described for single photodiode systems. Response to the IR and UV spectrum can be maximized by selecting cameras specifically designed for the purpose. See Figure 12.3.

12.3.5 Laser scan systems.

Laser scanning systems use laser light sources together with rotating mirrors and multi-facet prisms. The light beam is reflected by the mirror which causes it to track in a straight line as the mirror revolves, thus producing a scanning effect. The beam is directed onto a rotating background roller over which the product under examination passes. Light is reflected back from the product onto the mirror and thence to a single point photo-multiplier where the reflected light value is measured in terms of photons. In some applications the light is able to penetrate the product, making it possible to discriminate between good and unwanted material on the basis of the amount of light absorbed by the different products as opposed

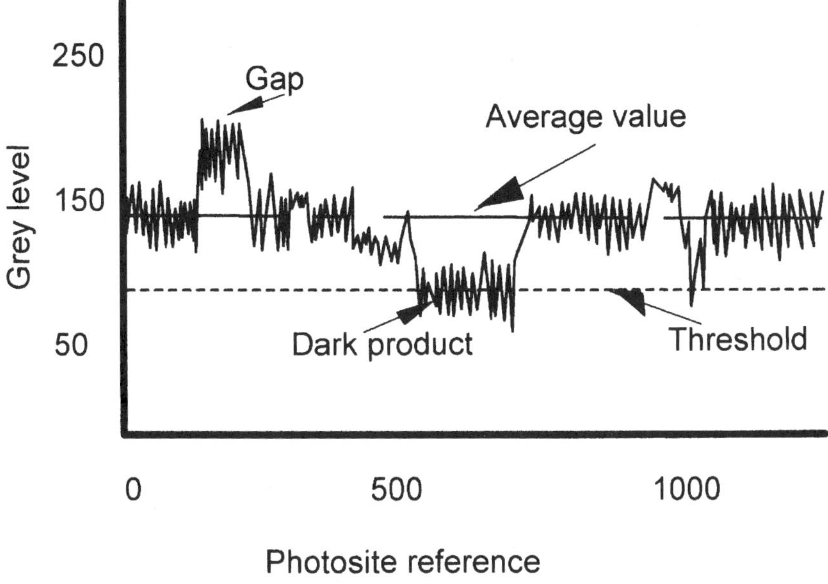

Figure 12.3 Line scan CCD camera output.

to the value of the reflected light. True colour inspection is based on the use of multiple lasers, each producing a different colour light with the proportional values of each colour being used to establish colour differences.

The background roller or drum is manufactured to have a colour equal to that of the ideal product. Where it is seen in gaps between the product, the information is used as a self-calibrating and monitoring signal.

The speed of operation of the laser scanning systems is limited by the mechanical engineering constraints of rotating the mirrors. In practice this equates to a minimum size definition of approximately 3 mm on a belt running at 1.5 m/second.

12.4 Image processing

While the function of the human brain in processing information is not understood, the human operator will learn to recognize exceptional or unwanted features of a product. Machine vision processors can be set to recognize some but by no means all exceptional or unwanted features of a product. Machine speed is limited by the speed computers can process the data. It is also true that the more complex the definition of the exception, the slower will be the speed of processing.

The difference between the combination of the eye and the brain compared to the camera and the computer is that the former is far more sensitive, judgemental and capable of continuous improvement through learning. The camera and computer are, however, much better at long-term repetitive work, particularly where the environment is uncomfortable for human beings.

The human operator has a series of outputs he/she can use when recognizing an exception, including manual removal, the operation of tools, the stopping of the machine and the voice. In most cases machine vision processor output is only capable of one output plus a record of the finding.

12.4.1 *Single-point colour sorters*

The information available from monochromatic single-point systems is the least complicated. Decisions on accept or reject will be made against a grey scale value with the background adjusted to match that of the good product. The latest 'self-learning' machines relate measurement of the product size made with the photodiode and the reflected light to eliminate the unwanted part of the signal, thus establishing the background match electronically.

When the system uses two or more diodes it is possible to make decisions based on a comparison of grey scale values. Each diode will produce a signal proportional to the light value it sees in the part of the spectrum it is selected to respond to. By comparing the relative values of two or more diodes it is possible to discriminate between products based on their proportional response. This technique makes it possible to separate pale yellow peas from green peas with white spots or reddish brown peas and dark green peas.

12.4.2 *CCD cameras*

The analysis of information derived from camera systems is a specialized subject. In the main most systems are monochrome, i.e. the object is seen in shades of grey. The sensitivity of the sensor or photosites is proportional to the number of grey levels that can be distinguished, normally 256 for industrial purposes, as well as the number of photosites in the scanned line or area.

The digital information produced by the cameras is converted to a form for image processing. The digital information derived from a line scan camera or a CCD camera defines the light value at a particular point of the object for computer processing. This is achieved by giving each individual photosite a digital light value [f] and a digital position value for a linear array [x] while in a matrix array it has two values [x:y].

Having defined each photosite or pixel, there are numerous methods of using the information to make decisions on the acceptability of product.

Thresholding is the simplest form of image analysis. This means defining a minimum grey level that must not be exceeded by any point or points in the image. The problem with this is that only a minimum can be used. For example, if it was decided that the minimum value was to be 75, anything with a value less than this can be rejected. If, however, the value was set to be the maximum, anything with a greater value, i.e. more transparent, would be rejected, but in practice this would mean that if any voids or spaces between items existed the whole would be rejected. Therefore on its own thresholding is not sufficient for many applications.

Image analysis beyond simple thresholding is a specialist subject and one which is still developing. Analysis techniques available include: smoothing edge detection, segmentation, texture analysis, perimeter measurement, axis measurement and measurement comparisons. These are only some of the techniques that have been developed. Their application calls for high levels of programming skills and hardware with very high speed processing capabilities. The ability of machine-based vision systems to duplicate the capability of the human eye is still limited by the hardware and the software available.

The output of the processors is electrical signals which are used to drive automatic rejection systems, and which are being used more and more as records of activity for 'due diligence' purposes.

12.4.3 *Laser systems*

The data available from the laser system can be used to establish colour differences in the same way as with any of the other systems, but as with camera-based systems the use of a controlled scanning system provides the same position data as that available from line scan camera systems, making discrimination by shape possible using similar image processing technology.

12.4.4 *Visual displays*

While rarely required in vision systems, the output of line scan cameras can be stored and used to produce a TV image of the product as it moves under the camera, each new scan adding to the last to build-up sufficient lines to form a picture. The output from a CCD camera can be directly viewed on a screen. These results are most useful if the result is to be viewed by an operator, but the principle idea of using cameras is to make the vision system automatic.

12.5 Rejection

Once an item has been recognized as undesirable it has to be removed from the line. Achieving this accurately requires fast acting reject devices synchronized to the movement of the product. The industry has developed special techniques, variations on the standard devices discussed in Chapter 10, to meet the specific needs of vision systems.

Multi-jet air blast systems are used to reject a discrete section from the width of the product. The operating principle is the same as that described in section 10.8.3 except that there can be 40 or more ejectors in a bank. These have to have a very fast response to operate with product falling under gravity.

Vacuum devices have been developed for use on the inspection of diced tomato, which is almost a pulp. This system uses a series of vacuum nozzles set across the width of the inspection belt which are individually lowered and activated as required.

For the precise rejection of glass containers, Heuft have developed and patented a special purpose rejection device which utilizes a series of independently activated fingers to reject the container without damage at speeds up to 1400 containers per minute.

12.6 Automatic vision systems

An automatic vision system will consist of one or more sensors or cameras and light sources, a product delivery system, and a reject system all controlled by a built-in computer system processing the information from the camera, controlling the reject system and sometimes the feed system, as well as producing information and records for quality control purposes.

There are four principal applications for foreign body detection:

- Single stream of product in a chute
- Wide stream of product on a chute
- Product supplied by a conveyor system.
- Container inspection

12.6.1 Single-stream systems: colour sorters

These are the first successful devices designed for the detection and removal of foreign bodies. A Sortex 3000 twin-chute colour sorter is shown in Figure 12.4. Figure 12.5 shows the principal components of a single-chute colour sorter. Product is fed into a hopper at the top of the machine. A vibrator feeds the product, at a constant speed, onto a series of inclined chutes. As the individual particles accelerate under gravity, they separate and pass into the inspection area. Figure 12.5 shows three single-point sensors arranged in a pattern to give all round view of the product. Data processing hardware linked to the sensors identifies any unacceptable particles. Air blast reject devices capable of operating at up to 600 times per second are used to divert any unacceptable particles from the stream. Throughput capacities up to 600 kg/hour can be achieved with a twin-chute system. Typical applications of this type of machine are in the sorting of beans and pulses, dehydrated vegetable flakes, nuts, and coffee beans.

The Sortex 3000 system is a bichromatic system to maximize the response to small changes in a particular part of the colour spectrum. As an option the unit can be manufactured to respond to the IR spectrum, which is particularly useful for detecting shell and some foreign materials.

The design of the machines incorporates automatic cleaning of the sensors, compensation for variations in illumination and auto-

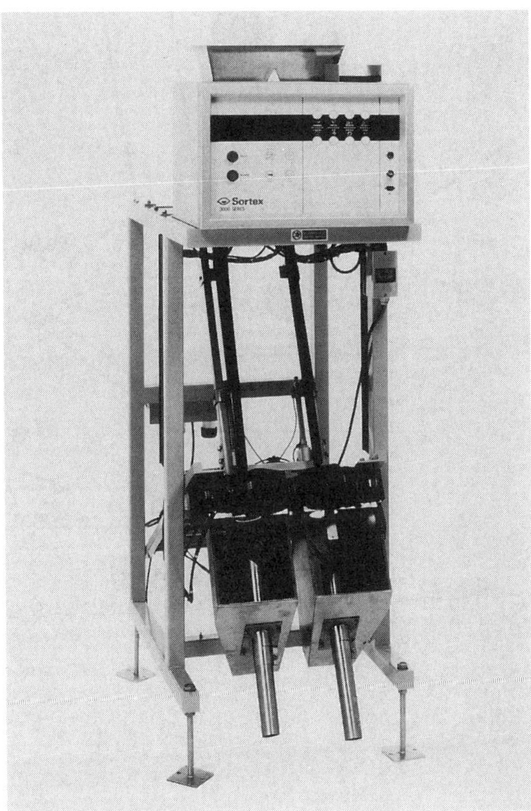

Figure 12.4 Sortex 3000 twin-chute colour sorter. (Courtesy Sortex Ltd.)

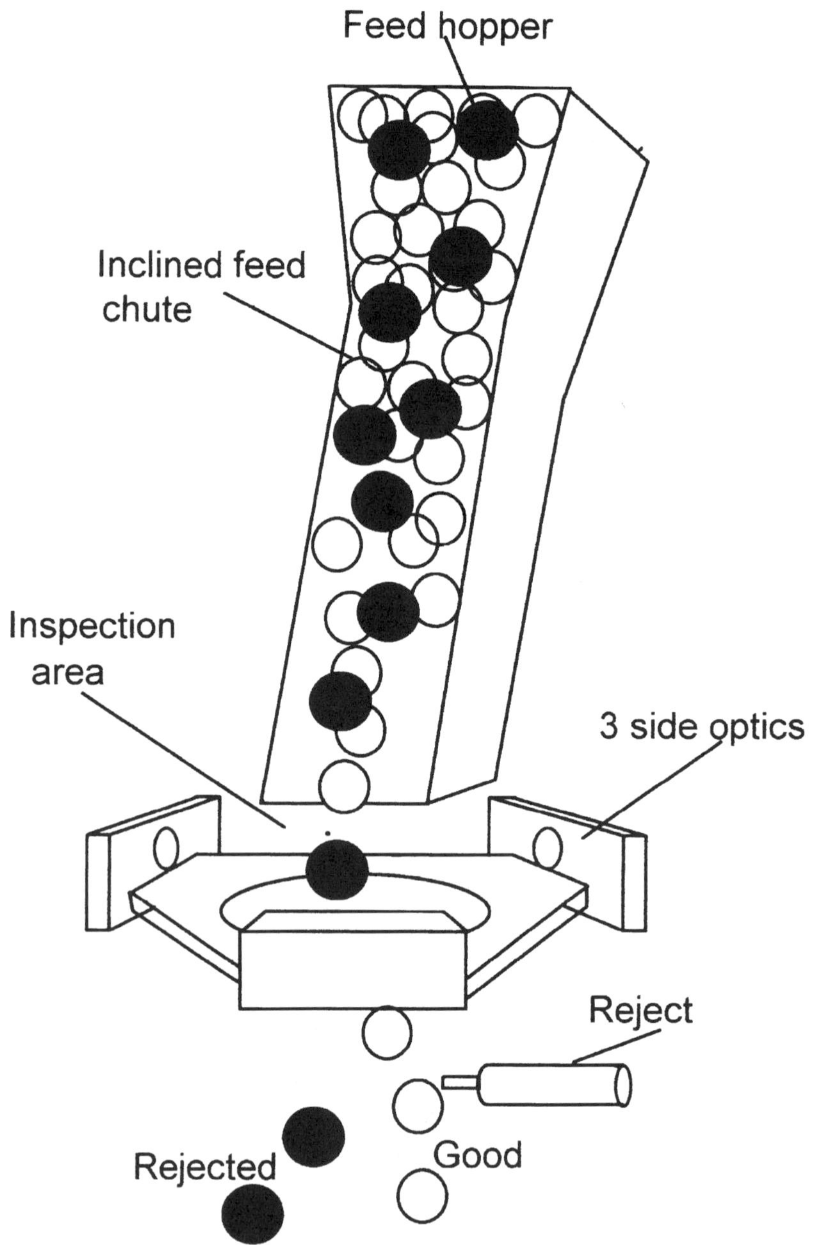

Figure 12.5 Schematic representation of a single-chute colour sorter. (Courtesy Sortex Ltd.)

matic reject systems. The latter are normally high speed air blast systems.

12.6.2 *Wide-chute colour sorters*

Wide-chute machines have been developed from the single stream machines in response to the demand for greater capacity. Figure 12.6 shows a Sortex 90000 high capacity colour sorter.

These machines use up to 1536 diodes and 96 ejectors, and are capable of handling up to 16 tonnes/hour depending on the material and the contamination problem. Inspection is carried out from two sides of the product stream.

The machines are equipped with automatic cleaning systems for the cameras, illumination calibration and compensation and automatic rejection systems.

12.6.3 *Conveyor system: colour, size and shape sorting using CCD line scan camera technology*

The increased use of mechanical harvesting of fruit and vegetables together with the introduction of more and more industrial prepa-

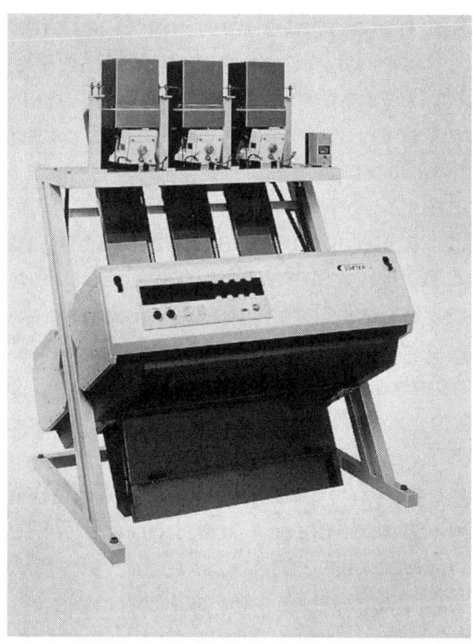

Figure 12.6 Sortex 9000 high capacity colour sorter. (Courtesy Sortex Ltd.)

ration of diced and prepared vegetables has led to a demand for automatic inspection methods to handle the increased volumes. The consumer has come to expect his/her food to be clear from all extraneous matter, and to be uniform in shape and colour. To answer this demand automatic optical sorting machines have been developed which use conveyor systems to deliver products which are not suitable for free-fall chute applications to the camera position. These systems are capable of recognizing undesirable particle sizes down to 1.0 mm – the exact specification will depend on the application.

Product is either fed from a hopper onto the belt, accelerated and spread into a single layer or delivered by conveyor with the relative speed of the two conveyors adjusted to give the same result. There are other ways of achieving the same result, such as using levelling bars. The setting of the relevant parameters is generally achieved by trial and error.

Once the product is separated into a single layer with each particle separated on the belt, it is allowed to fall from the end of the conveyor as shown in Figure 12.7. Product is normally inspected in free fall, although the systems can be arranged for the product to be inspected on the belt.

Figure 12.7 is a schematic diagram of a typical conveyor system. In this example only one line scan camera is mounted above the product stream to provide a view of one side of the product. Illumination is provided from above for reflected light. It could be from below when the product is transparent or the system could have cameras mounted above and below the product for a two sided view. Alternative versions can be produced using up to four cameras and IR as well as normal lighting.

The camera sees the product, and the information is taken and analysed in real-time by the processor; an output signal is then used to drive a reject system using air blast reject devices. Typical reject systems use 64 ejectors for a belt 624 mm wide or 128 for a belt 1248 mm wide.

The computer processors are capable of checking for colour as well as size and shape. For example, peas can be inspected for discoloration by colour, the presence of pods and stalks by shape and size, and foreign matter by a combination of both. Examples of detectable contamination are shown in Figure 12.8.

To achieve as close to 100% removal of contamination as possible, two or more systems can be used in-line. Where for some reason the batch is excessively contaminated by unwanted particles or there is a preponderance of difficult to detect particles, there are special purpose units designed to be inserted into the production line to take a sample automatically at a predetermined interval and to produce a report on the incidence of unwanted particles after cleaning. Where

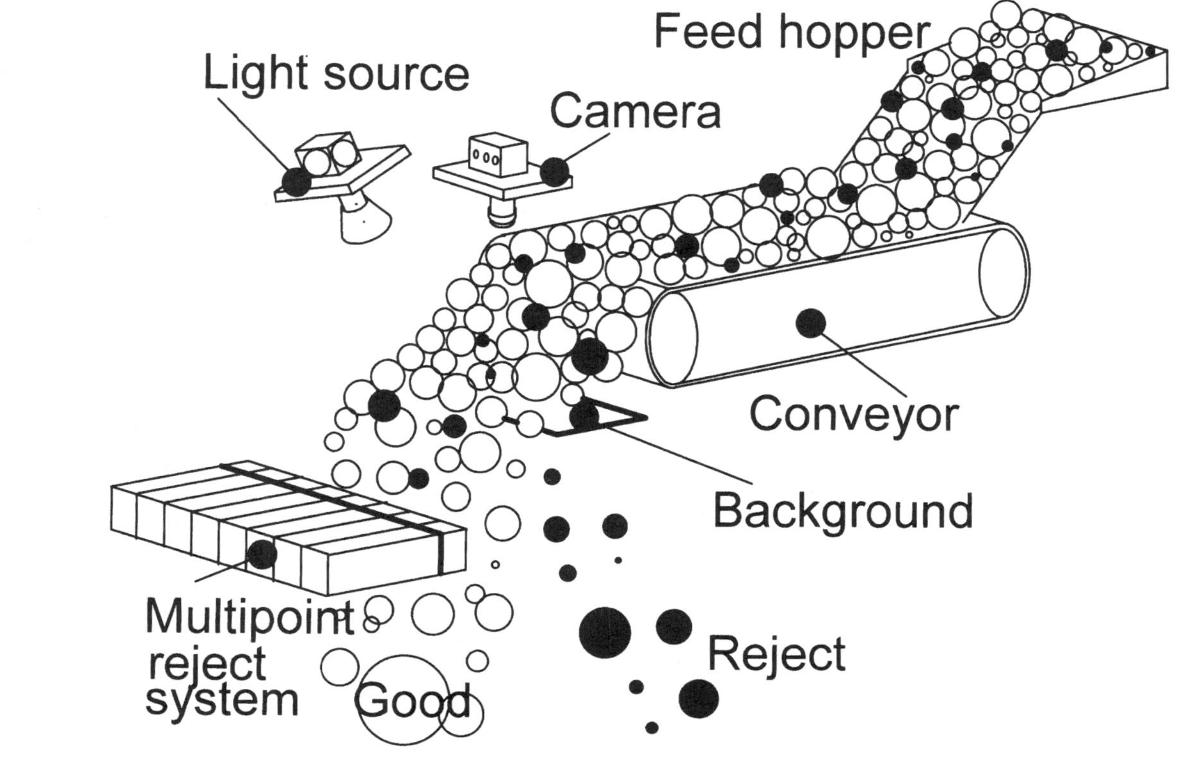

Figure 12.7 Schematic representation of a camera and conveyor system.

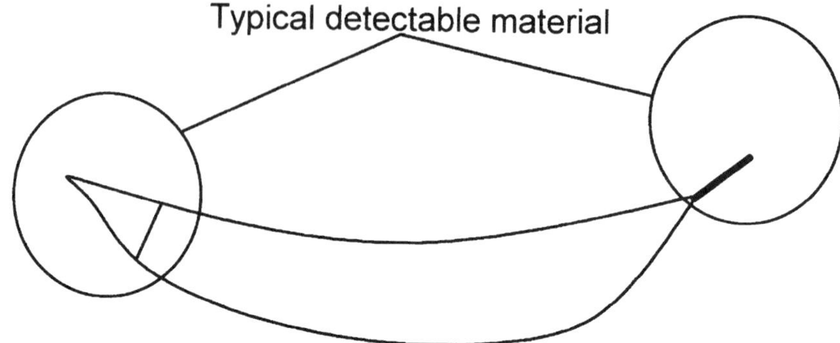

Figure 12.8 Schematic representation of detectable extraneous pea material.

this exceeds predetermined limits there is the option of re-inspecting the material by passing it through the system a second time. The equipment is designed with self-cleaning lights and compensation for changes in ambient lighting, or dust and dirt.

Laser systems are conveyor systems and except for the specific details of their optical systems are similar in principle to the systems used for CCD cameras.

(a) Special systems

Not all materials will flow freely when transported on a belt, and to overcome this problem Sortex have developed a patent delivery system which is incorporated into their Niagara machine (Figure 12.9). The material is delivered to the machine in the normal way and a horizontal conveyor is used to control the feed rate to the machine, material from this conveyor falls over the end onto a belt angled at about 60° to the horizontal. This belt controls the speed and separation of even the most difficult to handle materials ensuring they reach the same speed as the other product at the point they pass through the camera view. This ensures all material is inspected at the same speed and guarantees precise rejection no matter what the material. The system also allows the cameras to be mounted behind and in front of the material, not with one flowing above the camera, reducing the problems of keeping the system clean. Inspection uses line scan cameras and can be specified for colour and shape sorting. Rejection uses a 160 nozzle air jet reject system and has the additional facility of being able to sort into three streams, thus providing the opportunity to classify product into two groups as well as rejecting unacceptable product. Technology has been developed to ensure the air jet system of reject works on all product shapes.

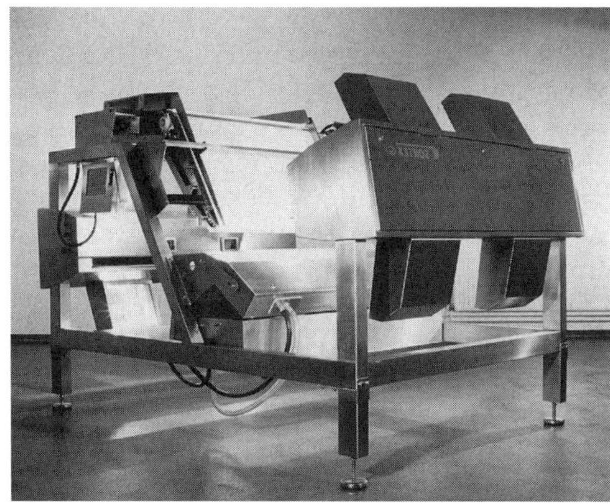

Figure 12.9 Niagra colour sorter and foreign body removal machine. (Courtesy Sortex Ltd.)

Other machines are available designed to control the quality of peeling. The systems deliver the material to an inspection point under a camera where the surface is examined and products with blemishes in excess of a predetermined size are rejected. These machines use rotating roller conveyors in order to rotate the material under the cameras in order that the whole surface is examined.

12.7 System capacities

The capacity of the various systems depends on the material to be processed, the amount of contamination present, the sorting task and the type of machine. The simplest machines have capacities in the range of 100–600 kg, while the wide belt conveyor systems are capable of achieving up to 25 tonnes/hour.

12.8 Container inspection

12.8.1 General principles

Bottle and glass container inspection using optical systems has developed rapidly since the first practical machine was developed by Heuft in 1982.

It is essential that before filling, containers used to hold food and drink are clean and safe. Even though the greatest care is taken with new containers, there is always the possibility of contamination entering the container during the manufacturing process, storage and transport. Glass containers are particularly susceptible to breakage, which can occur before and during the filling process.

Modern bottle manufacturing technology has overcome some of the problems associated with deformed bottles which interfere with the filling process, but there remains the hazard of 'spikes' which occur during the withdrawal of the plunger used in the moulding process and bird swings which may also break away leaving glass fragments in the product.

Glass containers are recycled. Bottles can be returned not only damaged but also with all manner of foreign bodies pushed into them. These may not be easily removed by washing or gravity, but it is essential they are removed from the container or the container removed from the line before filling. The washing process can also leave residual cleaning liquids in the containers.

A typical bottling hall layout is shown in Figure 12.10 for filling recycled bottles. The principles apply to the use of new bottles and jars in that the glass containers may need to be inspected prior to filling, which may include a washing point (liquid or air) prior to the inspection stage. The inclusion of an inspection stage to establish the correct size containers are on the line, stage 4 in Figure 12.10, is applicable to any line where there is the remotest possibility of the incorrect size container being loaded into the system as this has the potential to cause breakage within the process.

In the recycling process the activities are:

Stage 1 Crates and bottles are automatically inspected to ensure they are the correct type for the line. Usually in recycling this is the stage where other manufacturers' bottles are removed from the line. In a new glass container line this inspection point will be where the incoming containers are checked to make sure they are of the correct description for the subsequent process.

Stage 2 The crates are inspected to ensure the bottles are the correct colour for the line. The crate then passes to the unpacking position where the crate and the containers are separated.

Stage 3 The crates are passed through a washing line, and then inspected to ensure they are empty and that nothing is left in them which could cause filled bottles to smash when they are placed in the crate or to prevent them standing at the correct height to prevent breakage when the filled crates are stacked.

Stage 4 The empty bottles are sorted for shape, height, colour or damage. Bottles contaminated with solid detritus are emptied or rejected or returned to the line. The bottles then pass through an emptying station where any residual material is drained. The bottles then pass to the washing system and are transferred to the empty bottle inspection station.

Stage 5 Empty bottle inspection using automated vision techniques.

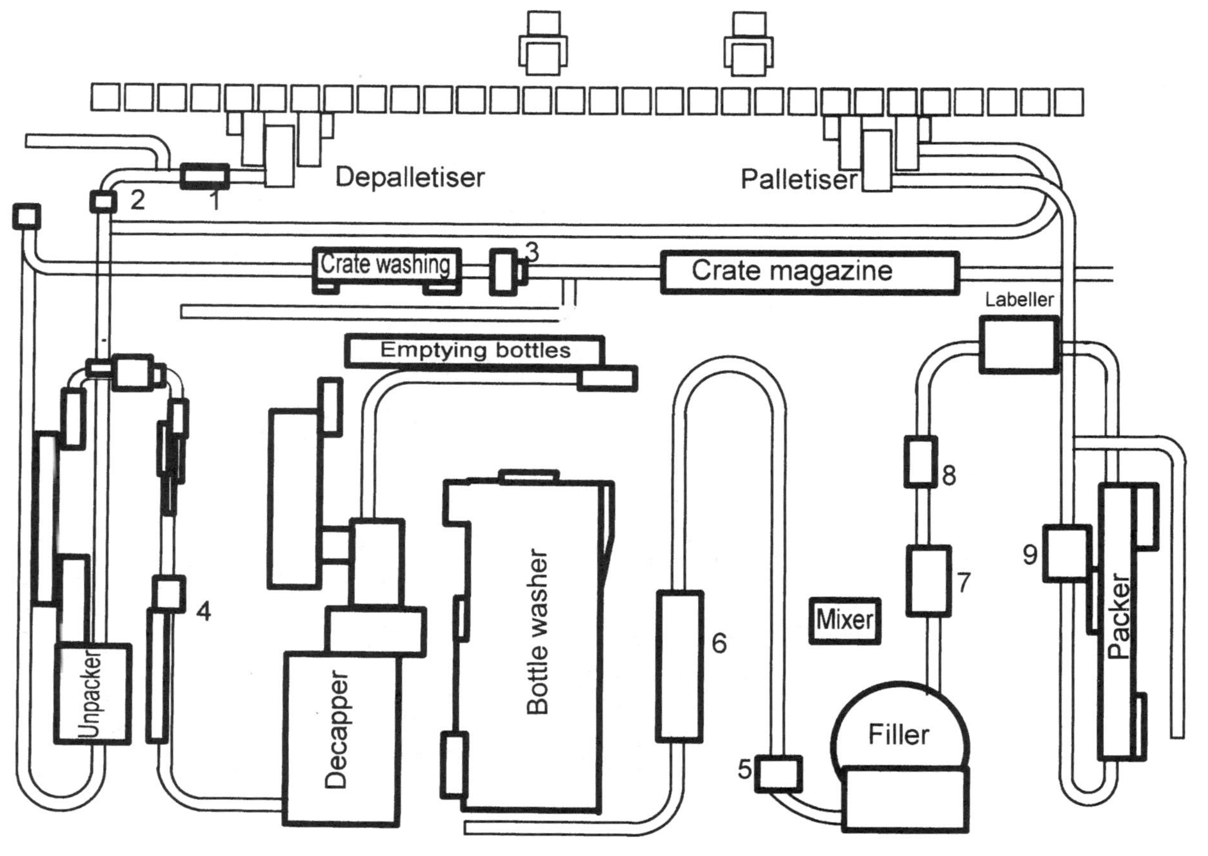

Figure 12.10 Niagara colour sorter. (Courtesy Heuft Ltd.)

Stage 6 Automated inspection for residual fluid where this is not incorporated into stage 5.

Stages 7–9 These follow the filling process and include checking fill level, labelling, and automated crate filling and check before passing to the palletizing or packing station. This stage may incorporate an X-ray system to check the filled containers for glass contamination from damage during the filling and handling process.

12.8.2 Container inspection

The automated inspection of glass containers will include all or part of the following checks.

(a) Base inspection (Figure 12.11)

The base of the container is inspected to ensure it is free from damage or faults either generated in manufacture or during use and transport in the case of recycled containers. At the same time it is inspected to pick out any contamination lying on the bottom of the container. The container is illuminated by a strobe light. (A strobe light flashes on and off for a predetermined time synchronized with the container movement. It provides the single frame image required for the image processing.) During the flash illumination the CCD camera and special optical module, in this case mounted above the container, takes an image of the base for the image processor. Control of the duration of the strobe light is critical in obtaining a sharp image for the best overall performance. Opaque contamination such as cigarette foil, drinking straws, etc., and some of the transparent contamination such as glass shards are detectable. By electronically manipulating the image to facilitate masking techniques, the image is compared with predetermined grey levels in the different areas, evaluated against standards and passed as a good or faulty container. This technique allows embossed marking and minor surface impairments to be accommodated.

The inspection process takes place after washing when the container is wet and there is a significant amount of water about. Techniques have been developed to clear water and any lubricants from the base of the container prior to the camera taking the picture.

(b) Side wall inspection

Side wall inspection is complicated by the potential for spatial contamination, i.e. contamination protruding into the bottle such as bird swings and transparent material adhering to the inner wall. The container may also have a permanent label on the external surface.

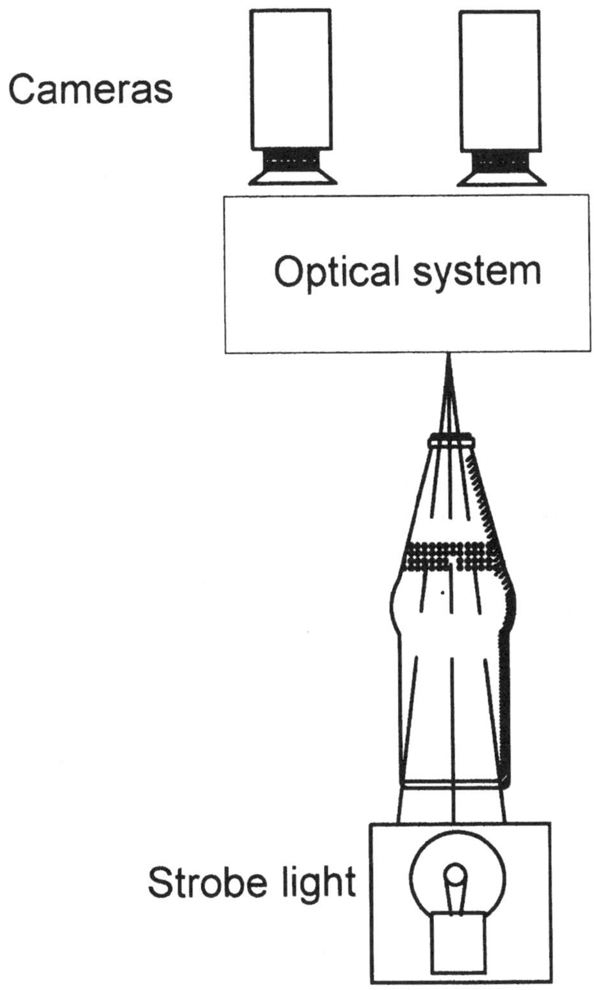

Figure 12.11 Base inspection. (Courtesy Heuft Ltd.)

For this reason the use of a side view of the container alone may not be sufficient to detect all the potential contamination and, therefore, it is necessary to examine the container both from the side and above. The same stroboscopic illumination technique is used in both applications.

To obtain images of better than 100% of the container when seen from the side, two side view cameras are used with the container rotated through 90° between exposure to each camera. This gives complete coverage of the container surface and interior as shown in the Figure 12.12. The image is seen by the camera via an optical module which optimizes the image information. Using masking techniques, the effects of external marking, labels and varying glass thickness as seen by the camera can be compensated for and processing decisions made against predetermined specifications. The images provided by the side view camera also provide the data required for measuring the degree of scruffing caused during repeated handling. Additional cameras and optical modules can be employed to detect the presence of mineral rings around the inside of the container.

Adding a third camera and optical system over the top of the container provides information on the condition of the interior of the container that may have been hidden to the side view cameras. This includes seeing bird swings, inner side wall faults and some contaminating materials adhering to the inner surface.

(c) Full thread check and neck examination (Figure 12.13)

Optical techniques have been developed to enable the condition of the thread around the neck of the container to be examined for damage or alternatively to examine the underside of the upper rim of a bottle for damage. This is not a foreign body check, but is important to ensure seal integrity of the sealed container.

(d) Cleaning solution

There is always a danger that some cleaning liquid will remain in the container after washing. Inspection to ensure all the liquid has been emptied from the bottle can be carried out using either optical images generated in the IR range or by the use of electrical signals generated and analysed by electronic capacitive devices.

Depending upon the nature of the residual liquid one of the techniques may be preferable. Figure 12.14 shows the relative sensitivity of a range of liquids to HF and IR identifying where there is a preferred technique.

The HF measurement is made by measuring the effect on a capacitive field by the container as it passes between the sensors. The results are shown diagrammatically in Figure 12.14.

IR measurements are made using the IR part of the spectrum generated by the base inspection strobe light. A special IR sensor measures the absorption behaviour of the container and compares it with the preset values of the standard sample container.

12.8.3 *Other applications*

While the emphasis in section 12.8.2 has been on the inspection of glass bottles, the same technology is applicable to other glass containers, although these are invariably new as opposed to recycled. Similar techniques have been applied to metal containers, particularly for the

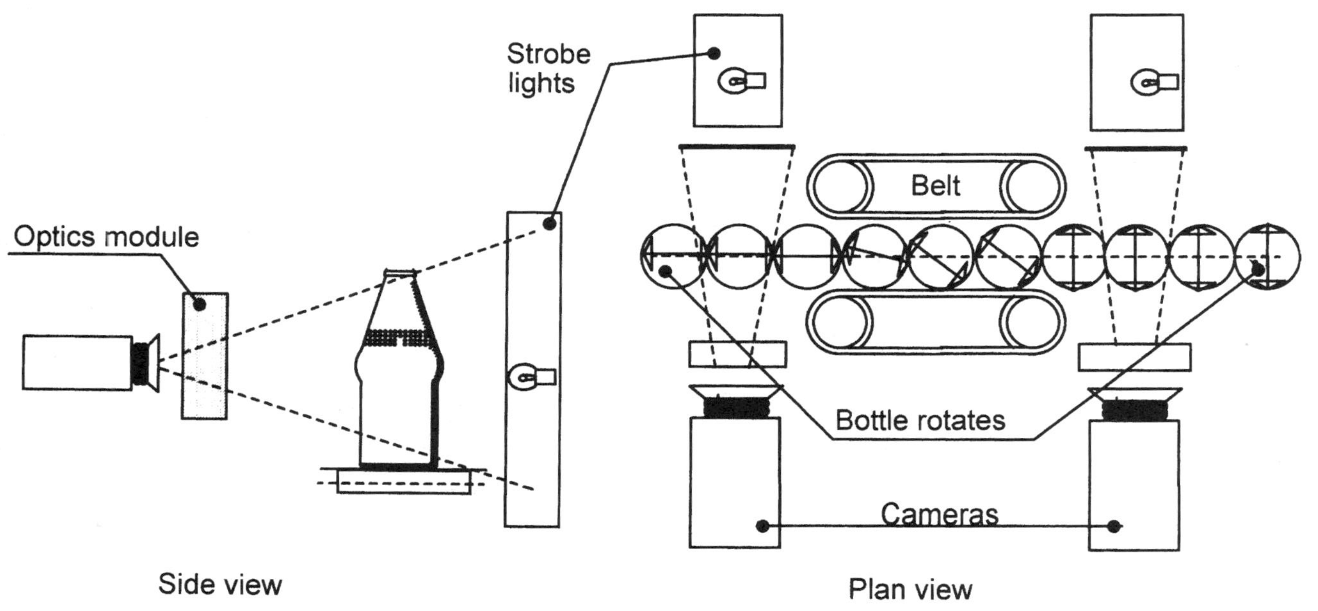

Figure 12.12 Principles of side wall inspection. (Courtesy Heuft Ltd.)

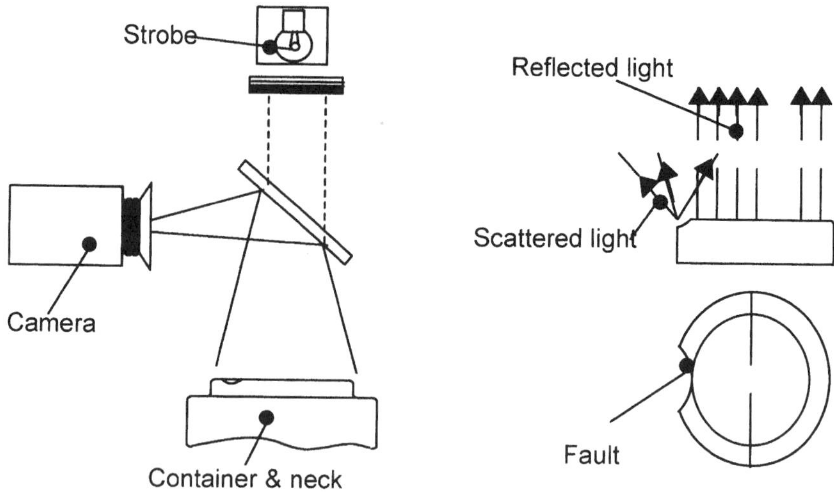

Figure 12.13 Damaged neck inspection. (Courtesy Heuft Ltd.)

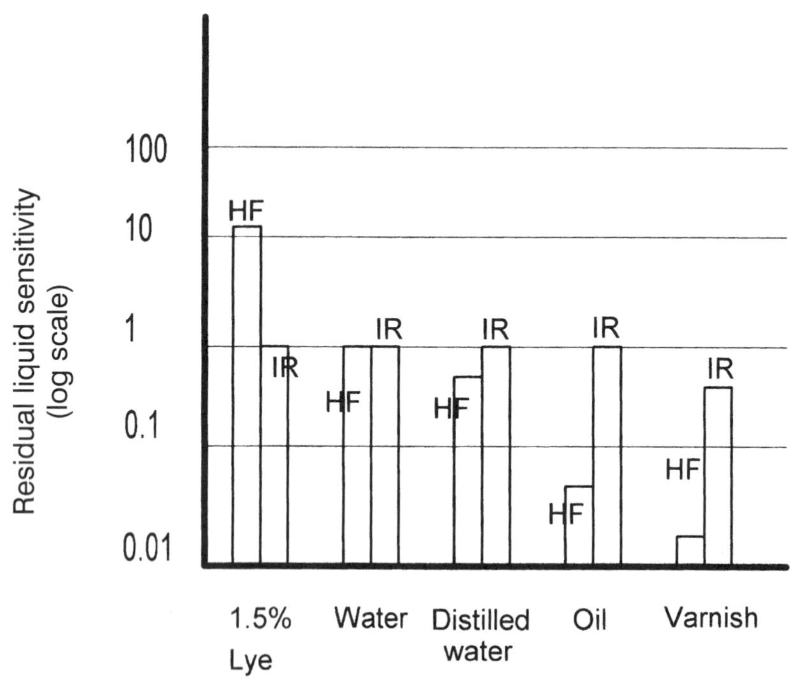

Figure 12.14 Residual liquid inspection. (Courtesy Heuft Ltd.)

examination of internal surface coatings using UV. However, the manufacture of metal containers has been developed to a very high degree and is a process which can be very precisely controlled, making the use of optical inspection systems generally unnecessary.

Metal containers need to be carefully stored to prevent the ingress of contamination between manufacture and filling, and they should be turned over to allow any solid material to drop clear after they have been removed from the transport/storage pallet. The use of an air washing process prior to filling may also be used.

12.9 Performance testing and records

12.9.1 *Self-checking and records*

The latest machines are equipped with a high degree of self-monitoring and compensation. Advances in computer technology have made it possible for machines to 'learn' the product and adjust the background to suit the application. Illumination values, including the ambient levels, are automatically measured and where necessary automatically compensated for by the system. Automatic self-checking of the various components of the system including the self-check system itself are available, ensuring long-term stability and reliability of the systems.

Dust and dirt obscuring the optical system can be compensated for to some extent and the use of automated cleaning of optical components is available.

The self-check systems are able to monitor the air supplies to the reject systems, although they do not monitor the actual functioning of the device in the same way as, for example, a metal detector (Chapter 9). Thresholds for rejection rate are set providing alarms when reject rates are outside preset values.

Depending on the manufacture and the machine specification, it is possible to obtain detailed records of machine performance and to download these to printers or central computers. Information of operation start/stop, rejection rate, faults, throughput, etc., is available. Machines are also able to store settings of specific products for instant recall and set up on product changeover. Test data is also recorded.

References and further reading

Chartered Institute of Building Services Engineers (1994) *Code for Interior Lighting*. CIBSE.

Fischler, M. A. and Firschein, A. (1987) *Intelligence, the Eye, the Brain and the Computer*. Addison Wesley, London

Fu, K. S., Gonzalez, R. C. and Lee, G. S. G. (1987) *Robotics*. McGraw-Hill, Maidenhead.

13

Foreign body detectors: testing, calibration and records

13.1 Introduction

Throughout industry all measuring and test equipment has to be calibrated to a known standard and monitored to ensure it continues to comply with that standard. Records of this information are central to quality control processes and essential to a 'due diligence' defence. This axiom applies to every industry, although the severity of the failure of measuring and test equipment on the end product and the user vary. The greatest dangers are in industries where death or physical injury are likely to occur as a result of failure in the quality system. The food industry is one of those industries.

The decision to use a specific type, or types, of foreign body detection machine will be taken as a result of an analysis of risk. The selection of the machine and its specification will have been developed and expressed in terms of the minimum size and type of particle the device can detect. In other words, a specification of accuracy and repeatability will have been developed.

Equipment calibration has two styles:

- The routine test (and where necessary adjustment) of the equipment to ensure it is capable of performing the specified task
- The regular detailed examination and calibration of the equipment to ensure that it is operating to the manufacturer's specification, together with the exchange of any components which have reached their predicted life

The three foreign body detectors which fall under this heading are:

- Metal detectors
- X-ray machines
- Vision systems

In many ways all these systems have similar test requirements and incorporate similar self-test and calibration features. In principle, they are all a combination of a sensor mounted on a transport system which in turn is fitted with a reject system to extract undesirable material. Similarly, they have very similar test and calibration requirements. For this reason the common features are discussed first, then the specific requirements of the individual systems.

13.2 Test pieces and test samples

13.2.1 General

The objective of all three of the systems under consideration is to detect unwanted material and to reject it. The minimum size of a particle and the repeatability have been specified. As has previously been discussed, none of the systems have the capability of detecting every contaminant – they are only capable of detecting particles of a given size, or larger, of a specific material. Therefore the first task in establishing a test procedure is to decide on the sensitivity required and to obtain samples which can be used to test that the foreign body detector is capable of detecting them.

The specification for sensitivity will normally be expressed in terms of metal spheres for metal detectors, although for some non-food applications this may be changed to cubes. The specification for the sensitivity of other devices will be based on the specified size, shape and material of predicted contaminants. In these cases, the sample has to be made or selected from available samples.

13.2.2 Metal detector test pieces

Metal detector manufacturers supply metal spheres of a known size and material, traceable to national standards, for use as test or calibration pieces. The manufacturers are now able to supply these spheres in ferrous, non-ferrous and stainless steel, in diameters rising in increments of 0.1 mm within the normal range used by the food industry.

The test pieces are normally mounted in plastic holders. This is essential to provide some means of identifying what they are and a means of handling them which does not have an effect on the metal detector.

Where the exact size required is not available, the manufacturer of the detector should be able to provide information which will allow a metal detector to be tested with a different size test piece from which the actual sensitivity can be calculated.

13.2.3 Other test pieces

Apart from glass, where some sizes are available as spheres, other test pieces have to be obtained by other means. The two most important factors are to be able to identify the material very specifically and to be able to quantify the size. For example, it is no use specifying a test piece as bone, it needs to be clearly identified by the type of animal, similarly glass needs to be identified by type as the lead content will have a bearing on its detectability by X-rays.

Where the test piece needs to be a regular shape, then it may be possible to manufacture it, e.g. a wire of a specific length and diameter.

Where the test piece needs to represent a naturally occurring object then either one needs to be found and preserved or a suitable alternative manufactured.

The important point is for a test piece to be available which is clearly identified, has a known specification and is available for use in calibration over a long period of time in order to ensure continuity of calibration and test.

The way the test piece is presented and how it is used will depend on the application. The selection, manufacture or other source of the test piece needs to be recorded.

13.2.4 Using test pieces

In all cases the detectability of the test piece will be affected by a greater or lesser extent on where it is positioned within the production material under test and in some cases by its orientation as it passes the sensor. The phenomena of product effect in metal detectors, aspect ratio in X-ray machines and other factors affecting detectability are discussed in the chapters dealing with each foreign body detection system.

The specification of the test piece will normally include details of how it is to be presented to the sensor, which has to be respected when using the test piece. With very few exceptions the test piece should be incorporated with the production material when it is used to check calibration of the system.

Ideally, a test sample should be produced which is a combination of the test piece and the production material, identified and reserved for test and calibration. Where the product is not subject to rapid deterioration and it is a single item or package, the provision of a test sample is straightforward. Where the product is subject to rapid deterioration, e.g. a frozen product, or loose or a liquid flowing in a pipe, the situation is much more complex and it may be impossible to completely provide a sample with the test piece in the material to meet the test specification. In these cases alternative solutions have to be found.

When testing liquids running in pipes it may be possible to enclose the test piece in a carrier that is neutral to the sensor, e.g. plastic in the case of metal detectors, and introduce this into the system. Where this is totally impractical an alternative solution has to be found, which may mean using another test sample presented to the sensor in some other way that can be demonstrated to equate to the production situation. In the case of pipeline metal detectors, for example, it is quite common for a metal test piece to be inserted in the space between the pipe and the aperture of the detector.

When testing powders in a free-fall situation with drop-through metal detectors or on line with vision systems, a sample may be put into the system and allowed to travel with the product to make the test, with the precaution of retaining the sample by a line to prevent it being lost in the product in the event it is not detected. With optical systems where the sample to be used to check the system incorporating a metal tracer without affecting the vision system is an ideal solution, then it can be allowed to flow freely providing a metal detector is available to pick out the sample should it be missed in the optical system.

Manufacturers of foreign body detectors have wide experience of the problems and are a good source of advice when designing a test sample. The critical factor is that the test sample used must be designed to duplicate the effects of the smallest specified contaminant the foreign body detector is specified to reject. When this is achieved and the test procedures are carried out efficiently the user can be certain that the system has performed as intended.

13.2.5 *Test samples*

(a) General

Having developed a test sample that replicates the desired test condition for the sensor, a procedure has to be developed to use it to test both the sensor and the rest of the system.

The test sample will have been designed to be clearly recognizable as a sample and it will carry markings identifying what it is. The sample, whatever its form, will normally be kept near to the machine, and the personnel using the system and those responsible for the testing will be trained in its use and storage. Where the sample is only a test piece in a holder, then the test procedure will specify how this is to be incorporated into the product. This information will be readily available to all personnel.

The objective of a performance test is to duplicate production conditions in order to verify that the complete system is capable of detecting and rejecting to the standard specified in the quality plan. Taking a sample and pushing it through by hand is not a suitable method. Safety devices and safety training prevent placing hands and arms in an X-ray machines. The human body and its clothing will affect the performance of metal detectors and vision systems, and must be kept clear of these and other devices. Therefore, the samples should be placed in the normal product flow and passage of the sample observed as it passes through the detection system to ensure that detection and ejection occur. Where there is any chance that failure to detect will cause the test sample to contaminate the batch, then precautions must be taken to prevent the danger of a test sample contaminating a batch. Mention has already been made of putting a metal tracer into a test piece for a vision system. Similarly, metal detector and X-ray systems can use samples which are gaudily coloured for easy visual recognition. Alternatively, isolate the machine from production temporarily so that any problems caused by the test can be readily dealt with.

(b) Long products

A product can be considered to be long when its length in the direction of travel through the detector is such that the position of a contaminant may cause it not to be rejected unless the time delay settings are specifically adjusted to ensure rejection no matter where the contaminant lies within the product.

In these cases the test sample should be made up with the contaminant located at one end which is clearly identified so that the test described below can be performed.

(c) The test procedure

The purpose of a performance test is to confirm the foreign body detector continues to perform to specification and that the associated systems are fully operational. The results are then recorded, which provide a permanent record of the performance of the unit which will be a valuable reference document should a situation arise where a complaint has to be investigated. Where the test shows the foreign body detector or its associated systems to be at fault, then this is recorded together with the action taken to prevent any product that has passed through the system since the last test being contaminated.

A performance test is made using the specified sample in the manner specified. The sensor will be observed to ensure that the test piece is detected, then the function of the rejection system will be observed to ensure the sample is ejected from the line into the reject container. Where circumstances require, the test may be repeated to check the detection of more than one sample when it is required. When the product is long it is recommended that the sample be passed through the sensor with the sample placed so as to present the test piece at the front and then at the back of the sample to ensure that it is rejected both times.

The results of the test are then logged manually or automatically depending upon the system.

13.3 Records

There are two types of records produced by foreign body detection systems. These are manual or automatic. The type of automatic record produced and the availability of central recording systems has been discussed in the sections dealing with the type of foreign body detector. Precise details of the systems will of course vary from manufacturer to manufacturer. Manual record systems will be designed to suit the requirements of each user and again will vary.

However, both systems have a common objective, i.e. to provide a permanent record of the performance of the system for future reference in the event of a complaint occurring. For these records to be most effective it is not enough for them solely to record that a test took place. They should include other relevant information so that if required the performance and efficiency of the foreign body detector can be demonstrated.

XYZ Speciality Foods ltd

Foreign Body Detector test report 1

Form No 1203
Issue 0005
Date 25.7.1997

Line reference						Foreign body detector identification 2			
Sample reference data 9									
			Settings 3				Test results		
Date	Time	operator	Air 4	Bin 5	Fault 6	7	Test 1	Test 2	Comments

Figure 13.1 Foreign body detector test report.

An example of the type of record and the points it covers is shown in Figure 13.1.

The heading of the form ① identifies the company and will normally have a reference or form identification number, part of the quality control system. Foreign body detector ② is where the type and reference information for the particular detector are entered. Sample ⑨ is the record establishing the references to the test samples. This may be a single item or multiple sample. Where relevant, it may also contain a reference to how the sample is used.

The columns headed date time and checker are self-explanatory.

The column headed settings ③ will be designed so that the condition of the essential settings before the test was made can be recorded. This provides a continuous record of the settings and conditions, highlighting either continuous satisfactory performance or when a potential failure has occurred. The design of these columns will depend on the application, although provision will be made here to record the product description where this is relevant unless the product never changes when this may appear in the heading area. Air ④, bin ⑤ and fault ⑥ columns are three common readings which will normally appear.

The final column contains details of the test result, good or not, and will often be for more than one test in order to check performance on different materials. The comments column is used to record the action taken in the event of the system failing, e.g. call maintenance or report to the line superintendent, which will then be able to be related to records held by other departments.

As stated previously, the precise design of the forms will depend upon the equipment, the application and the particular requirements of the organization, but will be designed to meet the objective stated initially.

A second form or additional columns may be used to record the number of rejects which have been taken out of the bin or otherwise identified by the system. This form should identify how they were disposed of. Ideally, this should be related to the system of investigation of complaints discussed in Chapter 14.

13.4 Frequency of testing.

There is a common idea that metal detectors should be tested every 20 minutes, which has tended to spill over into the ideas on supervision of other systems. This idea originated in the early days of metal detectors when they were relatively unstable and prone to drifting off setting. This was true in the days when the circuits included valves or in the very early stages of the development of solid-state systems. However, modern digital electronic equipment is intrinsically much more stable. Where any instability does occur, mainly due to the mechanics of the construction of the system, then the electronic circuits will automatically compensate for the instability.

Manufacturers provide information on the regular replacement or life of any components that deteriorate with use, e.g. the lights used with vision systems. This information should be built into the equipment test plan.

Equipment testing is in two forms:

- Routine testing by the operational personnel to ensure that equipment continues to be capable of detecting and rejecting to the prescribed standard
- Routine testing and calibration carried out by engineers trained to carry out calibration and to certify equipment is performing to the manufacturer's prescribed standards

The frequency of routine operational testing can be established empirically and then compared to the production process cycle. When equipment is new the manufacturer will normally recommend a frequency of operational testing. The results of this will be recorded, and can then be analysed and the information used to adjust the frequency of testing. It is a fact that the less often a test is carried out, the more thorough it will be and the more time there is economically available for the test to be made very thoroughly. When a test is required to be made three times per hour the work becomes a nuisance, particularly if each time the device is found to be operating correctly. Secondly, the test becomes careless as no one expects anything to be found, which leads to failures being missed. However, if each time the test is made adjustment is required then it will probably be carried out more thoroughly but at a cost which may not be economic and consideration to replacing the device should be given.

However, with modern devices that may well operate for days and even weeks without adjustment there is a maximum time which it is prudent to have between tests. This means that the practical maximum time between tests is that which is sufficient to prevent a contaminated product leaving the manufacturing plant. It is unlikely a situation will occur where the maximum frequency exceeds that of once per operational period or shift.

Routine testing and calibration is carried out by factory-trained engineers and includes the examination of the system to ensure all the automatic calibration circuits are operating within their range and that components are within their predicted life spans. The frequency of this work will vary depending on the type of equipment, but should be an annual inspection at the minimum. The record confirming the work has been carried out should also include positive confirmation of any critical values or component conditions. It is not sufficient for the report to confirm the unit was operating correctly and certain parts were changed. It must state the values or measurements taken which are critical to performance. Components examined for physical damage must be identified and a positive statement of condition recorded. This provides a positive basis for proving equipment is correctly maintained and operating to specification should the need arise.

13.5 System dependent features.

There are some specific points to be considered when setting up a testing and calibration procedure that are specific to the type of foreign body detector, these are summarized in this section. It is important to note that as technology develops these may change, and the advice and recommendations of the manufacturers should be sought before finalizing a procedure.

13.5.1 Vision systems

Vision systems are commonly used on continuous product flows making it necessary in many instances to halt the product flow before carrying out test and calibration procedures other than the passing of a test sample through the system.

All modern systems will have a system of monitoring the light value and compensating for changes in illumination caused by deterioration of the source or changes in ambient conditions. Where it is required to confirm the lighting profile is within tolerance, then the system has to be cleared of product and belts, etc., cleaned before the lighting profile measured. Depending on the sophistication of the system, this may need manual recording or it may be available electronically.

Many of the systems utilize multi-jet air blast rejection systems, which can make heavy demands on the air supply. A regular check of the operation of the system is required, as is care to ensure the air supply filters are regularly cleaned.

Where the systems record overloads, i.e. the material is carrying an excess amount of contamination generating an overload on the detection/rejection circuits, this should be alarmed and recorded with details of corrective action.

The frequency of these tests and examinations will depend on the application, and it is recommended that the manufacturer's advice be taken when establishing test procedures initially.

Units employing lasers will have specific safety legislation to adhere to and records of conformance to these, including any safety inspections, will be required.

13.5.2 X-ray machines

While the X-ray systems supplied today are designed to be safe in use and legislation requires the fitting of a range of safety features, in the UK all machines are required by legislation to be inspected and certified by a radiation protection advisor (RPA). Further, a radiation protection supervisor (RPS) will have to be appointed and trained. This training will cover all the requirements for safety testing of the machines and the requirements for recording the safe operation of the machines.

Other than the specific needs for safety, X-ray machines should be tested using the principles detailed in Chapter 13.1. As with any equipment, modern machines have much higher levels of self-calibration and monitoring, and are equipped with greater data delivery recording systems. Where the data is not captured and recorded electronically, then the test record required will be similar to that shown for a metal detector.

13.5.3 Metal detectors

The testing of metal detectors has been refined more than for the vision and X-ray machines because the body of experience with them is so much greater, as is the variety of applications.

In addition to the general points made in section 13.1, there are the following to be considered:

- The test piece should be placed in a test sample to test at the least sensitive position. The test piece should never be lain on the belt and, unless impossible to prevent it, should not be lain on the top of the pack.
- When the test piece is wire, care must be taken to ensure the orientation for test is as specified.
- When the system is subject to variable speed drive on the belt or stop start, the worst case scenario should be duplicated and tests taken at the extremes of speed conditions to ensure correct detection and rejection.
- Again, because metal detectors have been available for so long and the self-calibration features are so different, it is essential that the test procedure is developed to be for a specific unit as well as a line.

14

Human inspection

14.1 Introduction

It is human beings who are the final arbiters of what is acceptable. The objective of removing foreign bodies from food is primarily to protect the consumer from harm and secondly to prevent a product containing something that will be considered to be unacceptable.

Human beings have always been used in production processes to sort and clean the materials used. Large-scale industrial processing, made possible by the development of automation technology including cleaning and inspection machinery, has reduced the use of human operators and inspectors dramatically. However, there are still many situations where they are used. In the case of processing it may be because there is not a machine available, e.g. some de-boning operations. In the case of inspection it may be because there is no machine available able to perform the task, the cost of an inspection machine cannot be justified or it is the only solution to an immediate problem.

Where circumstances dictate the use of human inspection techniques for the control and prevention of foreign bodies, then as much thought and planning must be applied to what they will be expected to do as to the design of a machine. There is a branch of science specifically relating to this type of human activity, the science of *ergonomics*. The word ergonomics being derived from the Greek words *ergo* meaning work and *nomos* meaning law – in this case the relationship between human beings and work.

The objective of this chapter is to identify the principal factors which, if applied carefully, will lead to increased effectiveness of human inspection operations. It will also provide the basis for an understanding of the reasons human inspection is unlikely to ever attain 100% effectiveness. Much of the research work into the effectiveness of manufacturing and inspection tasks was carried out by the engineering industry during this century: Quality control and HACCP for the food industry have been developed from the work done in the engineering industry.

14.2 Human operators and inspectors – general considerations

Human beings are a disparate group. Some are short, some are tall – these are physical factors that affect reach, for example. Some are fit, some are not, which affects their ability to lift objects and, more importantly, will affect their ability to perform work at a constant level over a period of time. Some are young, some are old, bringing differences in motivation and sensitivity to the environment. Vision varies and colour blindness has to be recognized as a limiting factor to the ability to perform some inspection tasks. These and other factors have to be considered when setting up a process, whether in the context of the prevention of foreign bodies or any other operation. Human beings have to be considered individually not as a group with identical capabilities.

The major advantage of using human operators is their versatility in contrast to the fixed capabilities of a machine. Inspection machines in general will only look at one set of parameters and make accept/reject decisions based on predetermined levels of difference or contrast. Human beings have a judgemental capability and more than one sense available, which allows them to compensate for changes in the environment and the product which may occur during a production run.

The human senses most used in the detection and prevention of foreign body contamination in food are:

- Sight, used to 'see' contaminants in inspection and to locate items for removal in a cleaning process
- Touch, an important factor in a manual process facilitating the ability to pick up varying shapes and sizes

Sound, smell and taste are senses rarely used for the detection of foreign bodies in the manufacturing process, although they may be the sense used by the consumer in identifying the presence of a contaminant. It is the human ability to recognize differences which occur at random, which are unexpected or outside predicted parameters, which makes us so much more versatile than machines.

The human ability to recognize differences outside a specified range or to make judgements on acceptability without the need for close definition of rules is a positive advantage of human inspectors. This versatility means human inspectors can be moved around a process, undertaking a wide variety of tasks, something machines are unlikely to be able to do. Human beings learn by experience, build-up knowledge and are able to provide detailed information or feedback based on this experience.

The negative factors to the use of human inspectors or operators are their limited concentration span, susceptibility to interference and distraction and de-motivation. The engineering industry has found that in the worst cases the efficiency of manual inspection rates were as low as 35% and on average no better than 80%. Subsequent work to identify causes identified areas for improvement, but has not resulted in a method to guarantee 100% effectiveness, which is unlikely ever to be achieved.

To minimize the negative side of human inspection and to get the best efficiency from a manual operation the environment, both mental and physical must be optimized. This may seem to be an obvious statement, but so often the pressure to meet production deadlines or targets pushes proper consideration and preparation of a manual operation into the background. It is only when something goes wrong that we realize what could have been achieved if the operation had been set up with more care.

The main factors for consideration are discussed below.

14.3 Human factors

14.3.1 Age of inspectors or operators

When selecting personnel for manual inspection operations age in itself is not a factor. What is important is the physical and mental changes that occur with age and how these apply to particular individuals. For example, eyesight tends to deteriorate with age, but how badly it has deteriorated is not on a fixed scale. In any case, in most instances sight deterioration can be corrected by an optician. The important consideration is to select personnel for manual processes who are capable of the work. This may require some testing of physical and psychological attributes or careful review of performance to ensure the required performance levels can be achieved.

14.3.2 Concentration and fatigue

Probably the severest limitation to the effectiveness of human inspectors or operators in the production process is their concentration span. Most inspection tasks requiring human involvement are repetitive and boring. The result is that the mind tends to wander off into day dreams or the consideration of subjects of current interest, sport, relationships, money, etc., thus reducing concentration on the task in hand to the point where it is not performed efficiently. In inspection tasks faults or contamination are missed. Fatigue and concentration in most light industrial inspection tasks are one and the same thing for normal working hours. Where arduous tasks requiring significant physical effort are concerned the resultant fatigue can be measured and quantified. Fatigue from this level of physical exertion is unlikely to occur in the tasks concerned with foreign body prevention in the food industry.

When selecting a site for a manual inspection operation care should be taken to ensure that operator distraction is minimized. Locating a site close to a major gangway where people are moving constantly will tend to generate interference and reduce concentration. The site should not be isolated to the extent that the personnel feel divorced from the rest of the organization. In a workplace where sudden noise or other random bursts of activity occur, then every effort must be made to minimize the exposure of the operators to it. Equally, continuous noise will be found to reduce concentration.

The provision of music in the background can help to reduce boredom providing it is acceptable to everyone exposed to it. Where noise levels are high the provision of combined earphones and ear protection can be considered. Interest can be maintained or refreshed by the provision of fairly frequent rest periods and changing the task or position at suitable intervals.

Careful monitoring of the results will identify the best rest periods, task change and environment to optimize efficiency.

14.3.3 Vision

'Visual acuity' is a term used to describe the capability of the eye to see. There are three common types or measurements of visual acuity.

- The ability to see fine lines or small objects
- The ability to recognize space between objects
- The ability to recognize when one part of a line is slightly displaced

The degree of visual acuity is influenced by the level of illumination (although it should be noted that there can be too much illumination), the luminance of the object and the time available to see the object. Some drugs and alcohol can impair an individual's visual acuity.

About 6% of the male and 0.5% of the female population suffer from colour blindness. This usually means they are unable to distinguish between two colours, e.g. red with green or yellow with blue. It is rare to find someone who only sees in shades of grey.

Colour is a method of distinguishing a contaminant. Where a known contaminant will be expected to occur, then to improve detectability the contrast between the contaminant and the product can be maximized by selecting a specific colour for the light source to provide a greater contrast than normal lighting. There are light sources available commercially which can be switched to produce various colours of illumination. Experiments can be carried out to determine the best contrast.

It also assists recognition if the background colour of the inspection surface, or belt, is selected to provide optimum contrast. Conveyor belts coloured white, green, blue and black can be readily obtained.

Where visual acuity or the ability to recognize colour are important to the task, then tests can be readily carried out by professionally qualified persons.

14.3.4 Lighting

Lighting is probably the most important single factor affecting inspection tasks. Experience tells us that the brighter the light, the better we are able to see an object and discern the difference in objects. There is a law of diminishing returns to the effect that beyond a certain standard no significant improvement in performance will result.

The light effecting a visual inspection tasks has three components

- The light directed at the inspection point or surface
- The general lighting immediately surrounding the work area
- The light in the rest of the workplace

How the light is directed at the working point or surface is important. Glare must be prevented as this causes discomfort and distraction, reducing performance and concentration. Where there is natural light from windows measures must be implemented to prevent glare and reflections interfering with the inspection task even if this only occurs at certain times of the day.

The Chartered Institute of Building Services Engineers (CIBSE) recommend that the illumination in an inspection area should have three contrasting levels. The light falling on the inspection point given in Table 14.1 should be three times greater than that of the immediately surrounding area which in turn should be ten times greater than the lighting level in the rest of the workplace. A further CIBSE recommendation for inspection tasks in which colour plays a part is that lamps with a colour rendering index (R_a), based on Commission Internationale de l'Eclairage (CIE) specification 1A or 1B, be used. It is recommended that where an inspection area is to be set up on a permanent basis that specialist assistance in the selection and installation of lighting be used. Factors such as the glare index

Table 14.1 Recommended lighting levels for manual sorting

Task	Standard maintained illuminance (lux)	Limiting glare index
Slaughterhouses/abattoirs		
General	500	25
Inspection	750	19
Canning, preserving and freezing		
Grading and sorting of raw materials	500	25
Preparation	500	25
Canned and bottled goods		
Retorts	300	25
Automatic processes	200	25
Labelling and packaging	300	25
Frozen foods		
Process area	300	25
Packaging and storage	300	25
Dairies	300	
Bottling, brewing and distilling		
Keg washing, handling, bottle washing	200	28
Keg / bottle inspection	300	25
Process areas	300	25
Bottle filling	750	25
Edible oils and fats processing		
Refining and blending	300	25
Production	500	25
Mills		
Milling, filtering and packing	300	25
Bakeries		
General	300	22
Hand decorating, icing	500	22
Chocolate and confectionery manufacture		
General	300	25
Automatic processes	200	25
Hand decoration, inspection, wrapping and packing	500	22

shown in the table require specialist training for interpretation and application. Similar expertise or experimental results should be employed in the selection of specific correlated colour temperature light sources to maximize colour contrast.

Having established a satisfactory standard and specification for illumination, it is necessary to ensure that the standard does not deteriorate. Light sources have limited lives. Manufacturers of lights provide information on the expected life of their products, which is a factor that must be built in to a regular maintenance programme with changes of lights being recorded. Illumination provided by a light also deteriorates if the light source is dirty, therefore a comprehensive cleaning procedure must be written and records kept of the cleaning done.

Light sources must be selected bearing in mind the potential dangers from breakage. Glass bulbs and fluorescent tubes must be housed in shatter proof protective enclosures, protected as far as possible from accidental damage. Wherever possible, the light source should be mounted in such a way that even if breakage occurs the debris does not fall onto the product line.

Light sources and housings must be selected to meet the necessary IP standard to withstand the rigours of routine cleaning down.

14.3.5 *Heating and ventilation*

The conditions provided for manual inspection work have an effect on the efficiency achievable. Careful consideration must be given to the conditions the operators have to work under in designing a manual inspection station. Heating and ventilation have a direct bearing on performance. There are six main variables determining 'thermal comfort' for human situations:

- Air temperature
- Relative humidity
- Mean radiant temperature
- Air movement
- Metabolic rate
- Clothing

The American Society of Heating, Refrigerating and Air Conditioning Engineers (ASHRAE) defines thermal comfort as 'That condition of mind which expresses satisfaction with the thermal environment'.

There are standards published by ASHRAE and ISO setting out values to be applied to achieve thermal comfort and which provide a guide to environmental standards for human inspection tasks. The interpretation and the application of these standards is a specialized task to be undertaken by experts in the field. Consideration of the six factors noted above will include:

- *Temperature, radiant heat and air temperature.* There are requirements to be met under Health and Safety regulations applying to temperature which while satisfactory from a safety point of view may not apply to the conditions surrounding an inspection task. Inspection work stations should not be located near to the sources of heat such as ovens or at the lower end of the temperature scale near the outlets of freezers. The localized extremes can lead to discomfort and consequent loss of effectiveness.

- *Humidity*. A hot steamy atmosphere gives rise to excess perspiration which is uncomfortable. A very dry atmosphere dries out the nose and throat, which is again an uncomfortable condition to work in.
- *Air movement*. Ventilation is essential, stale air leads to drowsiness and loss of concentration. However, air flow must be controlled so that it does not generate draughts. The reaction to draughts will vary depending upon the person and wherever possible control of air flow or ventilation should be under the direct control of the inspection team.
- *Metabolic rate*. There is a difference in skin temperature and heat loss between men and women, particularly where the task is active as opposed to purely sedentary. This factor should be included in consideration of the effectiveness and motivation of inspection personnel.
- *Clothing*. The provision of adequate clothing where conditions are unavoidably cold is necessary, although every effort should be made to ensure inspection tasks are always carried out under comfortable conditions.

14.3.6 *Noise*

That noise has a distracting effect on performance is a subjective statement. As has been stated previously, sudden loud intrusive noises have a disturbing effect which may only be momentary but still sufficient to interrupt concentration and for a contaminant to be missed. Certain types of sound are more annoying than others, e.g. a relatively low level whine or the sound of dripping will annoy most people, affecting concentration and performance. The results of noise annoyance can be a severe drop in performance of an inspection task. As stated, what constitutes an annoying noise is subjective; however, where there is a complaint, then it should be accepted and acted on wherever possible.

14.3.7 *Other environmental factors*

Other factors relevant to the environment will affect performance and should be minimized or prevented as much as possible. Smells, for example – while we quickly build up a tolerance to some unpleasant smells their effect can be to reduce efficiency and to demotivate people. The general ambience of the site, the colour it is painted, the presence or absence of untidy stacks or of piles of boxes, the view, etc., all have an effect on operator performance. Every effort should be made to make the site of a manual inspection station as acceptable to the personnel working at it as possible.

14.3.8 Motivation

Motivation and leadership are two of the most complex factors in an industrial organization and are not a subject for detailed discussion in this book. However, without good management and a high level of motivation the efficiencies achieved by the personnel employed on an inspection task will be low.

Some obvious factors have been discussed which have an effect on motivation, good lighting comfortable surroundings, etc. The provision of background music may be advantageous, but this should be acceptable to the whole team – it is counter productive to have extremes of music at high volume forced on everyone. There are some other things that can be done to improve efficiency that are of a slightly different nature:

- Listen to what the operators have to say, listen to their suggestions and grievances, always ensuring that even if they are not acted upon they are not ignored.
- Watch the way individual members of the team work and where a preference is shown for a particular type of task always try to satisfy it.
- Inform those involved of the results of their work; let them see complaint levels even if these are only from the next stage of the process. Always strive to make everyone feel and understand their efforts have an influence on customer satisfaction.
- Where the inspection team identify a deteriorating drift in quality, acknowledge the information and let them know how their report is being used to correct the situation.
- Above all, listen and make every endeavour to build a team approach.

14.4 Training

There are two aspects to training where manual inspection processes are concerned, i.e. the training of the supervisors and the training of the operators.

14.4.1 *Training supervisors*

It is not sufficient to make an individual responsible for a manual inspection operation without proper training to carry out the task. Supervisors must be trained how to get the best from the staff as well as in understanding the technical side of the task. For this to be successful it also requires quite careful selection of the supervisor who must have the ability and the desire to take on the responsibility. Particular emphasis needs to be placed on the importance of keeping the designated records and the procedures to be followed when major process or quality faults are highlighted by the inspection team.

14.4.2 *Training operators*

The training of the personnel who will be responsible for recognizing and removing foreign bodies from food products is essential. The training should be documented, and carried out and repeated at regular intervals. The repetition process itself helps to improve quality as the practical experience gained will be discussed and then incorporated in the training programme for the future.

The prime objective of training operators in inspection and cleaning tasks is to clearly identify and differentiate between 'good product' and 'contamination', and the importance of the task. This can be achieved by discussion but needs to be supported by examples in order to establish common standards.

The secondary objectives of the training procedures will be to train personnel to recognize:

- *Excess levels of contamination.* Where these occur a review of the inspection procedures to ensure a satisfactory result can still be achieved or if a second pass or additional staff are required.
- *Errors in feeding.* Where the feed rate becomes excessive or the burden depth changes, inspection personnel must be trained to both recognize when these occur and in the corrective action to be taken.
- *Process faults.* Where the inspection takes place after a process, inspection personnel must be trained to recognize where the process has failed to achieve a known standard.
- *Equipment.* Personnel must be trained in the use and care of the equipment provided to assist with the detection and removal process and what to do in the event it fails. This covers not only tools but the equipment itself, e.g. conveyor belt condition or failure of a light source.
- *Storage and quarantine.* The personnel must be trained in all aspects of the disposal of foreign bodies removed by their activities, including the keeping of records where this is applicable.

14.5 Specifications

The various factors impacting on the efficiency of human beings in the production process, including inspection, have been discussed. Whatever these may be, they cannot be judged unless clear specifications of the task, the equipment and relevant records are available.

The decision to use a manual inspection station will have been taken to satisfy a need of the process in order to provide a safe final product acceptable to the consumer. Therefore, a general statement such as 'clean all the contaminants from the material' is unsatisfactory. The objective of the task needs to be clearly defined. As an example, manually inspecting dry kibbled onions could be defined as 'remove any particles which are darker than the samples provided'. This statement does not include the removal of metal contaminants derived from the drying belts or process as these would normally be removed by using a metal detector. It does, however, establish a specification for colour by reference to a fixed standard.

The basis for the definition of the specification should be recorded.

14.6 Equipment

Most benches and conveyors are provided with a working height of 840 mm. The statement 'Human beings are a disparate group' quoted earlier is particularly relevant when it comes to the choice and specification of equipment. To set standard equipment heights may be an attractive idea, but unless this can be accompanied by standard size inspectors it is impractical. This applies to both standing and sitting. Provision must be made for working heights to be adjustable to minimize discomfort and fatigue.

For any inspection operation that continues for more than a few minutes it is preferable for the inspector to be seated. Standing is much more fatiguing than sitting and, as previously stated, fatigue leads to loss of effectiveness. The design of the working position should be thought out. The seat needs to be properly designed and in good condition – an old decrepit stool is not sufficient for best results. Ideally the seat should provide even support across the buttocks and thighs, without digging in to the thigh, and allow the feet to rest naturally on the floor. Where the working height does not allow this, then foot rests which allow the foot to rest naturally should be provided. Where twisting or turning cannot be avoided in carrying out the task, then swivel chairs must be available. The design of seating is an area of ergonomics that has received much attention, as a consequence there are specialist suppliers able to offer a wide range of seating to suit specific applications whose advice should be sought. The seats, which will be in use continually for long periods, must be regularly inspected, maintained if possible, and replaced when worn out and no longer doing the job originally specified.

Where standing is essential due to the physical nature of the task, then allowance must be made for adequate rest periods if constant performance is to be achieved. Where footwear is provided, this must be comfortable as well as meeting hygiene requirements. Where the environment is wet, then the footwear must be waterproof and as wet usually goes with cold then the design of thermal insulation needs to be adequate for the conditions.

Clothing must be comfortable and non-restrictive. The normal rules for buttons and pockets must be applied. In some cases these are even more important on inspection processes as not only does the inspector sometimes need to reach over the product but there may be no subsequent inspection to spot something that has fallen into the product.

Tools and instruments used must be convenient and as light as possible to minimize fatigue. Wherever possible, tools should be chosen with the best ergonomic design, the easiest to control, most comfortable to handle and most easy to manoeuvre. Where the use of heavy tools cannot be avoided, then counterbalance supports are recommended to reduce fatigue. Tools used in the process are prone to fall into or onto the material or lose components. Records of tool issue, return and replacement should be kept, and procedures implemented to ensure no tool or component is lost in the process.

The design of work benches and conveyors must meet all the requirements of the machinery safety directives, with particular emphasis on design to prevent foreign bodies falling into the product from any part of the mechanism. Care must be taken to remove any structures, particularly those over the product that can be used to leave or deposit tools, pens, etc. The design of anything that is essential to be mounted over the product, side guides, levelling blades, etc., should remove or minimize the possibility of its components becoming contaminants, using welding instead of fasteners as much as possible. Where there is the slightest danger, then a recorded procedure should be introduced for regular inspection of the danger point. Particularly with conveyors, belt runs should be arranged to minimize the chances of components being picked up on the belt surface as it passes inside the frame of the machine.

As most inspection is a visual task, the design of the system must be such that the product is in a single layer. The single layer can be achieved on conveyor systems by the use of height control bars over the belt or by controlling the aperture of the discharge chute from a hopper.

Where the contaminant is part of the product or adheres to the product, then it will be necessary to rotate the product so that the whole surface is exposed. The forces acting on a round body on a moving conveyor will cause rolling to occur naturally in some cases. Roll-over can be induced by allowing the product to drop over a weir formed between two sections of conveyor or by having a contra rotating roller or contra travel belt mounted over the conveyor to impart a turning motion. A similar effect can sometimes be achieved with a vibratory conveyor.

A human inspector will have a natural restriction to the area of product to be inspected continuously. This applies particularly to moving belts. The size or length an inspector can handle will depend on the comparative differences between the product and the contaminant, the speed it travels at and the disruptive effect of the removal process. The ideal combination of belt speed and area to be controlled will depend on the application. Generally the inspector's area should be limited to about 50 cm of belt length and a width. The precise definition will need to be arrived at by experiment.

14.7 System supervision, review and testing

As with any quality control process, the concept of continual improvement is essential to manual inspection processes. As stated earlier, 100% effectiveness will not be achieved. The system has to be set up and the effectiveness measured, either by sampling or by analysis of complaints depending on the application.

Sampling is unlikely to be an effective tool for measuring the effectiveness of extrinsic contamination removal. The reason being that the random nature of the contamination would require an inspection sample of a size or volume very close to that of the production process in order to duplicate the potential distribution pattern. The recording and analysis of complaints will provide a better measure of effectiveness.

On the other hand, sampling may prove an effective tool when inspecting for intrinsic contamination which has a less random distribution pattern.

It is unlikely that a test of the system based on the introduction of known contaminants to the process will be an effective calibration tool. The supervisory activities surrounding the introduction and subsequent action to prevent their passing into the product will alter the normal activity level of the inspection personnel.

A constant review of reports from customers with the inspection personnel is essential to an improvement programme.

Records of analysis of risk, the definition of the control point, the training of personnel, the selection of equipment, the setting up of the lighting and other environmental controls, the maintenance of the equipment, and the regular review of complaints are an essential part of the process. The format of these records, their size and complexity, will reflect the scale of the business but they must exist.

References and further reading

Hammond, J. (1978) *Understanding Human Engineering*. David and Charles, Newton Abbot, Devon.

Osborne, D. (1982) *Ergonomics at Work*. John Wiley & Sons Ltd, Chichester.

Murrell, K. F. H. (1965) *Ergonomics*. Chapman & Hall, London.

15

Packaging material

15.1 Introduction

Packing materials play an important part in the food chain. They are used to deliver goods to manufacturers, and used by manufacturers for distribution through both the transport chain and by the consumer.

The manufacture of packaging, whether it be paper, board, plastic film, aluminium dishes, glass jars or bottles or metal containers is carried out by companies who supply other industries besides the food industry and who as a consequence need to be aware of the special needs of the food industry.

It must also be remembered that in many cases packaging is in turn delivered in protective packaging. Therefore, there is this continuous opportunity for foreign body contamination to be introduced to the manufacturing plant and the products via this source.

A further complication is that in many cases metal detectors and X-ray machines are used for final packed product inspection, and that any contamination contained within the packing material will be detected by these equipments which may lead to expensive product waste.

Finally, the choice of packaging material must always be considered in light of its suitability for passing through the various inspection devices that the quality control procedures specify for the product.

15.2 Packaging materials

A wide variety of materials are used for packaging. These include:

- *Paper and paper products*. Used for bulk outer containers in the form of corrugated board. Used as plain board for boxes to contain the products when it may be printed or coated with inks, paints, plastic, metal or metal vapour. Also used as paper for wrapping when it may be coated or printed in the same manner as board. The raw material may be clean new pulp or reclaimed materials.

- *Plastic.* There are literally dozens of grades of plastic available for packaging. Reclaimed plastic materials are commonly used. Produced in the form of film by a continuous extrusion process and often used in a laminated form where the special properties of different types of material are used to achieve specific results. Used in blow moulded form for bottles and similar products or injection moulded for semi stiff or rigid containers.
- *Aluminium.* Manufactured from new materials and reclaimed material. Used as film for wrapping, e.g. chocolate bars. Thicker films are used to manufacture aluminium trays as used for ready meals. Used in press extruded form for drink cans and similar products. Produced in a very thin film form and laminated with paper to produce special materials used for pouches and flow wrapping.
- *Steel.* Manufactured from reclaimed scrap but delivered to box makers from the steel mills in the form of various thickness strip metal. Can be coated with a wide variety of materials to prevent corrosion or to produce a surface suitable for printing.
- *Wood.* Used for packing some 'exotic' food products. Commonly used for the bulk shipping of raw materials, e.g. tea.
- *Cloth.* Used for packing bulk materials. This may be in the form of a woven cloth or open weave net. May be manufactured from a variety of natural fibres or plastics. Some exotic food products where a specific image is to be generated in the consumers mind are packed using cloth, e.g. herbs or jams. In net form used for packing fruit and vegetables for the consumer.
- *Ceramics.* Various ceramic products are used for the packaging of cheese or paté.

15.3 Raw material suppliers and transport

It is particularly important that the suppliers of the packing material be strictly controlled to ensure that general standards of hygiene are observed in their production processes. This will be readily understood by companies who specialize in the production of packing materials for the food industry, but may be a totally foreign concept to companies whose main market is non-food.

It must be ensured that the raw materials used are of the prescribed quality and that they are not contaminated by extrinsic materials that will be picked up by the detection equipment through which they will have to pass in the food manufacturer's process.

The storage of finished packaging materials must be controlled on the manufacturer's premises to the same standards as used in the food manufacturer's plant. Transport must also be controlled in the same way.

15.4 Reclaimed materials

Reclaimed materials are particularly liable to contamination from the recycling process. The raw material will have been treated as scrap when it was disposed of after it was used in its original form. It will have been stored without any control or protection at the collection site, and have been open to wilful tampering.

The recycling industry uses a variety of methods to clean its raw material and processes which ensure it is safe from a microbiological point of view.

The most common problems arise from the retention of very small particles of metal being carried through the process and remaining embedded in the finished product. A good example of this is corrugated cardboard. If one looks carefully at almost any piece of this material it is possible to see with the naked eye or with a low power magnifier minute pieces of metal glinting on or just below the surface of the material. Where the board is used for an outer container this is not of concern from a hygiene point of view, but if the container is to be passed through a metal detector it is. Because the cardboard will be closest to the walls of a metal detector where the sensitivity is greatest the presence of very small particles is easily detectable. In fact, if reclaimed board is used as a packing material which subsequently has to pass through a detector, the detector will need to be set to ignore contamination less than 2.5 mm Fe to prevent false rejection because of contamination in the board.

Plastic materials are also subject to the same problems. While in most cases this will not pass into the plastic packing material, it will cause damage to the moulding machinery by blocking the injection feed holes.

15.5 Materials presenting special problems

Some packing materials present particular problems to detection methods, particularly metal detectors:

- *Ceramics*. Certain grades of ceramics are manufactured from clays with a chemical composition that produces a finished product which generates a signal within a metal detector. Before committing to a specific source of ceramic containers, experimental work must be carried out to ensure the material is suitable for metal detectors.

- *Microwave boxes and metallized plastic films*. The very fine coating of metal that is used for these particular types of packaging is sufficient to be detectable by a metal detector, although it is transparent to an X-ray machine. The effect can be overcome by modifying the metal detector although some sensitivity is lost.
- *Plastics*. Some of the pigments used to colour plastics, particularly when used in injection moulded form, make the material electrically conductive. Carbon black in particular. When considering the use of heavily coloured materials, tests should be made to confirm suitability, particularly for metal detectors.

15.6 Material inspection methods

The major problem to be dealt with is the prevention or control of metallic contamination of the raw material. There are special purpose systems available for this purpose.

The conversion of plastic scrap into new plastic components is as follows:

- The scrap material is passed through a metal detector designed to detect relatively large pieces of metal which would damage the granulator used to break it down into small regular size chips.
- The chips are then passed through a drop-through metal detector before being passed through an extruder where the chips are reformed into a new plastic material. This may be used as a direct feed for a product or produced as a film for conversion into flake or into a rod for conversion into pellets for subsequent mixing with fresh raw material and further processing.
- The final material passes through another metal detector mounted above the final extruder or injection moulding machine.

The conversion of scrap paper into new paper or board utilizes a metal detector to ensure large metal contaminants are removed before the material goes into the paper-making process. This is a liquid flotation process which automatically has the benefit of losing a lot of metal contamination by specific gravity. The final product can be passed over a single-sided metal detector fitted with a counter to record the number of detections per unit of production from which material can be selected having a predictable contamination rate of whatever standard is set.

16

The investigation and handling of complaints

16.1 Introduction

Complaints arise from a variety of sources, which in the case of foreign bodies will be attributed by the complainant to a range of perceived causes. Any organization supplying manufactured goods, distributed items or a service must have a system in place to record complaints received, whether they are valid or not. In the case of foreign bodies the contaminant needs to be clearly identified. The resolution of the matter with the original complainant needs to be recorded and where the complaint has revealed a potential weakness in the systems used by the organization the remedial action should also be logged. Even when a complaint is clearly invalid, the matter must be investigated and records kept detailing the conclusions and reasons for them.

Glass inclusion during production provides a particularly good example of where the scrupulous handling of both internal and external complaints can result in huge improvements in quality at minimum cost. The series editor has personal experience where glass complaints were reduced by 84% following such an exercise that showed that most complaints arose in only two out of eight production lines where wrongly aligned transfer plates were seriously affecting jar integrity due to glass surface damage.

16.2 Sources of complaints

16.2.1 Complaints arising 'in-house'

Complaints arising from within an organization are often overlooked when a complaints procedure is considered. Faults and errors identified within the process by the manufacturer's own organization are of equal significance to continuous product improvement as those arising externally. The not uncommon practice of errors and faults occurring within a process being treated informally or even be ignored must be corrected.

When a failure is identified it must be investigated and corrective procedures implemented. In the case of foreign body contamination, particularly in food manufacture, it is essential that the results of the routine quality procedures applied to incoming raw materials are recorded and used as part of a vendor evaluation procedure. Equally, any foreign body contaminants discovered during the food manufacturing process, particularly those discovered by in-line quality control equipment such as colour sorters, metal detectors or X-ray machines, must be investigated, the cause identified, and where necessary quarantine and rejection procedures implemented to prevent contamination getting through to the consumer. Finally, the manufacture of packaging materials must be subjected to similar quality control procedures to prevent contamination being carried over into the product from the container. For example, in the case of glass containers there is always a danger present from broken glass or in the case of plastic pots and containers there is the danger of plastic scrap getting in to the container in the manufacturing process.

16.2.2 Complaints from outside sources

Complaints from outside sources will arise from the consumer. In this context, a consumer may be a member of the public, or a manufacturer or a caterer using the product. The complaint may come directly from the consumer, as defined, or through an agent, a retailer or wholesaler, a private label merchandiser, or an enforcement authority, government department or media opportunist. In the case of complaints from retailers, private label merchandisers, wholesalers and distributors, where the complaint has been raised by a member of the public and directed to them, it will almost certainly have already passed through their internal complaints procedure.

Wherever the source of the complaint, there must be a procedure in place to record the notification of a complaint and, depending on the company's policy, activate a method of acknowledging receipt of the complaint. In the case of foreign body contamination complaints, the procedure must then include identification of the contaminant where the contaminant is available, identification of the production process the product came from, and where possible the time and date of manufacture. How much of this can be achieved will depend on the nature of the complaint and the material received with the complaint.

An investigation will then take place to establish if the complaint is genuine with the identification of the foreign body. An assessment of the cause will be made. Based on this information, consideration of the potential for the complaint to be indicative of a greater problem or only an isolated incident will be made. Corrective action will be decided upon and implemented if applicable. Finally, the customer will be notified of the results in accordance with the company's policy.

16.2.3 *Complaints from UK (except Scotland) enforcement authorities*

In principle, written or verbal complaints received from enforcement authorities will be dealt with in the same way as any other complaint from an outside source. However, because the enforcement authorities have specific duties under the law, an additional procedure should be implemented in these cases. The main objective being to ensure the organization's legal position is not jeopardized in error.

Depending upon how the routine process of handling complaints fits in with company policies and the authority vested in those responsible for handling routine complaints, it may be necessary to have a system of notification to more senior management when complaints of this nature are received. It is essential that whoever is responsible for the handling of complaints from enforcement authorities is trained to understand the legal position, the limits and rules which the enforcement authorities have to adhere to, and is capable of conducting meetings and discussions with the representatives of the enforcement authorities. It is essential that anyone conducting these type of discussions is skilled in developing relationships, understands the company policy thoroughly and is well versed in the quality control and manufacturing procedures of the company. This does not mean they must know every minutiae of the details, but they understand the overall process and where and whom to use to fill in the gaps.

As discussed in chapter on the legal position, every effort must be made to make these discussions non-confrontational. The ability to achieve this will depend on the relationships built up over a period of time.

16.2.4 *Formal complaints from enforcement authorities with notice of intention to prosecute*

Where such a notice is the first indication of a complaint existing, then while the letter should be recorded in the log in the normal manner it should be treated in a different manner. The fact of its receipt should trigger a notification to the senior management and a team should be set up to deal with the response.

16.3 The investigation procedure

16.3.1 Objective

The objective of the investigation procedure is to establish the source and cause of the contamination, then using the information obtained implement an improvement to the process wherever possible. Secondly, the results of the investigation will be reported to the complainant in a manner consistent with the company's policy. The objective being to ensure that the company's reputation is undamaged and that the consumer will continue to purchase the company's products. In the case of a complaint from an enforcement authority having established the cause, a case will be made to demonstrate that 'all reasonable precautions' and 'due diligence' has been exercised by the organization in order to prevent wherever possible legal action being taken against the organization. How this objective is achieved will vary from case to case. Finally, in the case of a complaint identifying a major fault in the process, it is important that the necessary crisis action is implemented promptly and with a minimum of damage to the company's reputation.

16.3.2 The procedure

The flow diagram in Figure 16.1 summarizes the procedure, and demonstrates the 'feedback loops' and the way in which the results of the procedure play a part in a programme of continuous improvement.

(a) Registration of complaints

Ideally a central documentary system must be set up within the organization where all complaints are recorded.

In practice it may be impossible for one department to handle all the initial and final communications for both internal and external complaints. In this case there will be two or more systems operating in parallel. However, it is likely that the responsibility for the identification of the contaminant belongs to the quality control department irrespective of the source. It is also likely that the quality control department will be responsible for the recording of all internal 'complaints' or findings from the process. Other departments will be involved in investigating and identifying cause, deciding on the necessary action, and implementing the action agreed. Product dis-

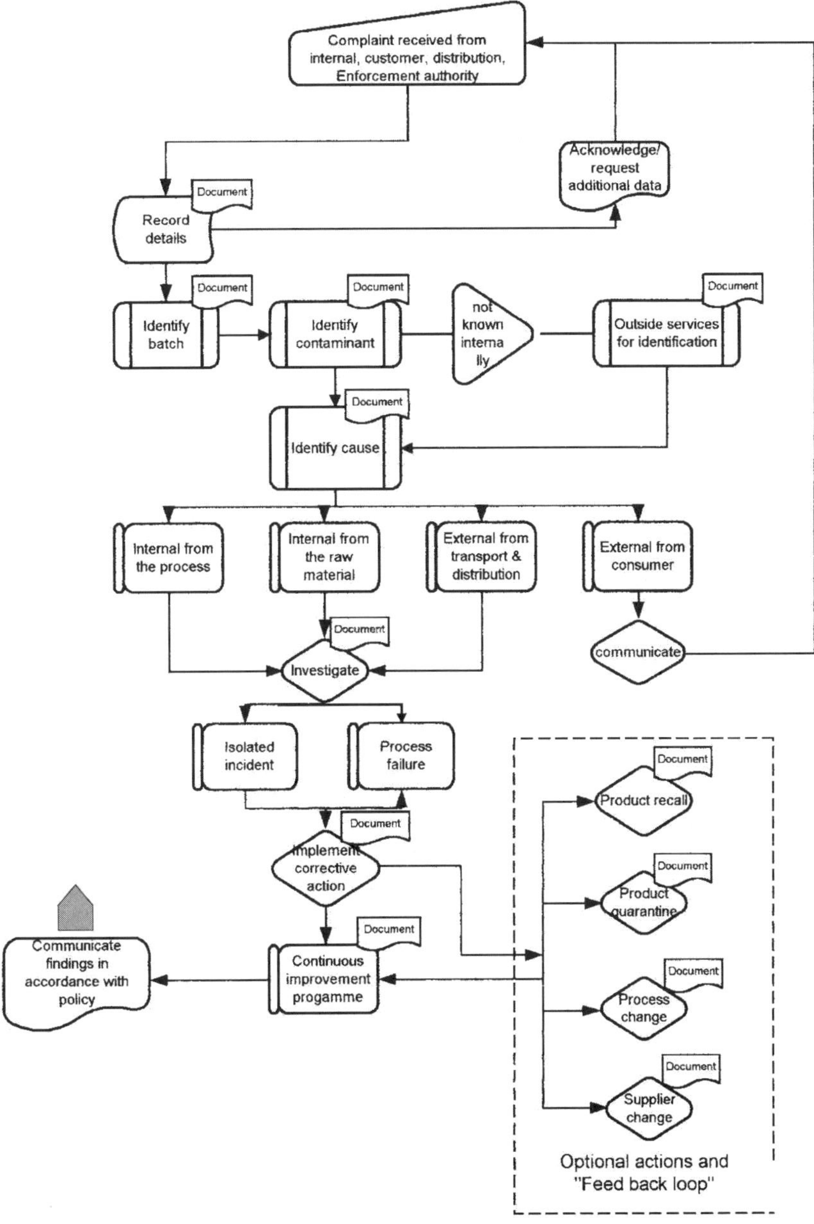

Figure 16.1 Complaints procedure flow chart.

posal and communication will also involve other parts of the organization.

Therefore, while there may of necessity be more than one register in use within the organization, because quality control will be the one department involved in all complaints, at the identification stage of the process, it is recommended that they have overall day-to-day supervision of the complaints procedure and the responsibility for keeping the whole organization informed of any matters pertaining to complaints on a departmental basis. They will also have a specific duty to bring any matters which may require product recall or involve the organization in legal proceedings to the notice of a nominated director or senior manager with the authority to authorize the necessary action.

Registration – External complaints
Complaints received from outside the organization should be recorded in a log kept by a specified department, e.g. the marketing department. This can be a handwritten log book, a loose leaf file with inserts or an electronic file. Whatever form is used, the complaints should be sequentially numbered with any cancelled numbers identified and the reason for cancellation shown. Its exact format will depend on the organization. However, it should include the following:

- Date complaint received
- Name of complainant
- Address of complainant
- Telephone and fax number where relevant
- Status of complainant – provision should be made to inform the rest of the organization whether the complaint is from an individual, a business, an enforcement authority or any other relevant information such as a pressure group if this is known
- Details of the complaint – express the wording of the complaint in a standard format so that it is clearly understood by all parts of the organization
- Product identification – identify the product and where possible batch number or lot number or any other information which will help in the investigation process; indicate if the package was received with the complaint
- Description of contaminant – a written description of the contaminant if possible or indicate if the contaminant was received with the complaint
- Identify where information has been requested to allow the complaint to be followed up, e.g. where the product has not been clearly identified request the information or ask for the contaminant where this was not received with the complaint
- Date to follow up the request for additional information
- Date the complaint was sent to the department authorized to communicate with enforcement authorities

- Date acknowledgement to enforcement authority
- Date the information was sent to the quality department
- Date an answer is required from the quality department
- Date the complaint was answered
- Details of the answer

Acknowledgement
When a complaint is received from outside the organization an immediate acknowledgement of its receipt should be made. This may include a date by which a full answer will be provided either in general or specific terms. The letter should be signed by someone trained and authorized to speak on behalf of the company. Dealings with some organizations will be dealt with on a formal intra company basis, where response targets are agreed contractually.

Where the complaint is received from an enforcement authority, the acknowledgement of its receipt must be dealt with by a specifically nominated person or department. It is only this department that is authorized to deal with this type of complaint. In preparing their acknowledgement, they may liaise with other departments ahead of the formal investigation procedure. However, this should not alter the fact that the initial complaint should be acknowledged prior to a full investigation and report.

Obtaining information
It is not uncommon for the complaint to be made without enough information being supplied to substantiate the complaint or to allow the matter to be investigated. In these cases it is essential that the information required to respond is obtained. This may be requested by the letter acknowledging receipt of the complaint, which will usually be the case if it is a consumer. In the case of another manufacturer, retailer or distributor, this information may be requested verbally – it will depend on relationships and agreed practice. However, without having access to the contaminant it will prove to be impossible to give a positive response. While business customers will understand this, it may require some tact to elicit the same from a consumer.

Registration – internal complaints
Complaints arising within the organization and the material rejected by detectors or cleaning processes should be received and recorded in a log kept by the quality control department. This can be a handwritten log book, a loose leaf file with inserts or an electronic file. Whatever form is used, the complaints should be sequentially numbered with any cancelled numbers identified and the reason for can-

cellation shown. Its exact format will depend on the organization. However, it should include the following:

- Date received
- Location within the process the complaint derives from
- Status of complainant – provision should be made to inform the rest of the organization whether the complaint is from the process, found in the raw material or from external sources; where there are special circumstances surrounding the complaint source these must be communicated to all those involved in the identification and investigation
- Details of the material supplier and batch information if relevant
- Product identification – identify the product and where possible batch number or lot number.
- Description of contaminant – to be completed by the quality department once the contaminant has been isolated; assistance of other departments and even outside resources may be required to complete this
- Date the information was sent for identification
- Date identification is expected

(b) Identification of the contaminant

The responsibility for isolating and identifying foreign bodies will probably rest with the quality control department. They will receive the rejected products from production and have the job of finding the contaminant. They will use various methods for this which will depend on the nature of the material and the contaminant.

External complaints received from the marketing department will be recorded in the same log as that used for internal complaints.

In all cases of foreign body contamination complaints identification of the contaminant is absolutely essential to the investigation and prevention of future occurrence. It is also true that where the contaminant comes from outside the organization greater care must be taken to obtain a positive identification than where the complaint is an internal one.

- *Internal identification.* Once the contaminant has been isolated, in most cases it is fairly simple to identify what it is when it has been found internally. The production department, together with engineering will usually be able to identify what the contaminant is. This information must be provided to quality control for entry into the central log. Where this cannot be done, then external sources are available.
- *External identification.* Where the contaminant has come from outside the organization, then unless identification is clearly obvious

consideration should be given to using outside resources for identification. It is possible to identify metals not simply in terms of steel or brass, but in much greater detail. It is also possible to microscopically examine fractures and identify probable cause. Insects can be identified and their probable source established. Plastic type can be analysed. Glass can be analysed and the type established.

Based on this type of detailed information it becomes possible to identify the source to a greater level of accuracy. This in turn helps to establish measures to prevent recurrence.

(c) Identification of the source

Once the contaminant has been identified the next step is to identify the source. This may be the raw material supplies. It may be a failure in the process, machinery breaking down or cleaning processes not operating efficiently. Contamination may be occurring in transport or storage, e.g. pest infestation or water damage. Finally, it may be the consumer at fault, either accidentally or maliciously. The identification of the contaminant is essential in achieving a reliable identification of likely source.

(d) Investigate

Having identified the contaminant and the source, the next stage is to decide if the occurrence is an isolated incidence or a process failure. Records will need to be examined to ensure the process requirements have been met and any incidents of breakages, accidents, etc., investigated to ensure they are not the cause.

- *Isolated incidence.* This may refer to an isolated incidence of contamination in raw material that the organization are satisfied is subject to the supplier taking all reasonable precautions to prevent. It may be an isolated incident in transport or storage that was either the result of an accident or for which all reasonable precautions are being taken to prevent recurrence. It may be failure of part of the process which is unlikely to occur again. Any of these isolated incidences, providing they do not have the potential for contaminating a large volume of product, should be recorded together with the basis for the decision that they are isolated.
- *Process failure.* This is the opposite of an isolated incidence in that unless changes are implemented it will occur again and indeed may have already done so. Examples are breakages of cutter knives, infestation from storage or transport under poor condi-

tions or using a supplier who does not have the capability to control product quality.

(e) Action implemented

Having identified the contaminant and its source, and decided if it was an isolated incident or a process failure, the decisions have to be taken on actions to be implemented to prevent further contamination reaching the customers.

Where the contamination has been identified internally, the decision is relatively simple. If it is raw material, changing supplier is one solution or alternatively the existing supplier can be persuaded to improve the process and for an interim period the organization implements its own inspection procedures of any deliveries from that supplier. Where the process has been shown to be at fault, then this can be changed and where a change will take time to implement, e.g. equipment delivery delays, the additional inspection processes can be temporarily introduced.

Where the investigation has revealed that a quantity of product is potentially contaminated, then the decision can be made to isolate the material if it is known to still be on the premises. Where there is a real likelihood of product in the distribution chain being contaminated, then the decision has to be to recall the product.

(f) Product disposal

Following product isolation or recall, the decision has to be made whether to scrap the affected batch or batches or to reclaim them. Destruction is always a possibility, but this is costly and wasteful. The alternative is to consider using a special inspection procedure. This may mean an additional metal detection check or X-ray inspection at an off-site test house. The options will need to be explored before a final decision is reached.

(g) Communication

Finally, having identified the contaminant and source and implemented action, the information has to be communicated to the complainant. In all cases the best way to do this is to tell the truth. How this is done is a matter of judgement on a case-by-case basis. What is essential to ensure customer satisfaction and to prevent a problem that could stay low key not getting blown up out of all proportion is to inform the complainant of the outcome.

Internally, any changes need to be communicated to all concerned. Where applicable, HACCP plans need to be revised and training modified if necessary. Purchasing need to be aware of how the suppliers are performing.

Lastly, the quality control log should be completed with a report on the identification of the contaminant and the source, the action taken and product disposal if applicable, and the completion of the communication.

The information is then returned to the relevant department for the information to be sent to the original external complainant.

17

The identification of foreign bodies

17.1 Introduction

Foreign bodies will be discovered by the quality control process machinery, foreign body detectors, customers and consumers. The material removed by cleaning equipment, washers flumes, etc., used in the process is normally disposed of automatically. Magnets, metal detectors, X-ray machines, visual inspection machines and human operators remove foreign bodies either as discrete items or in the form of a pack or sample of product available for investigation and identification.

The precise identification of contaminants returned by consumers in particular is essential. It is far too easy for an incorrect identification to be made of something found in food that the finder considers to be a contaminant and misleading conclusions drawn as to cause. Emotion plays a considerable part in this. A consumer may identify a clump of undesolved struvite or rock salt crystals as glass and react accordingly or the consumer may wrongly identify a piece of twig as being of animal origin and complain on this basis. It is only by precise identification of the material that the true description can be established. Precise identification also verifies if the material could have got into the product during processing or if it entered the product at a later date either accidentally or purposely. Two typical examples of this are have been reported by the Leatherhead Food Research Association.

- *Glass in a bakery product.* The sample was hard and amorphous, obviously a piece of glass. One original surface was seen – this was fairly smooth and flat. The other side of the piece had a small area of tightly concave surface which had a brown stain. X-ray microanalysis indicated a window glass and the brown stain appeared to be mostly iron. The appearance suggested a window and the rust deposit suggested a wire-reinforced window. An inspection of the factory showed that glass-reinforced windows were located above the processing line – these were intact but had been broken at the time of manufacture. It had transpired that during the time of manufacture pile driving was occurring next to the factory. This had loosened the glass which allowed the wire to rust, expand and force out the glass fragment.

- *Glass in a frozen dessert*. A piece of glass was found in a frozen dessert product. The shape of the piece of glass suggested part of the rim of a small bowl or drinking glass. The curvature was estimated by interference fringes to be in the range 7–9 cm diameter. X-ray microanalysis indicated kitchen or tableware glass. Thus the report concluded that the glass was derived from a drinking glass or small bowl. The local authorities were involved and reluctant to accept a domestic accident as the cause. After several weeks they agreed to inspect the complainant's kitchen and found two more fragments of glass in a cupboard. These were sent to the laboratory and they were not only a good match but fitted together with the original piece.

The first example clearly shows that the manufacturing process and building has to be reviewed, either by removing the glass from the roof or installing a suspended ceiling or cover over the line. The second clearly shows the value of careful analysis on which firm conclusions can be based being used to resolve a problem outside the control of a manufacturer.

Similarly it is important that the foreign bodies removed by the detectors in the process are identified and the information used to reduce or remove the incidence of similar complaints in the future. The information also serves to identify potential dangers of contamination in completed batches of product. This is arguably more important to achieving the highest possible level of freedom from contamination than the continued use of detectors as demonstrated by the first example.

Identification of contaminants is, therefore, an important part of the foreign body control and prevention process. It requires a mix of scientific disciplines to cover all the potential contamination that can occur as well as experience of the various fields. In this book it is impossible and impractical to discuss all the techniques available for the identification of contaminants, therefore the concentration is on the principles.

A designated point in the quality control department must be identified for the overall control of the reception, investigation, reporting and recording action taken, following the identification of a foreign body – whatever the source. There must be a system that ensures a foreign body cannot be lost, and that the records of the production department, customer service department and quality department cross-reference completely. This requires a central register, standard reporting and recording of the various stages of the identification process, followed by a record of the results and the action implemented. The size and complexity of the system will reflect the size of the organization.

17.2 Principles of the identification of foreign bodies

17.2.1 Reception

(a) Contamination identified within the process

Within the quality control procedures operating in any organization, a standard procedure needs to be specified to control the investigation of, action implemented and disposal of products identified as being contaminated. This procedure will include the action to be taken when cleaning processes, particularly magnets, reveal unusual contamination during the routine cleaning of the system.

This procedure will identify the route to be taken to deliver the contaminated product to the designated point where it will be logged and entered in the register. This will include provision to record the condition of the product, e.g. packed or unpacked, and the relevant batch, line, date and time information which is readily available when the contamination is identified within the process.

(b) Contamination identified by customers and consumers

The organization will have a procedure in place to ensure complaints from outside the organization are delivered to the designated point where it will be logged. The designated point in the quality control department will record details of the material received, e.g. if the pack is complete and what packing material if any was received. Any information relevant to the discovery, e.g. during consumption or on opening, should also be recorded.

17.2.2 Preliminary examination

The contaminated product will be initially examined by a designated department. In the case of complaints from outside the organization this will be a careful examination aimed at establishing the veracity of the claim as well as identifying the contaminant. The examination will be of everything that was returned to try and establish if there is any clear visual evidence to confirm or deny the truth of the claim.

Initially, this will be a visual examination using nothing more than a magnifying glass or a low power stereo microscope. It is directed towards narrowing down the options before a detailed examination is undertaken using expert and expensive resources. In many cases identification can be completed at this stage. Particularly when dealing with a consumer complaint, it is recommended that a photographic record be made of the material returned and at the various stages of separation, for future reference.

The following steps, in the form of questions, are a guide to the various stages of an initial appraisal:

- Can the product be identified as definitely originating from the organization.
- Where the packaging is returned:
  - Has the packaging been tampered with?
  - Does the packaging show signs of damage in storage?
- Where the product has been returned:
  - Does the product show signs of careless storage?
  - Is the contaminant still lodged in the product?
  - Can the contaminate be easily seen and removed from the product?
  - Is there a cavity or impression of the contaminant in the product?
- Where the contaminant only is returned:
  - Does it exhibit any obvious signs of having been in the material?
  - Is any product material adhering to the surface?
  - Is the identification of the contaminant obvious, e.g. a nut or bolt?
  - Is the contaminant an item previously identified as a contamination danger in a process

Where the contaminant cannot be easily removed from the product for detailed examination it will be necessary to separate it from the product.

There are various methods of achieving this. The quality laboratory may have an off-line detection device of the same type as the production line, in which case this will be used as far as practical to isolate the contaminant. Where a solid product is rejected by metal detectors this is achieved by progressively halving and retesting the contaminated section until the contaminant is revealed or the sample is too small to continue the process. Then the product can be dissolved and filtration techniques used to reveal the contaminant. A similar process can be used with loose products, gradually reducing the amount retested until the contaminant is revealed. Where the contamination is identified during processing it is always a good idea to examine the packaging separately to ensure this is not the source of contamination.

Similar techniques can be used with X-ray machines where there is no VDU to display details of the contamination. Where a VDU is available, the location of the contamination can be made using the information from the display.

Material rejected by optical systems will normally be visually inspected, although there are optical systems available designed for off-line use.

Alternatively it may be possible to use the process line equipment to carry out the same work.

It should be borne in mind that the separation of a contaminant, particularly those discovered by metal detectors, can be extremely laborious and time consuming. Some applications, e.g. liquids and slurries rejected by pipeline systems, are the most difficult and for this reason often ignored. This is a mistake and no matter how difficult it is to isolate the contaminant for identification it must be carried out.

17.2.3 *Results of the preliminary examination*

The results of the preliminary examination will often result in a clear definition of the contamination, the line and the batch from which it came. Where the contamination has been discovered internally, the information is then fed back to the process control system and controls and methods introduced, wherever possible, to prevent a recurrence of the contamination.

Where the contaminant has been reported from outside, then it is essential that the identification be used to assess the chances of it having derived from the process or in subsequent transport and use. This may require the use of sophisticated techniques to identify materials precisely.

17.3 The identification of contaminants

For the purposes of this section contaminants are broken down into the following general classifications:

- Intrinsic matter
- Metallic items
- Bird, animal, insect and reptile
- Glass
- Minerals
- Plastics
- Others

There are specialist sources for advice and assistance in identifying foreign bodies – in the UK the food research associations are experts in the field. Specialist resources of trade organizations such as Paint Research associations are available as are the services of other specialist organizations. There are guidelines available from Campden and Chorleywood Food Research Association which will assist in the identification of foreign matter.

17.3.1 *Intrinsic matter*

This heading includes any naturally occurring material that may have found its way through the process. Examples are stones (pits) in fruit, twigs and stalks, bones in meat and fish, and any other material that is normally removed by the processes applied to the raw material before it is converted into a food item. In some cases inclusion is virtually unavoidable. For example, prior to the advent of self-pollinating fig species, the fig wasp was an essential part of the pollination/fruiting chain; hence, it was inevitable that some wasps would die within the fruit and become 'foreign bodies'.

In many cases identification is relatively straightforward visual recognition unless the contaminant has been considerably altered in size and shape by the process. In these cases microscopy and other laboratory techniques are used to establish identification.

17.3.2 *Metallic items*

In many cases metallic contaminants are clearly recognizable, e.g. nuts or bolts, pins, paper clips, etc. Where they are not easily recognized, e.g. pieces of solder, dental fillings, etc., then the material can be very precisely identified by the use of scanning electron microscopes or chemical analysis.

Table 1.4 lists some of the sources of metallic contamination, not all of which will have originated from manufacture, so it is essential that clear precise identification be made.

Examination of the surface of the material for evidence of product adhering to it may require the use of microscopy by trained experts. Where a contaminant has no signs of the product on its surface it may indicate that it entered the product after manufacture. Metallic objects which have been trapped in food products may also exhibit signs of corrosion and staining; conversely a lack of these signs may mean the metal was not in contact with the food for any length of time.

Examination of the surfaces of the material will identify where the material has been sheared off and, rather like a jigsaw puzzle, provide clues as to its origin.

Where the material cannot be identified visually, clues as to its origin may be obtained by analysing the metal which can be done using scanning electron microscopes. Detailed examination of the trace elements of a metal sample also provides clues in relating, or otherwise, pieces of metal having the same specification but manufactured from different batches.

Identification will in some cases clearly indicate the source of the contamination as other than manufacture or it may indicate a fault in manufacture, e.g. a damaged machine or a substandard batch of raw material. The evidence can be made more conclusive by reference to other records of the process, e.g. the maintenance records.

17.3.3 *Bird, animal, insect and reptile*

Insects, birds and rodents are an inherent danger to the food processor. Chapter 3 discusses the measures which need to be taken to prevent this type of contamination. These living creatures are able to exploit the conditions which exist in food factories storage and homes to their advantage. Some specialize in living in food stores and many take advantage of the conditions in homes where there is not the same level of professionally supervised preventative measures in place all the time.

Food can become contaminated by small creatures during harvesting, transport storage and processing. Most of us refer simply to insects as a description of anything small with wings, legs and a hard shell. This is not a correct description. These small creatures are correctly classified as Arthropods – the most numerous and widespread group of animals on the planet. The group includes such diverse forms as insects, crustaceans, spiders, millipedes and centipedes, all of which are characterized by an external skeleton and jointed limbs. The exception to this rule is the subgroup of velvet worms classified as Onychopora which occur in the southern hemisphere.

There are literally thousands of species of these animals. There are over 1 million insect species, including the group Apterygote of which Thysanura (silverfish) is just one species. There are 6500 species of millipedes, 26 000 species of crustaceans and in the Arachnida (spider) subgroup Opiliones, which includes the Daddy Long Legs, there are 3200 species.

While whole or complete insects can sometimes be identified by the naked eye or with the help of a low power microscope, based on experience or reference to specialist publications, the species is so vast that identification may need the assistance of specialist centres, e.g. the Natural History Department of the British Museum. Positive identification will establish not only the type but the lifecycle and natural habitat, which provides valuable information in identifying the source.

Fragments of insects are more difficult or impossible to identify, almost certainly specialist advice should be sought immediately if a fragment of an insect is under investigation. Note, if part of an insect is found by the control system during manufacture, the question which has to be answered is where is the rest of the insect? This should be answered satisfactorily and then the possibility of there being more than one insect present investigated before the batch is released.

Having identified the insect and the stage of its development, it is often possible to narrow down how and where it got into the product. Many insects have a natural habitat in a specific region and are unable to survive in other climates – knowledge of which narrows down identification of the source. Some insects only exist in a particular stage at certain times of the year – knowledge of this may be useful in identifying the source by reference to time. Some insects feed on specific foods and ignore others. This can be used to identify whether contamination occurred in storage or not, pointing to contamination occurring at another stage. An enzyme test can be carried out to ascertain if the insect has been heated (cooked). Because the result can be affected by the type of product and its effect on the enzyme as well as secondary affects caused by bacteria or moulds, the application of the test and interpretation of the results is a job for a specialist laboratory experienced in the field.

Contamination by birds or animals is a comparatively rare occurrence. Identification may be simply visual or it may require more detailed laboratory analysis. As with insects, identification of the animal or bird provides clues as to its origin. Tests can also be made to establish if the remains have been heat processed by examination of the tissues and collagen.

17.3.4 *Glass*

Glass is arguably the most common cause of consumer complaints. Finding a piece of glass in a food product is upsetting and almost certainly will result in a complaint being made either to the manufacturer the store or the authorities. However, as Table 17.1 shows, glass contamination mainly occurs in the home.

Fragments of glass are chipped off containers, glasses, cooking dishes, etc., during storage and handling in the home. It is often these shards which are the cause of complaints.

Table 17.1 Glass contamination sources (%)

Domestic	39.8
Heat resistant	27.8
Container	25.4
Domestic/container	2.3
Other	4.7

Glass identified during the production process has to be identified and the cause identified. The result then provides information which is used to modify the process, alter cleaning processes, change the fabric of the building or implement new controls to raw materials.

Therefore, it can be seen that the positive identification of glass is important. Fortunately, glass is not made to a single composition. The composition of glass varies sufficiently for the types to be identified using X-ray microanalysis. Analysis of the elements and their proportions contained within a sample can be compared with known data to identify the type of glass. This technique is fast and non-destructive, which is very important when the contaminant is the subject of legal proceedings.

Fragments of glass received as complaints can also be visually examined in the same way as metal particles. Their shape can be analysed and related to specific items based on the shape and radius of any curves present. The surfaces can be examined for product adhering to it and so on. An experienced investigator can readily identify glass shards as having come from specific articles based on shape, moulding marks, surface damage and scratching.

17.3.5 *Minerals*

Harvested materials are naturally exposed to mineral contamination, stones, etc. They are collected during the harvesting process and should normally be removed by the cleaning processes.

Identification is important in establishing the source when complaints of this nature are received from outside the organization. Fortunately, stones and minerals can be classified and identified as coming from a particular geographical location.

Identification may be carried out visually. It may require a section to be polished for microscopic examination or it may be analysed using X-ray microscopy. This process also eliminates materials often identified as stone by the consumer but which are in fact man made materials, such as ceramic tile shards or pieces of tooth or tooth crowns.

17.3.6 Plastics

The increased use of plastics and the indiscriminate disposal of them has resulted in them becoming a more common source of complaint. Visual examination will give some information on the item based on colour, markings if any and shape. Precise information on the type of plastic can be gained by Fourier transform (FT)-IR microscopy or measuring the IR spectrum.

Many plastics are laminates, not only work surfaces but packing materials. The resultant information from detailed analysis can then be used not necessarily to identify a source, but to exclude some potential sources.

This group also includes conveyor belting, which is a laminar construction, and fibre reinforced plastics, which can often be visually identified and related to particular locations within a process.

Solid plastic items include pieces from the special plastic conveyor belting manufactured from interlocking segments and using moulded plastic drive train components.

17.3.7 Other

There are many other types of contamination that will occur either during the process or be reported from on outside source.

These can include black or dark smears resulting from grease on machinery or black particles of burnt food. These can also include accidental carry over from previous crops, e.g. potatoes in onions, etc. Where visual examination fails to identify material of this nature, then X-ray microanalysis is a valuable tool in identification. Experience and detailed knowledge of the process is often the best source of clues to identification, which can the be confirmed by standard chemical analysis or staining techniques.

Careful adherence to the rules itemized previously will help towards achieving an identification. Magnifying glasses and optical microscopes are invaluable for examining the contaminant and will quite often be sufficient to make an identification.

References and further reading

Edwards, M. 1995. *Food Manufacturer*, Miller Freeman, London.

18

Future and emerging technologies

18.1 Introduction

When projecting into the future one has to look back a number of decades to observe how technologies have developed. When one does this it becomes apparent that there have been major changes and significant advancements. Most of the fundamental principal technologies utilized in the food industry for inspection machines were actually discovered many years ago. The major developments have taken time to be implemented, and the reason for this elapsed time between the discovery and use of the technology has been because of some of the following factors or issues:

- Ability to apply the technology
- Cost reduction (awaiting natural decline in component costs)
- Improvement in technology performance
- Time taken for the food industry to accept the technology
- A 'real' need for improved technology
- Changes in legislation
- Consumer, retailer, food manufacturer – perceptions and attitudes
- Increased knowledge of causes of contamination

To develop a new technology to a point of making it commercially available is both costly and also takes a considerable time. There are many potentially emerging technologies, some of which are described below.

18.2 Developments in X-ray technology

The area of X-ray technology, although talked about much, is one which has not taken off in the food industry. Although it provides a much superior technical solution than metal detection systems, its cost is still considerably higher. Therefore, the major advancements that could assist the food industry in producing safer foods would be the availability of X-ray systems at metal detector prices.

X-ray technology is reviewed fully in Chapter 11, but is an area of research activity attempting to improve the technology and reduce the costs. The progress from photography-based systems to real-time systems is now well developed. The areas where there is continuing research activity which could benefit the food industry are in the detector and image processing technologies.

18.2.1 Image generation or capture

The generation of X-rays is relatively straightforward; however, the detection systems which allow one to visualize an image are more complex. To date, the most widely used method is that of absorption, which has limitations when a contaminant has similar absorption characteristics to that of the product. However, there are ways in which this could be improved, but also there could be more effective methods such as X-ray scatter. Technologies are being developed that in a number of ways could help to improve the quality and resolution of images.

One development that would improve the resolution is that of producing smaller photodiodes – in being smaller, one can use more photodiodes in the array and, therefore, increase the resolution of the system. This allows the development of more detailed images, allowing smaller objects to be identified or finer details of larger objects to be examined. Work is also going on to produce an alternative miniature X-ray detector to the coated photodiodes. One company is using a 3 × 3 mm $CdWO_4$ scintillator. These type of scintillators can be arranged in an array similar to that of photodiodes. The signals from these receivers can be multiplexed and operate at very high speeds (up to 1000 lines of data can be collected per second). This will allow high speed processes to be inspected.

18.3 Image processing

Once an image or data has been generated and captured, it then has to be interpreted to evaluate whether the object(s) (food product) under analysis is acceptable or not. The method of interpretation is one that can be very difficult because under X-ray analysis many objects that could be good or bad look similar and it is how to differentiate which is more complex. Sometimes the absorption can be very similar, and therefore the contrasts are very slight and almost indistinguishable. A method of magnifying this contrast could provide an improved resolution.

If a clear X-ray image is presented to a human, it can be determined whether it is an acceptable product or not based on that person's cognitive skills which have been learnt by observing many good and bad examples of the product. This method, although reasonably effective, is expensive as someone has to be used all the time to observe the images. Another drawback with manual interpretation of images is that the concentration spell for humans is not long (approximately 30 minutes). It takes a considerable amount of computing power in order to automate and reproduce this type of human cognitive sense in a computer, and would at present be prohibitively expensive.

However, by reducing this approach down to a lower level it is possible to utilize some of the elements and techniques that people display. Probably one of the most effective techniques is that of key feature recognition. The use of specific features reduces the amount of analysis required and, if the correct features for a specific product or contaminant material are chosen, it can provide an effective means of inspection. Some types of features which could be characterized include:

- Sphericity
- Shape
- Specific colour
- Texture
- Number of substituents

This type of approach can be low cost and effective for specific contaminant detection. However, the approach is not so suitable if one wishes to screen a large number of products for a wide range of contaminants.

18.4 Nuclear magnetic resonance (NMR)

18.4.1 Introduction

The recent developments in NMR systems for the medical industry has provided some major breakthroughs in the use of such a technology in recent years. It is interesting to note that NMR has been used for many years and was first used in 1940. One of the major advantages that this technology could provide for the food industry is the provision of lower cost components which could result in an affordable system. Magnetic resonance spectroscopy as a technique has been developed and used extensively for many years in the laboratory with great success. For food products, it is routinely used for the determination of molecular structures.

18.4.2 The technology

The technique is based on subjecting a sample of material to a high magnetic field in order to achieve a high resolution spectrum, thus enabling spin–spin couplings and chemical shifts to be determined. As the nuclei of atoms in different compounds require different magnetic field levels to reach resonance, the NMR spectra can be utilized to identify different compounds.

The magnet employed within a typical NMR system is usually of the order of 10 000 gauss but is dependent on the particular application. The magnet is normally an expensive part of the system as it has to be very stable and provide a homogeneous field. The magnetic field is required to cause the axis of the spinning nuclei to tilt as they spin. This has a similar effect to that observed with a gyroscope. A gyroscope when placed in an external field will not only carry on spinning around its own axis but will also tilt and commence a secondary rotation. This secondary effect is called precession.

The second field around the x-axis is the alternating radiofrequency field – the frequency is specific to each element (e.g. so for hydrogen it is 60 MHz). If the second field oscillates with the same frequency as that of the nuclei, then energy can be transferred from the oscillator to the nuclei. If the nuclei becomes out of phase with the oscillator they will lose their energy and return to a lower angle of precession. The effect causes some of the nuclei to 'wobble' (resonate); however, not all will appear to 'wobble' because of the cancelling out effect of some nuclei being raised to higher precession while others simultaneously return to lower precession levels. It is this resonance that can be detected and utilized to identify the compound(s) under examination.

18.4.3 Current developments

For use as an on-line system, both the design of the NMR magnet and the radiofrequency excitation coil are important as well as the final cost of these components. One of the initial drawbacks with NMR was that it could not be used on-line because of the magnet homogeneity requirement. In the medical field developments have been made which allow more information to be obtained but at a high cost.

In order to reduce the cost and allow on-line use, a number of research teams have investigated utilizing other data which can be obtained when food compounds are subjected to a high magnetic field. Probably the most useful is the free induction decay signal in the relaxation time constants. It is also possible to utilize a radiofrequency excitation coil in addition to the magnetic field.

Different foodstuffs provide distinctive NMR signals, particularly those containing fat, oil, water and solid material, which includes many processed foods as well as natural food ingredients. It is also possible to measure the bulk effects within the product such as the fat/oil/water ratios, texture, porosity, moisture, temperature, etc. The technique is also suitable for on-line use because the time taken for the compounds to resonate in the field is very short (of the order of 10–100 milliseconds), which will allow reasonable line speeds to be inspected. It is not necessary to utilize imaging or spatial localization because a bulk measurement is sufficient for most applications.

Investigations have been made in this area and prototype systems developed. Figure 18.1 shows a diagram of a potential on-line NMR system that could be used to detect foreign objects in foods.

The prototype systems that have been developed have often maximized benefits by combining foreign body detection with the detection of moisture. The basis for this technology is that a food product is placed on a conventional belt and passed through a magnetic field. A high radiofrequency source is applied for a short duration, usually just a pulse, and when turned off the nuclei release energy. This radiofrequency energy pulse relates to the properties of the food and can be interpreted on-line as described above. The system will look not dissimilar to that of a metal detector.

18.4.4 *Future developments*

The technology requires further development in order to make it available for use in a food factory. The cost is still high, but if a market develops this is likely reduce over time. One of the major cost factors has been that of the magnets.

18.5 Ultrasonics

There are two main types of ultrasonics, i.e. low and high intensity. Low intensity has been used traditionally for echo sounding, body scanning and material inspection. High intensity has been used for cleaning purposes, deburring, welding plastics and sono chemistry. The frequency spectrum shown in Figure 18.2 shows that ultrasound occurs at a frequency of between 10^4 and 10^{11} Hz.

Below 10^4 Hz, sound waves are audible. The intensity of a wave can be defined by the equation:

$$I = P/A = W/A$$

where I is intensity (W/m^2), P is power (W) and A is area (m^2).

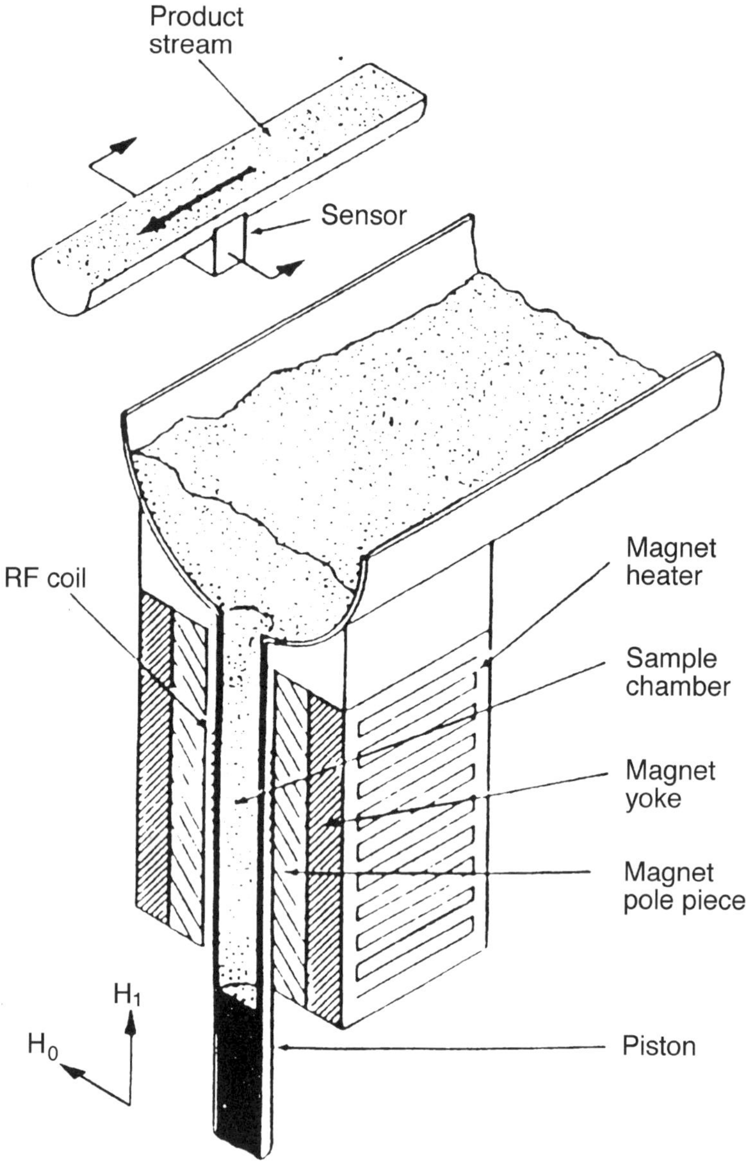

Figure 18.1 A typical NMR system. (Courtesy of C.I. Nicholls and A. Delos Santos.)

The medical industry has been provided with ultrasonic systems and probably the best known imaging system is the 'baby scanner'. This technology uses low intensity ultrasound. The baby scanner is the closest use of the technology to the application of foreign body

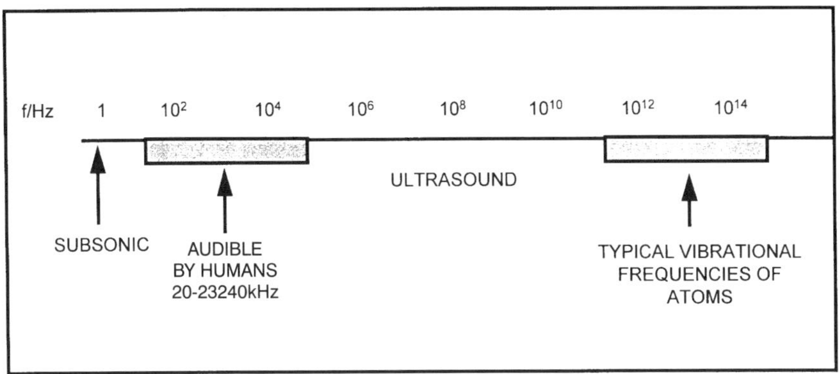

Figure 18.2 Ultrasonic frequency range.

detection. These type of ultrasound systems are able to build up an image of the object under observation. The image can be of a high quality. The quality does tend to be variable due to a number of factors. The ultrasonic imaging systems available tend to emit quite a narrow beam of ultrasound and the angle of the beam is critical in order to achieve a good image.

18.5.1 Generation of ultrasound

The ultrasound system works by first generating the sound wave, and this is done using a signal processor which produces an electrical pulse of a specific frequency and amplitude. A transducer, usually a piezoelectric device, converts the electrical signal into a sound wave of a specific frequency and amplitude corresponding to the electrical signal generated. The piezoelectric device is such that two parallel faces of thin layers of piezoelectric material are coated with silver and when a voltage is applied to the plates the thickness of the plates changes according to the voltage applied. The frequency of the alternating voltage causes a sound wave to be produced from the surface of the plate.

The power of the ultrasound is measured in decibels. The sound wave can be reflected by a material or transmitted. This attribute can be utilized to great effect in measuring liquid levels as the time the reflected ultrasound takes to be transmitted back to the transmitter can be used as a measure of tank level. However, ultrasound is attenuated – attenuation being the reduction in intensity per unit of distance. In liquids the velocity of sound is 1500 m/second and the attenuation is not very great. The impedance of ultrasound in air is very high and the attenuation is very high, thus only enabling penetration of a few millimetres possible. When ultrasound is transmitted through animal cells, the attenuation is far greater than that of water and it increases linearly with frequency.

18.5.2 Ultrasound images

When an ultrasound beam encounters a material which has a very high impedance, such as stones, glass or bones, the majority of the ultrasound is reflected. Therefore, it is possible to use the reflected ultrasound as a means of providing an input. As mentioned, the ultrasound is generated from the piezoelectric device; however, this device can also be used as a receiver and, therefore, converts the reflected ultrasound signals into a signal. This technique is similar to that used for radar and depth measurements, and is commonly referred to as a pulse–echo system.

A number of different types of scans have been developed in the medical field and these are briefly described. The A-scan system emits a pulse of ultrasound and waits for the amplified echo back from which the distance the ultrasound has travelled can be measured if the speed of sound through the material is known. The B-scan system allows an individual spot to be shown on a cathode ray tube and as the transducer is moved it allows an image to be built up. The most appropriate ultrasound system for the food industry is the real-time scanner, where a linear array of transducers are utilized to develop an image within a few milliseconds.

Therefore, one of the major limitations of ultrasonic imaging for food applications is the fact that one has to have a contact medium between the object and the ultrasonic emitter. The reason for this contact medium, which can be water but in medical fields is usually a gel, is that it is used to transmit the ultrasound as air is a poor transmitter due to its very low acoustic impedance. Although the limitation does not prohibit the use of the technology, it does have severe limitations as only materials which are wettable can be inspected and the shape of these can also present a problem.

Other similar applications of ultrasound have been made in the food industry to detect density changes and voids. Quality parameters have been measured using sonic or ultrasonic pulses, which can be utilized to measure the ripeness or texture of fruit and vegetables such as melons, tomatoes or peaches. One specific application project which is closest to foreign body detection was an investigation into detecting hollow hearts in potatoes.

The technology does have advantages in that it is safe, non-destructive, relatively low cost and hygienic. Further developments and advances could adapt it and make it a viable means of foreign body inspection.

18.6 Infrared (IR) and near-infrared (NIR)

NIR technology is a versatile and adaptive technology. It is presently utilized in the food industry for a number of different applications such as colour, moisture, fat, protein and density measurements. There is an opportunity to develop this technology further, and research has been carried out to investigate applications such as the detection of stones in cherries using NIR light transmission and an image analysis system.

It would appear that NIR has the ability to be used to detect certain surface defects, but is not so well suited to the internal inspection of products due to its lack of penetration. The lack of penetration may limit the possible future application of an overall screening method for foreign body detection.

18.7 Microwave and 'millimeter' waves

According to the wavelength of electromagnetic waves, microwaves have the ability to penetrate food. As everyone is aware, the wavelength of microwaves is such that it can cause products to heat up. In the field of military defence, various technologies are used to locate objects that are both visible and invisible. These techniques are used in tracking missiles, submarines or warships. More recently, the techniques have been adapted to locate underground buried items such as pipes. Although the technology has not been specifically applied to searching for foreign objects in food, it could be used for this task if further developed and adapted.

18.8 Image analysis and software

18.8.1 General

There are now many different means by which an image can be produced (such as ultrasound, X-rays, microwaves or NIR as discussed above). Once the image has been produced or captured there is a common requirement to interpret that image and extract specific information relating to it. In the majority of cases it is important that a good clear image is produced because that is likely to yield the best results from any image analysis to be carried out. Camera technology has improved significantly, therefore enabling an improved transfer of the image into an electronic format that can then be manipulated and interrogated. Figure 18.3 shows the basic building blocks of a typical advanced image acquisition system.

A limiting factor for optical images is still the level and type of lighting required, along with the effects of hygiene, humidity

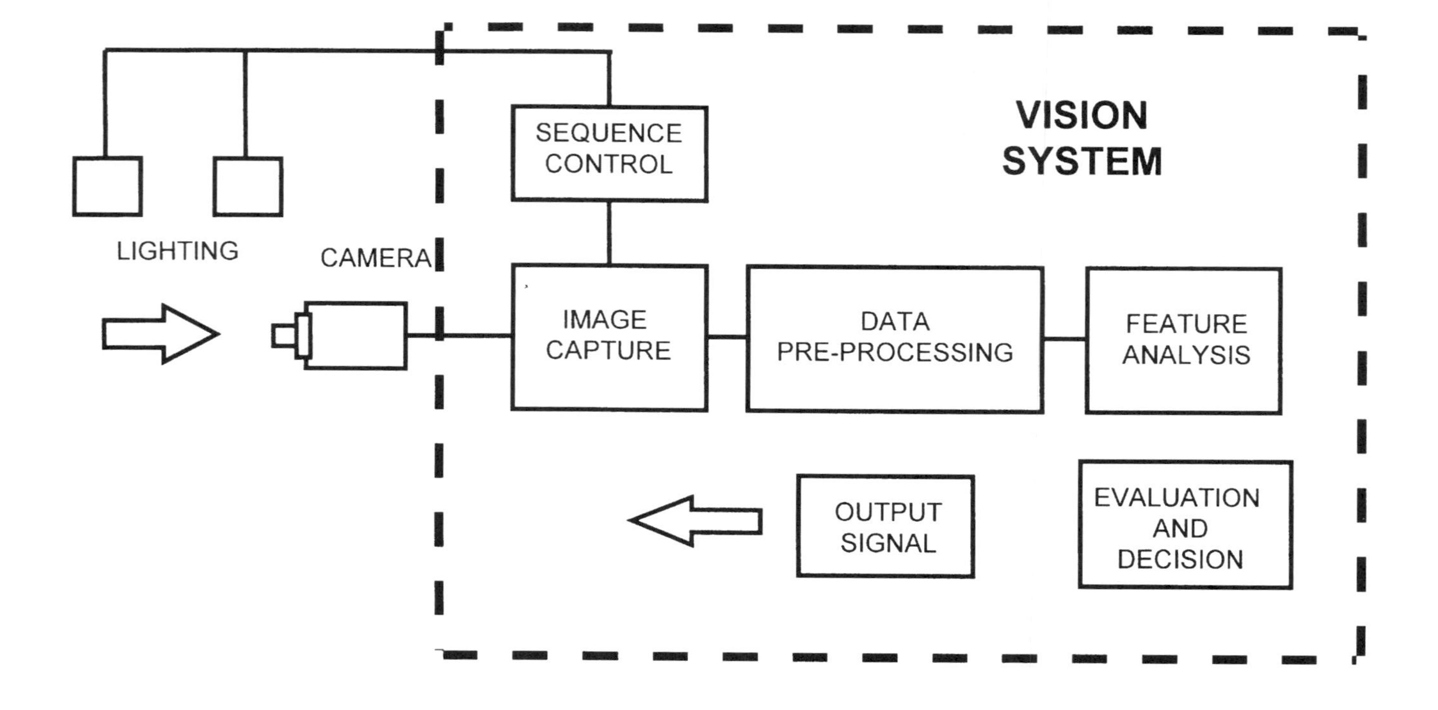

Figure 18.3 Typical image acquisition system.

changes, etc. Some equipment companies have overcome this by a 'black box' or 'sealed box' type approach which allows one to control the environment of the camera and the lighting by passing the product through an integrated inspection machine as opposed to under an unprotected camera.

In order to take the image converted into a digital format and process that data very quickly and efficiently a new type of electronic chip was developed. This digital signal processing chip (DSP) is now commonplace as a component of many image processing systems. It allows image data to be handled and processed at high speeds. The image analysis or data interpretation is the next stage in the process, which is more complicated as it is dependent on the specific application.

The development of neural network software analysis tools allows a different approach to conventional statistical and mathematical analysis or filtering of data. This type of analysis method allows more imprecise data to be analysed. It is more suited to the areas of pattern recognition where one is not looking for an exact measurement but whether a product is acceptable or not. Neural networks have been utilized in many image analysis systems because of their ability to be trained to recognize patterns.

18.8.2 Neural networks

A neural network is such that is can be trained on data sets, which it can then build up to establish a system of linkages which have different weightings and these weightings can be used to represent the overall shape or pattern of the data. The linkages are between what are called neurons (because of the similarity to human neurons). The linkages are shown in Figure 18.4 by the interconnecting lines between the layers of neurons.

Once the network of neurons has been trained to recognize the links or patterns, it can then be used to overlay these links on other new data and a comparison made. The level of likeness can allow one to determine whether there is a match or how similar the sets of data are. This type of technique could be used to identify any abnormalities in foods by training the neural network to recognize good products and, therefore, identify bad products.

This type of system can be used where it is not possible to model or use straight statistical or mathematical functions. It can be a low cost option as the system software can be used on a PC-based platform. Some interfacing is required and maybe pre-processing or data handling. The system can be very quick once a network has been established. One drawback at present is that a network has to be trained, which takes time and has to be carried out for each product.

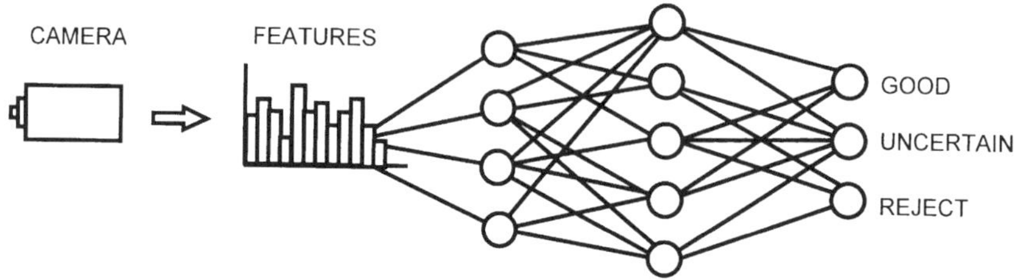

Figure 18.4 Typical neural network configuration.

18.8.3 Advanced algorithms and filters

New algorithms and advanced filters, which are methods of mathematically processing data to give a solution in a set number of steps, have been developed. These include the use of local Fourier transforms, and Gabor and Law filters, which are specific mathematical and data processing methods. Other filters that are available are based on standard mathematical functions or algorithms. This form of data processing allows one to extract or attenuate more specific attributes of the data, thus making it easier for subsequent analysis. Most have been developed for general applications rather than specifically for the food industry. There is, therefore, scope to develop more advanced and focused algorithms for specific food categories or products.

The Gabon type of filter is an example of this, as Gabon filters have a texture format similar to that of mammalian cortical cells. They could, therefore, help to characterize surface texture of specific products and thus allow abnormalities to be more readily identified. This has been attempted by using a technique to discriminate between textured and smooth regions of chicken skin.

Colour inspection has been utilized successfully in many food applications (Chapter 12). However, the use of colour could be greater utilized. Its use to date has been for applications where colour matters to the consumer, such as peas, carrots, etc., although in addition it does sort foreign bodies from the produce. Colour systems have been expensive and, therefore, not widely applied. They could be used to identify more surface defects of products. There has been a lot of work to apply the technology for inspecting poultry and the grading of birds.

18.9 Laser systems

Lasers can be used as a source of light for inspection systems. Research has been carried out relating to quality inspection of fruit and measurements of ripeness. Helium–neon (He–Ne) laser beams have been used to study the quality of meats. The scatter of the laser beam from the surface of the meat has been investigated. Tu *et al.* (1995) have investigated the ripeness of tomatoes and apples. They used a low power laser (3 mW) and a wavelength of 670 nm. The results obtained looked promising and they suggested that different power lasers could potentially reveal more information regarding the produce under the skin. If this proves promising there could be scope to use the techniques for foreign body detection.

In the medical field lasers are being used for mammography with some most promising results. Although these systems are relatively expensive, the prices are likely to reduce. Other new developments in the use of lasers is that of 'T-rays'. These are electromagnetic waves which have a wavelength in between that of IR and radar, and a frequency in the terahertz range, hence the name. In the medical field they have shown potential to give clearer images than X-rays. It is claimed they could have a resolution down to 1 mm. The rays are created using a titanium–sapphire laser which is pulsed for a fraction of a second. The laser beam is split in two and then one half passes through the object under examination whilst the other passes directly to the detector. The two input data sets can then be analysed and compared. Although in its early days, this technology could provide a major advancement.

18.10 Multiple sensor systems

Most systems used in inspection are based on a single sensing technology. The major reason for this is that the inspection company has specialized in a specific technology.

There is an opportunity now to combine technologies within one machine. This approach could potentially provide many benefits. It has partially been exploited with the combination of an in-line weigher with a bar code, and this has generated some cost and performance benefits.

One application one can think of is the combination of an internal inspection technique (such as X-rays) and a surface inspection technology (such as vision). The combination of these two techniques could provide a system which enables the interior and exterior to be inspected by the same machine. This type of intelligent advanced inspection system could be used to grade products and simultaneously inspect them for quality attributes.

18.11 Information technology

The use of information has increased significantly as the ability to process data has increased not only in speed, but also in cost. There is a considerable amount of information produced in a food factory and from other sources such as customer complaints which can be of importance in reducing the possibility of contamination of foods. The type of information that could be useful in detecting abnormalities in a factory includes:

- Machine condition monitoring
- Quality monitoring
- Statistical process control
- Maintenance
- Power consumption

Comparative analysis and variance techniques can be powerful. These methods involve building up standard, performance or criteria data which can be used as a comparative measure. In comparing the actual processing data to a standard or base signature, any deviation or variation from this norm can identified. It is also possible to investigate in order to determine what caused the deviation. This approach often will allow a warning to be given prior to a production problem occurring.

In a milling or size reduction operation, this technique could be used to identify if a higher level of power was being consumed to that normally consumed for a particular product or material – this could indicate if other material or a contaminant was being processed. Pressure drops in flow lines for liquids could be used as an indicator to identify abnormal flow. The pressure drop could be an indicator that the product had congealed in the line, burnt or lumps had formed.

Therefore, through analysing key parameters it is possible to detect whether there is anything abnormal and one can also look at the trends in parameters to see if they are drifting. Limits can be set of the drift such that alarms will be sounded if there is a change in trend.

Another technique called multivariate analysis is a new technique which has been developed specifically for monitoring processes which are complex and have many interacting variables. This type of technique enables many variables to be analysed simultaneously and any deviation from the norm detected. It is then possible to detect which variable or variables have contributed to the deviation and investigate why the variable has departed from the normal level.

A company will often obtain information from customers who complain about specific problems relating to its product. Through the use of information technology it is possible to trace back through the system rapidly and find out what problem had occurred and what had caused the specific problem. Following the identification of the problem, one would then make any modification to ensure that it did not re-occur. Tracking of products back to a specific date, time and production line/machine is made possible in most factories by coding the product as it is produced. The code will often include the date, time (to nearest minute) and the production line it was manufactured or packaged on. If the factory is controlled using a supervisory control system (SCADA), a manufacturing execution system (MES) or a similar system it is possible to log the manufacturing data encoded with the time of manufacture. This data can then be replayed to establish what process was running at the time and all the variables that were logged, along with the names of operators and quality assurance staff on duty at that time.

The major advancement of this technology is the speed at which the information can be made available. In many factories it would also be possible to link back to the ingredients that went into the specific batch of product and even in some cases back to the field where the raw material was grown. This correlation of data and the speed at which it can be accessed can allow problems and contamination issues to be resolved very quickly, and can limit product recall or unnecessary damage to the organization.

18.12 Advanced diagnostics

With the advances in computer technology there are now many diagnostic tools that can be used to check that processing, cleaning and packaging equipment is performing correctly. This type of software monitoring system allows operating parameters to be monitored and analysed.

There is more advanced software being developed which allows multivariate simultaneous analysis. This is where many inter-related variables are monitored simultaneously such that if there is any major changes in the range of data and their inter-relationship it can be identified, and the major contributing parameters identified and addressed. This type of monitoring allows many 1000s of variables to be monitored automatically and any major deviation from the normal brought to the attention of the operator. This wider monitoring of the operations allows faults to be detected quickly before any potential contamination has occurred.

18.13 Electromagnetic inspection

For some products there are specific requirements to inspect foodstuffs for foreign bodies. One example is parasites in fish. In Alaska an experimental system has been developed and that found that there was a change in current flowing around the parasite which could be detected by a change in the electromagnetic field strength.

The electromagnetic field they used was generated using a 120 V, 1.4 mA, 100 Hz signal. The system showed that the parasite exhibited a much greater electrical impedance to the flow of current than the healthy fish tissue did. Therefore, the research indicated that this type of inspection technology was possible. At present the approach has just been used to investigate parasites but it may be that the technology could be utilized to detect other foreign bodies.

18.14 Capacitive systems

Capacitive systems have been developed and utilized in the food industry – primarily to detect missing parts or products in packs. One of the first companies to exploit this technology was described by Faruq of Laetus Systems Ltd. They developed a system for inspecting closed packs of products.

The system works by conveying the product to be examined through a detector which has a transmitting electrode on one side and an array of sensing electrodes on the other. The early systems had up to 256 electrodes which were used to sense changes in capacitance, their output being transmitted every second as a set of data from the array. The line of information is sent to the data processing system which can then assemble a two-dimensional image. The line speed on the belt has to be synchronized with the data acquisition. Figure 18.5 shows a diagram of the system.

The resolution is limited to the size of the sensors, which in the case of the systems described was 2 mm and it allowed for pack sizes up to 500 mm in length.

This technology could be utilized in order to detect foreign bodies and it could well provide an opportunity to be combined with other technologies to provide a more comprehensive inspection system.

18.15 Development in farm systems

Over recent years there has been a move towards controlling the complete food chain to ensure quality and reduce the risk of contamination. On the farm there were very few systems employed to detect or remove foreign objects. Most traditional systems are centred around grading of produce. Now that consumers are more conscious of foreign objects and much farm produce is being sold direct through major retailers, there is a requirement for improvement of farm systems. Some of these systems are being developed so they can be incorporated in the harvesting machine. These types of intelligent harvesting machines will be able to selectively pick, sort and grade products.

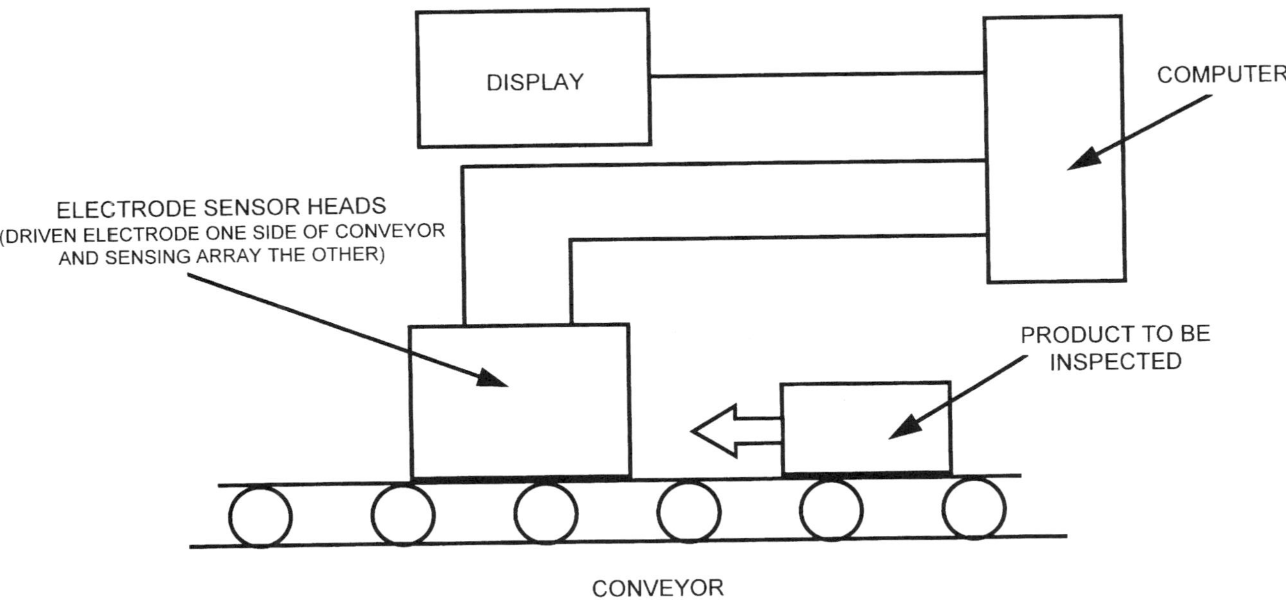

Figure 18.5 Example of the Laetus capacitive system.

18.16 Developments in magnets

Most magnets that are used are either electromagnets or rare earth magnets. Many companies have realized that with their technologies, whether it be NMR or magnetic separation, there is a requirement for lower cost magnets which can provide improved performance. There has been a search to find alternative materials such as rare earth types that are of lower cost but could also provide this improved performance. Electromagnets and superconductors are being researched to provide a cheap source of magnetic fields. One of the limiting factors in such developments has been achieving the appropriate field strengths for the size of food products that require inspection.

References and further reading

Faruq, A. (1991) Closed pack contents inspection – without X-rays. *Sensor Review*, 11(4), 26–27.

Tu, K., DeBusscher, R., De Baerdemaeker, J. and Schrevens E. (1995) Using laser beam as light source to study tomato and apple quality non-destructively. In *Proceedings of the Food Processing Automation IV Conference*, 3–5 November 1995, American Society of Agricultural Engineers, pp. 528–536.

Appendix I: Manufacturers of food inspection and sorting systems

X-ray systems

ASH, Advanced System House SpA, via Carlo Capelli 93, 10146 Torino, Italy.

EG&G Instruments, 100 Midland Road, Oak Ridge, TN 37830, USA. Tel: (+1) 615 482 4411; Fax: (+1) 615 481 2427.

Elbicon NV, Industrieterrein Nieuwland, 3200 Aarschot, Belgium. Tel: (+32) 16 56 06 11; Fax: (+32) 16 56 59 65.

Grasby Product Monitoring Ltd, Vale Road, Windsor, Berkshire SL4 5JX, UK. Tel: (+44) 1753 869351; Fax: (+44) 1753 840079.

Intelligent Manufacturing Systems Ltd, 45 Roman Way, Coleshill, Birmingham B46 1JT, UK. Tel: (+44) 1675 466111; Fax: (+44) 1675 467111.

Lixi Inc., 1438 Brook Drive, Downers Grove, IL 60515-1025, USA. Tel: (+1) 708 620 4646; Fax: (+1) 708 620 7776.

Par Technology Corp., New Hartford, NY 13413-1191, USA.

Pulsarr Industrial Research BV, Ambachtsweg 19, 5627 BZ Eindhoven, Holland. Tel: (+31) 40 421955; Fax: (+31) 40 427754.

Metal detectors

CEIA SpA, Zona Industriale Viciomaggio, 54/G 52040 Arezzo, Italy. Tel: (+39) 575 4181; Fax: (+39) 575 418296.

Cintex Ltd, 12 Trident Industrial Estate, Blackthorne Road, Colnbrook, Slough, Berkshire SL3 0LX, UK. Tel: (+44) 1753 685261; Fax: (+44) 1753 681814.

Detronic A/S, Th. Eriksensvej 7, 9640 Farso, Denmark. Tel: (+45) 98 63 1911; Fax: (+45) 98 63 1844.

Grasby Product Monitoring Ltd, Vale Road, Windsor, Berkshire SL4 5JX, UK. Tel: (+44) 1753 869351; Fax: (+44) 1753 840079.

Krones UK Ltd, Westregen House, Great Bank Road, Wingates Industrial Park, Westhoughton, Bolton BL5 3XB, UK. Tel: (+44) 1942 840044; Fax: (+44) 1942 841414.

Krones AG, Böhmerwaldsraße 5, 93068, Neutraubling, Germany. Tel: (+49) 94 01 700; Fax: (+49) 94 01 70 24 88.

Lock Inspection Systems Ltd, Neville Street, Oldham OL9 6LF, UK. Tel: (+44) 161 624 0333; Fax: (+44) 161 624 5181.

Loma Systems Ltd, Southwood, Farnborough, Hampshire GU14 0NY, UK. Tel: (+44) 1252 540346; Fax: (+44) 1252 513322.

MDL Boekels, Barnfield Industrial Estate, Tipton, West Midlands DY4 9DW, UK. Tel: (+44) 121 557 2104; Fax: (+44) 121 522 2013.

S+S Metallsuchgeräte und Recyclingtechnik GmbH, Regener Straße 130, 94513, Schönberg, Germany. Tel: (+49) 85 54 3080; Fax: (+49) 85 54 2606.

Safeline Limited, Montford Street, Salford M5 2SN, UK. Tel: (+44) 161 848 8636; Fax: (+44) 161 848 8595.

Total Quality Corp., PO Box 1075, Branford, CT 06405, USA. Tel: (+1) 203 483 7447; Fax: (+1) 203 483 7449.

Magnets

Boxmag-Rapid Ltd, Chester Street, Aston, Birmingham B6 4AJ, UK. Tel: (+44) 121 359 5061; Fax: (+44) 121 359 3501.

Eclipse Magnetics Ltd, Unit 3B, Nunnery Drive, Sheffield S2 1TA, UK. Tel: (+44) 114 225 0555; Fax: (+44) 114 225 0525.

Eriez Magnetic Europe Ltd, Bedwas House Industrial Estate, Bedwas, Newport NP1 8YG, UK. Tel: (+44) 1222 868501; Fax: (+44) 1222 851314.

Goudsmit Magnetic Systems BV, Postfach 18, 5580 AA Waalre, The Netherlands. Tel: (+31) 40 221 3283; Fax: (+31) 40 221 7325.

Magnetic Separations Ltd, 14 Meadowside Road, Cheam, Surrey SM2 7PF, UK. Tel: (+44) 181 642 4413; Fax: (+44) 181 642 9476.

Master Magnets Ltd, Magnet House, 251 Alcester South, Kings Heath, Birmingham B14 6DT, UK. Tel: (+44) 121 444 4266; Fax: (+44) 121 443 3511.

Vision and colour systems

CR Technology, 27752 El Lazo Road, Laguna Niguel, CA 92677-3914, USA. Tel: (+1) 714 448 0443. Fax: (+1) 714 448 0445.

Filtec Inspection Systems Ltd, Filtec House, Walkmill Business Park, Walkmill Way, Cannock, Staffordshire WS11 3XE, UK. Tel: (+44) 1922 416604; Fax: (+44) 1922 412255.

ESM UK Ltd, Building 41, Satake, Bird Hall Lane, Cheadle Heath, Stockport, Cheshire SK3 ORX, UK. Tel: (+44) 161 491 4775; Fax: (+44) 161 491 4776.

Elbicon NV, Industrieterrein Nieuwland, 3200 Aarschot, Belgium. Tel: (+32) 16 56 06 11; Fax: (+32) 16 56 59 65.

Heuft Ltd, Unit 26, Innage Park, Holly Lane, Atherstone, Warwickshire CV9 2HA, UK. Tel: (+44) 1827 717002; Fax: (+44) 1827 716146.

Inex Vision Systems, PO Box 95, Atlantic Street, Altrincham, Cheshire WA14 5EW, UK. Tel: (+44) 161 928 6344; Fax: (+44) 161 928 8758.

Key Technology Inc., 517 N. Elizabeth, PO Box 8, Milton-Freewater, OR 97862, USA. Tel: (+1) 503 938 5556; Fax: (+1) 503 938 7346.

Pulsarr Industrial Research BV, Ambachtsweg 19, 5627 BZ Eindhoven, Holland. Tel: (+31) 40 421955; Fax: (+31) 40 427754.

Radix Systems Ltd, Premier Centre, Abbey Park, Premier Way, Romsey, Hampshire SO51 9AQ, UK. Tel: (+44) 1794 830240; Fax: (+44) 1794 830143.

Sortex Ltd, Pudding Mill Lane, Stratford, London E15 2PJ, UK. Tel: (+44) 181 519 0525; Fax: (+44) 181 519 5614.

Sieves and screens

Bühler AG, 9240 Uzwil, Switzerland. Tel: (+41) 71 955 11 11; Fax: (+41) 71 955 33 79.

Fareygreene Ltd, Molesey Business Centre, Central Avenue, West Molesey, Surrey KT8 2QZ, UK. Tel: (+44) 181 941 9155; Fax: (+44) 181 941 9166.

Hosokawa Micron Ltd., Rivington Road, Whitehouse Industrial Estate, Runcorn, Cheshire WA7 3DS, UK. Tel: (+44) 1928 755100; Fax: (+44) 1928 714325.

Kason Corp., 1301 E. Linden Avenue, Linden, NJ 07036, USA. Tel: (+1) 908 486 8140; Fax: (+1) 908 486 8598.

Locker Process Solutions, PO Box 161, Warrington, Cheshire WA1 2SU, UK. Tel: (+44) 1925 651 212; Fax: (+44) 1925 636 290.

Pascall Engineering, Gatwick Road, Crawley, West Sussex RH10 2RS, UK. Tel: (+44) 1293 525166; Fax: (+44) 1293 536214.

Russell Finex Ltd, Russell House, Browells Lane, Feltham, Middlesex TW13 7EW, UK. Tel: (+44) 181 818 2000; Fax: (+44) 181 818 2060.

Filters

DCE Ltd, Humberstone Lane, Thurmaston, Leicester LE4 8HP, UK. Tel: (+44) 116 269 6161; Fax: (+44) 116 269 3028.

Pall Process Filtration, Europa House, Havant Street, Portsmouth PO1 3PD, UK. Tel: (+44) 1705 303303; Fax: (+44) 1705 302506.

Ronningen-Petter, 9151 Shaver Road, PO Box 188, Partage, MI 49081-0188, USA. Tel: (+1) 616 323 1313; Fax: (+1) 616 323 0065.

Appendix II: Sources of specialist assistance for the identification of foreign body contaminants

The following is a non-exclusive list of organizations who may be able to offer direct assistance or be able to advise on specialist resources from among their members for the identification of contamination. In addition the manufacturers of detection equipment may be able to assist in identification and detectability.

British Disposable Products Association	Rivenhall Road, Westlea, Swindon, Wiltshire SN5 7BD, UK. Tel: (+44) 1793 886086	Non-wovens, paper products
British Glass Manufacturers Association	Northumberland Road, Sheffield, South Yorkshire S10 2UA, UK. Tel: (+44) 114 268 6201	Glass
British Museum (Natural History)	Cromwell Road, South Kensington, London SW7 5BD, UK. Tel: (+44) 171 589 6323	Insects
British Textiles Technology Group	Shirley House, Wilmslow Road, Didsbury, Manchester M20 2RB, UK. Tel: (+44) 161 445 8141	Textiles
Building Research Association	Garston, Watford WD2 7JR, UK. Tel: (+44) 1923 894040	Building materials

Campden and Chorleywood Food Research Association	Chipping Campden, Gloucestershire GL55 6LD, UK. Tel: (+44) 1386 840319	General
Central Science Laboratory	London Road, Slough, Berkshire SL3 7HJ, UK. Tel: (+44) 1753 534626	Pests
Institute of Food Science and Technology	5 Cambridge Court, 210 Shepherds Bush Road, London W6 7NJ, UK. Tel: (+44) 171 603 6316	General
Institute of Packaging	Syonsby Lodge, Nottingham Road, Melton Mowbray, Leicesteshire LE13 0NU, UK. Tel: (+44) 1664 500055	Packaging materials
Leatherhead Food Research Association	Randalls Road, Leatherhead, Surrey KT22 7RY, UK. Tel: (+44) 1372 376761	General
Paint Research Association	Waldegrave Road, Teddington, Middlesex TW11 8LB, UK. Tel: (+44) 181 977 4427	Paint
PIRA International	Randalls Road, Leatherhead, Surrey KT22 7RU, UK.	Paper
Public Analyst	See local telephone directory	General
RAPRA Technology Ltd	Shawbury, Shrewsbury, Shropshire SY4 4NR, UK. Tel: (+44) 1939 250383	Plastics and rubber
Rentokil Ltd	Felcourt, East Grinsted, Sussex RH19 2JY, UK. Tel: (+44) 1342 833022	Insects

Appendix III: Available methods of prevention and control

Key to codes in the tables:

1	Metal detector – magnetic field system	Chapter 9
2	Metal detector – balanced coil system	Chapter 9
3	Magnetic grids/permanent magnets	Chapter 8
4	Separation – air	Chapter 6
5	Separation – liquid	Chapter 6
6	Vision system – colour opacity	Chapter 12
7	Vision system – shape	Chapter 12
8	Sieves and filtration	Chapter 6
9	X-ray	Chapter 11
10	Human	Chapter 14

List of tables:

This material is reproduced from Campden and Chorleywood Food Research Association, Guideline No 5: *Guidelines for the Prevention and Control of Foreign Bodies in Food.*

Table AIII.1 Harvesting and initial preparation of primary food products

Food material	Foreign body													
	Ferrous metal	Non-ferrous metal	Insects	Glass	Animal/bone	Dirt debris	Fabrics	High density rubber and plastics	Plastic films	Wood	Paper	Oil	Stones	EVM
Cereals and dry pulses	2,3,9	2,9	4,6,8	4,6,8,9		4,6,8,9	4,8	6,8,9	4,6,8	6,8	4,6,8	6	4,6,8	4,6,7,8
Fats and oils	2,3,9	2,9	5,8	5,8,9		5,8,9	5,8	8,9,10	8,10	5,8	5,8		9	
Fish (including fillets)	1,9	2,9	10	9	9,10	10	10	9,10	10	10	10	10	9	
Shellfish	+2,5	+5		+5	+5	+5		+5					+5	
Fruit	2,3,9	2,9	10	4,6,9,10		10		9	10	10	10		9,10	10
Dried fruit				+5,8					+4,5		+4		+4,5,8	+4,5,6,8
Nuts			+4	+7		+4	4,10	+10	+4		+4	10	+4	+4,6,7
Soft fruit				+5		+5			+5				+5	+4
Top fruit (apples, etc)			+6	+5,8		+5,8				+5,8			+5,8	+5,8
Meat (red and white)	2,9	2,9	10	9	9,10	10	10	9,10	10	10	10	10	9	
Milk (raw)	2,3,9	2,9	9	8,9	8,9	8,9	8	8,9	8	8	8		8,9	
Tea and coffee	2,3,9,10	2,9	8,10	4,8,9,10		4,8,9,10	8,10	4,8,9,10	4,8,10	4,8,10	4,10		4,8 9,10	4,8,9,10
Vegetables	2,3 9,10	2,9	10	5,8,10	5,6,10	5,10	10	5,8,10	5,8,10	8,10	10		5,8,10	5,6,10
Dried vegetable materials			+8	+4,6,9		+4,6		+9	+4	+4	+4		+4,9	+4,8
Non-root vegetables		+4,5,10	+5,8	+4,9		+6		+9		+5	+8		+6,9	+4,9
Root vegetables		+10	+5	+9		+8				+5	+8	10		

Table AIII.2 Manufacturing operations

Food material	Foreign body												
	Ferrous metal	Non-ferrous metal	Insects	Glass	Animal/ bone	Dirt debris	Fabrics	High density rubber and plastics	Plastic films	Wood	Paper	Oil	Stones
Biotechnology (Including fermentation)	2,3,8,9	2,5,9	5,8,10	5,8,9	5,8	5	5	5,8,9	8	8	4,8	6,10	4,5,6,7,8
Coating (including crumbing)	2,3,9	2,9	8,10		9	6	6	5,6,8,9	4,8	8	4,8	6,10	
Filling (including solids)	2,9	2,9	10	9	8,9,10	5,8	5,8	6,8,9,10	4,8	8	4,8	6,10	9
Dry			+8										+8
Liquid			+8										+8
Hydrogenation	2,3,8,9	2,8,9	8	8,9	8	5,8	5,8	5,8,9	4,8	8	4,8		8,9
Infusion (including injection, marinading, pickling, steeping)	2,3,8,9	2,8,9	8	8,9	8,9	5,8	5,8	5,8,9	4,8	8	4,8	6,10	8,9
Mechanical forming (including compressing, extruding, forming, massaging, moulding)	2,3,9	2,9		9	9	10	10	5,8,9	4,8	8	4,8	6,10	9
Mixing	2,3,9	2,9	8	8,9	8	5,8	5,8	6,8,9,10	4,8	8	4,8	6,10	8,9
Emulsifying	+8	+8											
Product transfer (including conveying)	2,3,9	2,9	8,10	8,9	8,9,10	6,8,10	6,8,10	6,8,9,10	4,8	8	4,8	6,10	8,9
Bagging	+8												
Dispensing	+8	+8											
Pumping	+8	+8											

Table AIII.2 Manufacturing operations (*continued*)

Food material	Foreign body												
	Ferrous metal	Non-ferrous	Insects	Glass	Animal/ bone	Dirt debris	Fabrics	High density rubber and plastics	Plastic films	Wood	Paper	Oil	Stones
Separation (including centrifuging, churning, coning, destoning, extraction, peeling, pressing, stripping)	2,3,4,5,9	2,4,5,9		4,5,9	4,5,8,9	4,5,8	4,5,8	4,5,8,9	4,5,8	8	4,8		4,5,9
Size reduction (including comminuting, dicing, flaking, homogenizing, mashing, milling, pulping)	2,3,9	2,9		9	9	5,6,8	5,6,8	5,6,8,9	4,8	8	4,8		9
Purée	+8	+8		+8									
Thermal processing (including baking, blanching, boiling, cooling, freezing, frying, malting, microwaving, proving, roasting, smoking, steaming, sterilizing)	2,3,9	2,9	8	8,9	9	6,7,8, 9,10	6,7,8 9,10	6,7,8 9,10	4,8	8	4,8	6,10	8,9
Drying	+8	+8			+8								
Pasteurizing	+8	+8			+8								

Table AIII.3 Packaging systems

Packaging material	Foreign body											
	Ferrous metal	Non-ferrous metal	Insects	Glass	Animal/ bone	Dirt debris	Fabrics	High density rubber and plastics	Plastic films	Wood	Paper	Oil	Stones
Composites	2,9	2,9	10	9	9	10	10	9,10	10	10	10	10	9,10
Glass	2,4,5,6,9	2,4,5,6,9	4,5,6	4,5,6,9	4,5,6, 9,10	4,5,6,10	4,5,610	4,5,6 9,10	4,5,6,10	4,5,6,10	4,5,6,10	6,10	4,5,6 9,10
Laminates	2,9	2,9	10	9	9	10	10	9,10	10	10	10	10	9,10
Metal	9	9	4,5,7	4,5,9	4,5,9,10	4,5,10	4,5,10	4,5,9,10	4,5,10	4,5,10	4,5,10	10	4,5,9,10
Steel	+4,5,6	+4,5,6											
Aluminium	+1,4,5,6												
Paper and board	2,9	2,9	10	9	9	10	10	9,10	10	10	10	10	9,10
Plastic (flexible)	2,9	2,4,9	4,10	4,9	4,9	4,10	4,10	4,9,10	4,10	4,10	4,10	10	4,9,10
Plastics (rigid)	2,9	2,4,9	4,10	4,9	4,9	4,10	4,10	4,9,10	4,10	4,10	4,10	10	4,9,10

Appendix IV: UK prosecutions and penalties

Table AIV.1 Examples of prosecutions and fines or damages awarded by UK courts April 1994 to July 1997

Category	Type of food	Foreign body	Detail	Fine (£)
Bakery products	apple pie	rubber		500
	beef and onion pie	plastic		7000
	bread pudding and buns	dirt/debris		40000
	cake	insects	ant	1000
	doughnut	metal	spring	5000
	eccles cake	dirt/debris	cigarrette end	700
	loaf	animal	feather	350
	loaf	animal	feathers	350
	loaf	dirt/debris	medical plaster detectable type	750
	loaf	insects	moth	300
	loaf	metal		1000
	rolls	Insects	slugs	6500
	loaf, sliced	string		350
	vegetarian pizza	animal	chicken meat	1000
	cheese and ham flan	metal	pin	5000
	pasty	insects	blue bottle	NG[a]
Chocolate confectionery		insects	grubs	2500
		plastic		1000
		rubber		1000
		rubber		1000
		rubber		2000
Dairy products	cheese	metal	blade	4000
	milk	glass		5000
Meat products	burger	insects	beetle	2000
	cold meat	metal	injection needle	3000
	sausage	metal	wire	2500
Pickles		glass		2000
Prepared food	sandwich	dirt/debris	plaster	500

Category	Type of food	Foreign body	Detail	Fine (£)
	baked beans	wood	splinter	6000
	fries	metal	wire	1000
	fries	metal	wire	1500
	restaurant meal	animal	worm	730
	restaurant meal	metal		4000
	restaurant meal	plastic		4000
	sandwich spread	glass		4000
	potato salad	glass		2500
	shepherd's pie	metal	wingnut	2000
Snack foods	pop corn	metal		5000
	crisps	metal	blade	NG[a]
	crisps	metal	copper pipe	1500
	nuts	insects		2500
	nuts	metal		2000
Soft drink		cleaning water		6000
Sugar confectionery		metal	blade	25000
		metal	ferrous clip	600
		wood		4000
Tea and coffee	tea bags	dirt/debris	condom	6000
Tomato juice		glass		1500

Source: *Food, Drinks and Drugs Industry Bulletin*. The data is not comprehensive as the proceedings of magistrates courts are not reported to a central register.
[a] Not given

Table AIV.2 Examples of prosecutions and fines or damages awarded by UK courts April 1994 to July 1997

Foreign body	Detail	Category	Type of food	Fine (£)
Animal	chicken meat	bakery products	vegetarian pizza	1000
	feather	bakery products	loaf	350
	feathers	bakery products	loaf	350
	worm	prepared food	restaurant meal	730
Dirt/debris		bakery products	bread pudding and buns	40000
	cigarrette end	bakery products	eccles cake	700
	condom	tea and coffee	tea bags	6000
	medical plaster (detectable type)	bakery products	loaf	750
	plaster	prepared food	sandwich	500
Glass		dairy products	milk	5000
		pickles		2000
		prepared food	sandwich spread	4000
		prepared food	potato salad	2500
		tomato juice		1500
Insects		snack foods	nuts	2500
	ant	bakery products	cake	1000
	beetle	meat products	burger	2000
	blue bottle	bakery products	pasty	NG[a]
	grubs	chocolate confectionery		2500
	moth	bakery products	loaf	300
	slugs	bakery products	rolls	6500

Category	Type of food	Foreign body	Detail	Fine (£)
Metal		bakery products	loaf	1000
		prepared food	restaurant meal	4000
		snack foods	pop corn	5000
		snack foods	nuts	2000
	blade	dairy products	cheese	4000
	blade	snack foods	crisps	NG[a]
	blade	sugar confectionery		25000
	copper pipe	snack foods	crisps	1500
	ferrous clip	sugar confectionery		600
	injection needle	meat products	cold meat	3000
	pin	bakery products	cheese and ham flan	5000
	spring	bakery products	doughnut	5000
	wingnut	prepared food	shepherd's pie	2000
	wire	meat products	sausage	2500
	wire	prepared food	fries	1000
	wire	prepared food	fries	1500
Plastic		bakery products	beef and onion pie	7000
		chocolate confectionery		1000
		prepared food	restaurant meal	4000
Rubber		bakery products	apple pie	500
		chocolate confectionery		1000
		chocolate confectionery		1000
		chocolate confectionery		2000
String		bakery products	loaf, sliced	350
Water	cleaning water	soft drink		6000
Wood		sugar confectionery		4000
	splinter	prepared food	baked beans	6000

Source: *Food, Drinks and Drugs Industry Bulletin*. The data is not comprehensive as the proceedings of magistrates courts are not reported to a central register.

[a] Not given.

Index